IAN WHITE

Bachelor of Science, Diploma of Naturopathy,
Diploma of Botanical Medicine

Ian obtained his Bachelor of Science from the University of New South Wales and graduated from the New South Wales College of Natural Therapies. For the last twenty years, Ian White has been practising successfully as a naturopath and homoeopath. Ian is a fifth generation Australian herbalist. Both his grandmother and great grandmother were early pioneers in researching and discovering the medicinal properties of Australian plants and as a boy Ian spent a great deal of time with his grandmother in the bush learning from her.

Since 1987 Ian has travelled Australia extensively, researching and developing a range of sixty-two specific remedies using native flowers from such diverse areas as the Northern Territory wetlands, Kakadu, the Olgas or Katajuta, the Kimberley, South Australian deserts, south-west Western Australia, Victorian heathlands and Sydney sandstone region.

These remedies are used by naturopathic practitioners, medical doctors, pharmacists and ordinary people to assist in healing the emotions. It is a well known and proven principle that when emotional balance is restored true healing occurs.

Ian is also the author of the book *Australian Bush Flower Essences* (Bantam), and regularly contributes to well known Australian publications such as *Wellbeing* and *Nature and Health*. He is also a regular guest on television and radio talk shows. Ian also teaches at the major Australian naturopathic colleges and runs his own workshops on the Australian Bush Flower Essences regularly throughout Australia, North America, South America, Asia and Europe. These workshops are attended by a wide range of people, including lay people, natural therapists, medical specialists and people with an interest in healing, nature and metaphysics.

AUSTRALIAN

Bush Flower
– Healing –

IAN WHITE

BANTAM BOOKS
SYDNEY • AUCKLAND • TORONTO • NEW YORK • LONDON

AUSTRALIAN BUSH FLOWER HEALING
A BANTAM BOOK

First published in Australia and New Zealand in 1999 by Bantam

National Library of Australia
Cataloguing-in-Publication entry

White, Ian.
Australian bush flower healing.
Bibliography.
ISBN 1 86325 212 6 (hardback)
ISBN 0 73380 053 X (paperback)
1. Wild Flowers– Australia– Therapeutic use.
2. Materia medica, Vegetable– Australia. I. Title

615.3210994

Bantam books are published by

Transworld Publishers,
a division of Random House Australia Pty Ltd
20 Alfred Street, Milsons Point, NSW 2061

Random House New Zealand Limited
18 Poland Road, Glenfield, Auckland

Transworld Publishers (UK) Limited
61–63 Uxbridge Road, Ealing, London W5 5SA

Random House Inc
1540 Broadway, New York, New York 10036

Edited by Sarah Baker
Cover design by Liz Seymour
Cover photographs by Ian White
Text design by Trevor Hood
Photograph of Freshwater Mangrove by Kim Brennan;
other photographs by Ian White
Drawings by Kristin Coburn
Typeset by Midland Typesetters, Maryborough, Victoria
Printed in China
Produced by Phoenix Offset

10 9 8 7 6 5 4 3

—Contents—

——Acknowledgements——

As in my first book I would initially like to thank Spirit for all the tremendous love, light and protection and not to mention the unseen help offered to me. I am also greatly indebted to Chris Andreas; my Office Manager of the last ten years; and all the staff at the Australian Bush Flower Essences for their wonderful work and support.

There are some very special people I would like to take the opportunity to thank for their invaluable assistance which helped me to research and write this book.

Firstly, both Kerrie Redgate and Louise Anderson for their contribution to the astrology chapter and the latter for her case history I have used in the book. Also to everyone else's case histories I have used in this book, especially Mrs Dorothy M. Johnson. To Erik Pelham for his Devic Analyses and research into the correlation of the Bush Essences and their related working on the Subtle Bodies. To Zoe Hagon for allowing me to use her survival checklist for practitioners. And to Bernard Jensen for his kind permission to use his Iridology chart. Dr Jensen's chart is available in Australasia from Jeni Edgley and Friends, telephone (07) 5533 7733.

I would like to especially thank Marie Matthews for her dedication and commitment in helping me collate the emotional repertory and upgrading the physical repertory. Not to mention her willingness to leave her family for weeks at a time to come to Sydney, take my dictation, thrash ideas around and to make sure I got around to finishing the manuscript!

Carol Dingo, Mark Skinner, Tom Reeve and Mary Anne Leary, all very dear friends, who at various times have accompanied me on flower essence expeditions. Special thanks to Tom for his help in the making of Alpine Mint Bush. To all of my Bush Essence distributors, Insight group and workshop co-ordinators in Australia and overseas who have greatly helped in getting the essences out there! Not to mention all the people around the world taking and prescribing the Bush Essences and especially those ones who took the time and trouble to record and send us their case histories and insights.

To the many people who have been great teachers to me consciously or unconsciously. In particular Anthony Robbins, who inspired and motivated me to end my inertia and procrastination in writing the book. He helped me to realise that I prefer to work with people rather than be typing away by myself. As a consequence I gladly took up Marie Matthews' longstanding offer to help transcribe this book.

Thank you to one and all.

—Introduction—

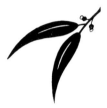

In the eight years since the publication of the first edition of *Australian Bush Flower Essences* there has been tremendous change and expansion within the Bush Essences. During this time twelve new remedies have been added to the original fifty and they are now all being used widely throughout the world by families and practitioners, and in hospitals as well. They have also gained great respect and a wonderful reputation for being incredibly fast acting and producing very powerful results on the physical level, not just on the emotional and spiritual levels.

Today these remedies—which are totally safe for everyone—are used in a cosmetic range; incorporated with aromatherapy and added to massage oils and oil burners; and sprayed in classrooms to enhance children's learning ability and decrease their stress at exam time. Landscape architects utilise the plants from which the Bush Essences are made in their designs so as to incorporate the healing and harmonising qualities of the essences into the environments of their clients; Bush Essences are used in hospitals in Europe and South America as a viable, effective and safe alternative to hormone replacement therapy without the increased risk of breast or cervical cancer and elevated cholesterol levels. Flight and cabin crew take them to negate the effects of air travel. The scope of Bush Essences is quite unlimited.

One of the unique features of the Bush Essences is that they can easily be combined with all other healing modalities, whether it be homoeopathy, allopathic medicine or chiropractic, to name but a few. Practitioners from virtually all the different modalities—not to mention individuals who simply want to use the remedies for themselves and their families—have constantly asked me for an emotional repertory of the Bush Essences as well as an expanded physical index. Finally their needs have been met for both are included in this book, and the book certainly fills a previous very large gap in the available Bush Essences knowledge. In the Repertory of Emotional, Mental and Spiritual Conditions, under each category you will find a detailed description of every essence in relation to the theme being discussed. Although I have also added a chapter giving an update on the original fifty remedies, many subtle distinctions between the Bush Essences can be found in the Repertory.

This book also contains chapters on iridology, pregnancy and goal setting along with two case histories that show both the scope and practical application of the Bush Essences. In addition there are detailed descriptions of each of the twelve new essences that were not contained in the first edition, although half of them had already been made up by the time of publication of that book in 1991. At that time I did not feel that these new essences had been used widely enough and that perhaps we did not have the fullest picture of their healing qualities. Absolutely no such doubt exists today!

This has always been my process with the Bush Essences, whereby from time to time new remedies will come through and their healing qualities made available. In November 1998, after five years of research, I finally prepared an essence from the Monga Waratah. Even though I am very familiar with the healing properties of this essence I decided not to include the Monga Waratah in this book as there are not enough case histories or people familiar with and working with this essence at this point in time. I imagine that it will be fully described in my next book! It is sufficient to say that the Monga Waratah (*Telopea mongaensis*) addresses issues of disempowerment; neediness and dependence on others; the fear that you can't do it by yourself, that you need others as well to help you; and that you are not strong enough to do it by yourself. This remedy helps you to reclaim your spirit and find your inner strength, and to let go from unhealthy relationships.

These new twelve essences covered in this book very much address spirituality at a very high level in the qualities they bring with them and the areas in which they work, and very much reflect the tremendous shift in human consciousness that has occurred in the last ten years. These new essences include remedies such as: Angelsword—to access previously learnt skills and abilities as well as to establish clear communication with one's higher self; Boab—working at a very profound level by breaking the negative emotional patterns that have been, for centuries, passed down from one generation to the next; Mint Bush—to assist a person going through the spiritual trials and tribulations immediately prior to initiation, when they feel they are being tested, often to their limits; or Green Spider Orchid—to assist a person in working with telepathy and attuning them to be more receptive to other people, as well as to other species and kingdoms.

Since 1996 there has been a marked and exciting shift in my experience in making the mother tinctures.

Whereas previously I would simply tune into and listen to the plant and its deva to determine the healing quality, I now find myself being able to actually merge into and become the plant. Sometimes at the completion of making the essence I would merge into the mother tincture as well.

Such experiences have allowed me to more fully understand the inherent healing qualities, mysteries and nature of the plant and its essence. These mergings have also broadened my scope of what is possible when working with both Spirit and Nature.

But it's not only humanity that has been evolving—so have the planet and the plants. Two years ago, while replenishing my Mother Tincture supply of Bush Fuchsia, I was surprised to find that its healing qualities had greatly expanded, that it was now able to help an individual to become far more in touch with the rhythms of their own body and the earth and to be in tune with the seasons and changes in the vibrations and energies of the earth. The plant did not have these qualities twelve years earlier when I first made it up. What surprised and fascinated me even more was that the original Bush Fuchsia Mother Tincture had also equally evolved, and now possessed these same new healing qualities— while in its glass container!

When I first started making the Australian Bush Flower Essences I was working very much with the personality and characteristics of the plant— what we could call the consciousness of the plant, at its current point of evolution. My understanding was that each of the Bush Essences— whether as Mother Tincture, Stock or Dose—contained an equivalent of one drop of pure Source or Spirit and that this was the highest amount with which human consciousness, at that time, was able to bear. But now, as a result of our expansion of consciousness, the equivalent of three drops of Source can be tolerated and incorporated into each Bush Essence remedy.

Not only has the information about how to make all the new Mother Tinctures so that they contain this incredibly higher added potency and strength come down to me, but also how to work with all the old, existing Mother Tinctures to bring them up to this higher level. It is comparable to when computers were first designed: they were then, by modern standards, huge, very cumbersome, slow and limited in their action, whereas today they are incredibly fast, smaller and more efficient, and with each succeeding 'generation' improving upon the previous model.

The way I am now making my essences involves working with that very sacred part of the plant, the soul of the plant, where all its knowledge and wisdom from its earliest origins, when it was brought through from Source, is contained. Just as humans have changed through the ages—their structure, personality and adaptations to the changing environment—so have the plants. So when I now make the Flower Essence I am accessing, with its permission, all the plant in its entirety, all the knowledge and wisdom of the plant that has ever existed before, in all its different forms. So in bringing through the essences now, we are obtaining a greater wisdom and strength which can do more subtle and powerful things. With Angelsword in its new form, for example, not only does it still help to cut any attached cords of energy from one's feeling centre, but it now also brings with it an understanding of the cause behind why that cord was attached in the first place. People who are now coming to work with the Bush Essences will be able to reach a different part of themselves and they will be able to receive further truths, for through the plant we are now accessing a doorway to the ancient energies and wisdoms.

This current generation of children mark a major transition from the road humanity had previously been travelling. In this generation we have the forerunners of the spiritual seers, psychically open and intuitive ones who will primarily operate from their feeling centre and inner knowing, not from their intellect. And the higher vibration now present in the Bush Essences, although it will still be beneficial for the adults of this and previous generations, is specifically designed for today's children and even more so, *their* children, so that they will be able to go back and access so much more of the intuitive knowledge, memories and ancient wisdoms that are stored in the feeling centre.

Many cultures have predicted that a thousand years of peace will soon envelope the planet and next century, numerologically, it can be seen that everyone will be born with at least a single two in their birth date. Two is the number for intuition, sensitivity and co-operation. I have always seen the Australian Bush Flower Essences as a catalyst and 'midwife' to assist the planet and its people in their birth from a third to a higher dimension, and help to deal with any associated labour pains. Although they will always work to improve the quality of our lives, they have a much larger role to fill in human destiny. These new generations will be made up of very sensitive souls and the Bush Essences will help them adjust to a very rapidly changing society where the values that these generations contribute—sensitivity and intuition—will be more and more valued, appreciated and honoured.

How to Prepare and Take Australian Bush Flower —Essences—

Preparation Methods

Use flowers that have grown in an environment away from pollution and power lines. Sensitivity and a degree of reverence are necessary. Without directly touching them, place the flowers in a bowl of water and leave this in the sunlight for several hours. Remove the flowers from the bowl, preferably with a twig or a leaf from the same plant. This Mother Essence water is preserved with an equal amount of Australian brandy to make the Mother Tincture. Seven drops of this Mother Tincture are added to any size bottle up to 30 mL, containing two-thirds brandy and one-third purified water, to form the concentrate, or stock bottle.

Stock Bottle Use

Dosage bottles are prepared by taking a dropper bottle of any size up to 30 mL, filled with three-quarters purified water and one-quarter brandy as a preservative and adding seven drops from the stock bottle. Several essences can be combined in the one bottle, but it is generally suggested that the number combined be limited to four or five.

After the stock has been added, the dosage bottle can be lightly shaken or tapped to release its energy. Alternatively, some people energise their essences with a prayer or invocation, or with a visualisation such as surrounding the essences with white or gold light, although none of these is essential. Affirmations can also be used very effectively with the essences.

Dosage Bottle Use

Flower essences are taken from the dosage bottles morning and night by putting seven drops under the tongue or by adding the seven drops to water. They are usually taken for a two week period. They can also be applied topically by adding them to lotions and salves, or to bath water (a very effective method).

Choosing and Administering the Essences

Often the excitement or amazement people feel on initially reading about the properties of the Bush Essences is quickly overtaken by their absolute conviction that they need to take at least half the remedies instantly, because they identify with them so strongly. This is a very common and normal response! It demonstrates one of the beauties of the essences— namely, their simplicity. Not only can you see yourself in the remedies, but also your aunty, cousins, best friend, next-door neighbour and your parents! All this instant insight is available to you without years of formal training, just a basic understanding of human nature. There are many ways to choose the most appropriate Bush Essence or combination of essences: you can simply read the descriptions of the individual essences and select the one most relevant to your situation or personality; you can choose the flower to whose appearance you feel most drawn from our *Flower Insight Cards* or the photos in our books; you can use Kinesiology to pinpoint the right essence; or you can select a remedy based on your numerological or astrological chart. A question to ask yourself that will help you choose an appropriate remedy: what do I most want in my life? The answer to this question will lead you to the essence that is most relevant to your life at that time.

So, now you have chosen a few remedies that seem appropriate, what's the next step? Well, you have the option of taking either a single essence remedy or a number of essences combined. Generally the effect is finer, more powerful, faster acting and longer lasting if you take an individual remedy. The mixing of two or more unrelated essences can produce more of a physical action in the body. Therefore, you may decide to narrow your choice to the one remedy that most completely addresses the issue, situation or emotion with which you wish to deal. However, certain combinations work exceptionally well—in fact, just as well as a single essence—as long as the essences in a combination all address different aspects of a particular condition or situation.

—Affirmations—

I have included this section on affirmations because they can be very useful tools for further empowering the actions of the Bush Essences. Affirmations can be written, spoken, sung or listened to. They are positive statements which help to program the subconscious mind for particular goals or in particular directions, and they are very easy to use. I have found writing affirmations to be the most effective method, for then you can do two things at once—you can say the affirmations while writing them.

You can use an affirmation anywhere and at any time, though it should be used when you can really focus on it. An affirmation works well if it is used at the same time as taking the corresponding Bush Essence remedy, that is, either on rising or retiring, or at both times of the day. Writing your affirmation once a day for a week is usually sufficient time for it to work.

If you want to create your own affirmations or to modify the affirmations provided in this book, you can either phrase them so that the statements are in the present ('I am now ... '), or so that they have a sense of 'becoming' ('I am now becoming ... '). For example, simply writing 'I am a loving person' will most likely bring up a lot of resistance in the subconscious mind and will be easily rejected. However, the affirmation 'I am now becoming a loving person' will be accepted far more readily by the psyche, which will make the affirmation more powerful.

A highly recommended technique to incorporate into your affirmations is to refer to yourself in the first, second and third person. 'I, Ian, am now beginning to love and accept myself' is an example of using the first person in an affirmation. I would write this out ten to twenty times, and after each affirmation I would write my response to it. For example, 'If no one else does, why should I?' What the response represents is the negative pattern or belief that is held in the subconscious. As you use affirmations, old garbage from the subconscious is revealed, and by writing out those old messages you are helping to eliminate them.

After writing in the first person, change the affirmation to the second person: 'You, Ian, are now beginning to love and accept yourself.' Putting the affirmation in the second person will help to clear negative beliefs that have come about from others speaking to you directly. For example, being told, 'No one loves you'. This leads to the belief, 'I am unlovable'. After writing these ten or twenty times, go to the third person: 'He, Ian, is now beginning . . . ' This will cover those beliefs that have arisen from overhearing someone talking about you.

Your response to affirmations can give you valuable insights into some of your unconscious beliefs. You are likely to find that the intensity of their negativity decreases as you write out your affirmations and responses. Sometimes you may get to the point where you basically have no response at all. But, remember, when writing out affirmations do concentrate on them.

At the end of each Bush Essence entry a couple of affirmations appropriate for that essence have been provided. These have been compiled by Amanda Davey of Melbourne, creator of the Balance for Life program, Russell Sharpe, owner of Just for Love, Sydney's premier florist, and Gina Vanderhage. You can choose an affirmation that you are drawn to, to accompany a specific remedy, but don't feel that you have to use the affirmation in that particular form. If an affirmation doesn't feel totally right, then change its wording. You can tell when you find the form that is right for you.

There are many other ways in which affirmations can be used. They can be listened to on a tape recorder, they can be said while looking in the mirror, or they can be read aloud from the fridge or bathroom door. Take a dose of Turkey Bush, be creative and discover other ways of using them.

Twelve New —Essences—

ALPINE MINT BUSH

(Prostanthera cuneata)

Every now and then go away, have a little relaxation, for when you come back to your work your judgment will be surer; since to remain constantly at work will cause you to lose power of judgment.—Leonardo Da Vinci, in Susan Hayward (ed.), A Guide for the Advanced Soul

The Alpine Mint Bush grows in exposed rocky sites in alpine and sub-alpine areas of south-eastern Australia and Tasmania. The essence was made up in the Snowy Mountains region, a very famous skiing area in New South Wales. It belongs to the Labiatae family which is found throughout the world, especially in the Mediterranean region. It is a spreading shrub up to 1 m tall. At high elevations it is found as a semi-prostrate plant while lower down it is seen as a very compact shrub of between 30 and 40 cm. The stem is erect and branching with a densely textured crown. The flat, opposite, obovate to orbicular leaves are dark green and highly aromatic, being 4–7 mm long and 3–5 mm wide. The white to pale mauve tubular 10–15 mm long flowers occur

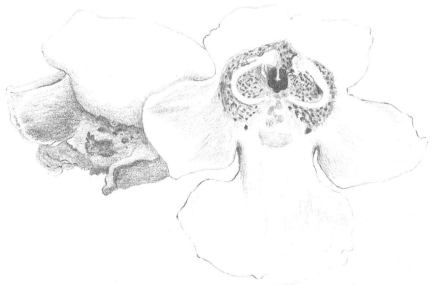

in dense clusters towards the ends of the branches. They have five petals that form a three-lobed spreading lower lip and erect two-lobed upper lip. Contained within are four stamens and a multitude of delicate golden and purple spots.

A very distinct Doctrine of Signature of this plant is that it usually grows with two buds. One will come out first and when that one starts to fade and is past its peak the second will come into full bloom. My first sighting of Alpine Mint Bush came after a very difficult and painful crossing of the Snowy River in March 1993. On this trip I was accompanied by a good friend, Tom Reeves, who had been living in the mountains for many years. Halfway across the icy river my legs began to cramp and the pain was intense. I wondered if I would be able to make it to the other side. It was mainly as a result of Tom's cajoling and encouragement that I eventually succeeded in getting across. I'd like to say that Tom was nurturing and caring towards me during my crossing, but I think he was more amused at my expense! As he helped me to a resting spot I was engulfed by the rich scent of the highly aromatic Alpine Mint Bush. Its penetrating perfume instantly had a calming and uplifting effect on me. I found myself instinctively taking deep breaths of its scent and it very quickly alleviated any remaining discomfort. This was helped also, I must admit, by a few carob-coated bananas!

Soon after this at South Ramshead, with two eagles riding the thermals high above, we made up the essence. When Tom was tuning in, praying over the bush, the energy was so intense that he was almost blacking out. Later on, as we walked back down the mountain, carrying with us the precious Mother Tincture, Tom had a very strong sense of reconnecting with his spirit guides and returning to the Source and was filled with tears of joy. Altogether it was a very replenishing experience.

The healing quality of this essence is to rejuvenate those people in service or who care and take responsibility for other people. It is for those who work in caring jobs, giving much of themselves both physically and emotionally, and who are in danger of burning out. It revitalises and induces in them a renewed enthusiasm and joy in what they do.

This remedy is very good for health practitioners or counsellors who are listening to people's problems, whether emotional or physical, all day long, day in, day out, needing always to stay very focused, intuitive. They are constantly in the position of making decisions which they know will seriously affect the lives of others, and of having people rely on their expertise and knowledge.

I know an English medical practitioner who uses the Bush Essences extensively and he told me the story of how his last patient one Friday afternoon was a man with a long history of domestic violence who was feeling furious with his wife and worried that he might do something destructive and brutal to her. The patient wasn't able to go to a safe space to let these very aggressive feelings pass. The doctor knew that he couldn't have this man locked up or retained for observation unless the man actually committed some act of violence, nor did the patient want to admit himself. You can imagine the dilemma in which the doctor found himself. He gave his patient Dog Rose of the Wild Forces, intuitively trusting that this essence would resolve the situation. At the same time he had the man agree to ring him if necessary over the weekend, no matter what hour, and made an appointment for him to come back first thing on the Monday morning. Dealing with situations such as this on a regular basis really takes it toll. I doubt very much if many people could just go home that night and watch TV or play Monopoly and forget all about it. The doctor would be wondering what his patient was doing at any given moment, or whether he had made the right choice of treatment.

Alpine Mint Bush is also highly appropriate for people who are working in roles where they have to make choices that affect the welfare of others, but from a more detached position than the caregivers and counsellors. This could be, for example, a social worker, or a hospital administrator responding to budget cuts by closing down a certain number of beds in the hospital. There would be all the agonising over where to make the cuts—intensive care, labour ward or cardiac. People in these positions constantly have to juggle with and make decisions that will greatly impact on the lives of other people.

This is also an especially beneficial essence for someone looking after a family member on a caring basis who is always on call 24 hours a day. This may involve looking after a handicapped or invalid child, a partner who has become a quadraplegic or paraplegic, or attending to an elderly parent with Alzheimer's disease. A good friend of mine has four children all under eight, two of whom are autistic. There is a constant demand on both him and his wife, especially on the latter who spends most of her time at home with the children and who can become drained and weary from the unremitting caring. People in situations such as this can commonly suffer from varying degrees of compassion burnout sooner or later.

There are some health practitioners, such as home birth midwives, whose job also necessitates working and being on call all hours of the day, and for long periods, in a very intense emotional arena. In hectic times, they often must go straight from one birth to another. While all this is occurring, they still need to look after and maintain their own family and personal lives, even though they may not see their partner or children for days at a time.

Alpine Mint Bush is wonderful for anyone in any of the above categories who is tired, weary and feels that their life has lost its joy and is repetitious, or who may be feeling disillusioned or wondering 'why bother?'. This essence works on the mental and emotional level before there is physical exhaustion. It can revitalise these people and bring about a renewed enthusiasm, joy and spring in their life for what they do.

This essence can be extremely helpful when used in a preventative way before there is physical exhaustion, and ideally long before there are any signs of mental and emotional burnout. Alpine Mint Bush, however, is not appropriate for the weariness of a shop assistant, labourer or waitress, for example, whose tiredness at the end of a day is purely of a physical nature.

There are very few disciplines within medicine, healing or counselling where a system is in place to provide individual practitioners with support, regular checking, counselling and appraisal of their emotional and mental wellbeing by a mentor or colleague. Transpersonal Psychotherapy and Trauma Therapy does offer this in an attempt to guard against practitioner burnout. One of Australia's leading trainers of therapists in this combined field, Zoe Hagon, has compiled a survival checklist for practitioners which is designed to improve the quality of both their personal and professional lives. Some of the key and salient questions on Zoe's checklist are as follows:

• How comfortable are you in saying 'no'?
• Do you have structured time/supervision for unloading?
• What types of clients—if any—will you not work with?
• Are you willing to go past your limits for someone in crisis?
• Do you have clear limits around fees/money?

- What are your limits around self-destructive behaviour?
- What are your limits around telephone calls?
- What is your comfort level around intense affect and content?
- How much of your personal life do you share in a session?
- What are your limits on reading clinical material?
- Does your work ever disturb your sleep, or enjoyment of life?
- Do you discuss your work in social situations?
- Do you start and end sessions on time?
- How aware are you of your own personal boundaries and limits?
- What are *your* particular signs of stress?
- What are *your* particular signs of burnout?
- How do you tend to your spiritual needs?
- Does your work impact on your spirituality?
- How much do you trust your intuition during sessions?
- Do you look after your physical wellbeing? Exercise? Rest? Eat properly? Play?
- How comfortable are you in saying 'yes' to yourself?

You can see from this list that Flannel Flower—to help establish healthy boundaries—and Fringed Violet—to help guard against having your energy drained by those you are caring for—along with Alpine Mint Bush would lead to a greater vitality and wellbeing for the majority of lay or professional carers and healers.

On a personal note, this essence was made up a month prior to a three month teaching tour in the northern hemisphere which would mark the end of my fifteen year career as a full-time practitioner. I was finding it harder and harder to fit in clients as my teaching schedule, research work, making the essences and overseeing the staff and business took increasingly more and more time and focus. In order to be able to see my patient within what I thought was an appropriate time for a follow-up consultation, I had to book them in later and later on the nights I was practising—way past my normal last appointment time, because sometimes the next available appointment wouldn't be for two or three months. The making up and taking of the Alpine Mint Bush enabled me to make the realistic decision to let go of one of the 'hats' I wore and to stop seeing patients on a one to one basis and, instead, focus on training other practitioners so the Bush Essences could be used to treat many more people.

Negative condition

•

mental and emotional exhaustion

•

lack of joy

•

weight of responsibility

Positive outcome

•

revitalisation

•

joy

•

renewal

The Universe now provides me with all the joy and strength I need to do my work.
My life is rich and exciting.
I am divinely guided in all my decisions.
I choose everything that happens in my life, and I am never given anything I can't cope with.

ANGELSWORD

(Lobelia gibbosa)

Seek always
for the answer within
Be not influenced
by those around you,
by their thoughts
or their words—Eileen Caddy, in God Spoke to Me

Angelsword belongs to the Lobelieae family which contains approximately 1120 species from twenty-nine genera. This family is widely distributed throughout the world, with the main centre of diversity located in America, from California to Brazil. There is a secondary centre in the Hawaiian Islands. Australia has over fifty species in six genera. Lobelia was named in honour of Matthias de l'Obel (1538–1616), the French botanist and gardener who was physician to King James I of England. He was also the author of an important Flemish herbal widely used in its day. Angelsword is a native of all states of Australia, preferring light soils in an open sunny position. It is drought and frost resistant which explains why it can be found in the sub-alpine forests. It is an erect fleshy annual, 15 to 40 cm high, which flowers in autumn when it carries several deep blue to purple labiate flowers 12 to 18 mm long on a terminal one-sided raceme. The sepals are very narrow. The deep blue corolla has two upper lobes which are shorter, narrower and more pointed than the three thick lower and in-curved lobes. The anthers are all tipped with short tufts of gold pollen-stained bristles. The few alternate and lanceolate dark green leaves are often withered at flowering time. The species appears to be

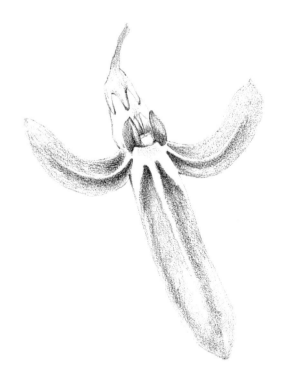

composed of a complex of hybrids while its name, *gibbosa*,
derived from the Latin, means humped, which refers to the
shape of the fruit capsule.

I found this amazing flower growing below the treeline
in the alpine regions of the Snowy Mountains in south-east
Australia. This essence was made on the same trip as Alpine
Mint Bush. On this particular morning I set off intending to
explore around the higher regions. But while still at lower
altitude, basically at the foot of the peaks, I was drawn by
the strong calling of the Angelsword. I pulled the car over,
hopped out and started walking through the bush, clamber-
ing over huge rock boulders and intuitively following the
guidance I was receiving. After a few hundred metres I
finally found why I had been led there. In a large clearing
by the side of a fast-flowing icy stream, bathed in dappled
light, I had my first sight of Angelsword.

Viewed from one aspect the purple Angelsword flower is
sword-shaped like a fleur-de-lis. When the flower is viewed
the opposite way it resembles a Merlin-like monk in purple
robes. That image is accentuated by the yellow stamens
marking the third eye area. This plant is stunning in its Doctrine of Signatures.

In the month before finding the Angelsword, I had

received in meditation a particular spiritual exercise which I had been performing before going to sleep each night in order to develop and deepen my sensitivity for earth energy healing. It was stressed to me the importance of closing-off psychically on waking each morning before my normal daily interactions. This closing-off process entailed visualising myself fully cloaked in a purple robe and placing a symbol over each chakra. I think that the nature and spirit kingdoms must have enjoyed both this cosmic joke and the look of shock on my face after they led me to Angelsword. For this flower, in its shape and colour, was an exact replica of the visualisation—symbol and all.

As often happens on the day an essence is made, the immediate area was easily discernible as being highly charged with energy and vibrancy. This, I feel, is the emanation from the presence of all the nature spirits, angels and light beings who have gathered to assist in the spiritual alchemy of the creation of a new essence. Rarely have I experienced the same degree of vibrancy in these locations at any other time. The quality of the light is different also. There is a real sparkling present on an essence day which is noticeably absent at other times. Often there has been a strong presence of an animal at times when I have been preparing an essence. Nearly every time I have made an essence at Terrey Hills, which is north-west of Sydney and where I grew up as a boy, a large, majestic, 1.5 m long monitor lizard has appeared and has stayed, stealthily striding through the nearby undergrowth in close proximity to the bowl, until the essence has been decanted. I have never seen it on any of the many other occasions I have been in this area—never when walking or photographing in this familiar and well-loved bushland.

Its distinctive fleur-de-lis shape has given rise to its common name Angelsword (Angel-sword). This essence brings out and enhances the quality of discernment, allowing a person to cut through with the spiritual sword of discernment to find what is their own spiritual truth. At this point in time many people are giving their power away by accepting the validity of spiritual messages, teachings or books without questioning, especially if their source is seen to be channelled from a being not on the earth plane. These people believe that because the beings are not of the earth they must be far more evolved than we humans, struggling along in the third dimension. However, it is a real privilege to be incarnated here in a physical body at any time but particularly at this moment in time. There is hardly any-where in the universe where there exists the same oppor-tunity for rapid growth and learning of lessons as on the earth right now. Very often we are far more evolved than the channelled entity bringing down the information to us. It has been said that on a good day 80% of a channelling is accurate. Assuming the book or message was brought through on a good day, how do you then determine the 80% from the 20%? What if it were a bad day? Also people are at different levels, so what might be a truth for someone at one level may not be for you if you are above or below that particular level. And just because it is written in a book doesn't mean it is true!

So you can see that Angelsword's quality of discernment is an invaluable gift. It clears and removes confusion and misinformation and allows us to perceive with our heart and inner knowing. For many of us our most important teachers will not be obviously discernible as teachers, rather they can appear in many different guises and we won't be able to rely on feeling their energy or vibration, as it is not their nature to project out and attract us to them in this way. Instead, they cloak their essence and leave it as a test for us to feel them in our heart and in our knowing.

This essence assists in establishing clear communication with your Higher Self, to really listen and tune in. Many people prefer to speak of this essence as Angels-word as opposed to Angel-sword. But both are totally appropriate. As the Angels-word it does allow you to hear the words of the angels and also the word of your own angel—your Higher Self or inner guidance. The Angel-sword cuts off and removes from the psyche mischievous or negative entities or other sources that interfere with reception of clear com-munication from your own Higher Self, or who attempt to feed in false information. This can be extremely dangerous, as well as confusing as can be seen in many schizophrenics who describe hearing voices inside their heads, telling them to hurt or even kill themselves or others. The Angelsword has repeatedly brought about major healings of these people by clearing the negative entities providing those destructive messages that are attached to them.

While Fringed Violet works to repair damage to the aura, usually in specific places, Angelsword works more on the aura and energy fields as a whole. At the same time it releases any energies that entered while the aura was open. It is a very powerful but gentle essence. Many spiritual healers have expressed great gratitude in being able to have an essence that assists their work so effectively. Many had always felt that there would be a companion to help Fringed Violet complete the work the latter had started. The Fringed Violet, they knew, was brilliant at healing the aura, but by itself it didn't release what had been picked up while the aura was open. The aura is opened when there is a loss of consciousness such as with a general anaesthetic, drug taking, getting drunk, or severe physical shock and trauma. Some people, especially if there are many twos in their birth-date, but even more so if they are very open psychically, can take on negative energies quite easily, particularly if they are unaware of, or not practising, closing themselves off. The consequences of this can range from just feeling drained and tired to the other extreme of being possessed and commit-ting violent acts. Currently it is even more imperative to regularly practise closing off and ensure at all times that any psychic protection you do is adequate.

Angelsword can also cut and unplug the energetic cords that are frequently formed between and attaching us to family members and others to whom we have been inti-mately connected. These cords function as viaducts of energy between the people who are connected. If one person is low and needing energy, they can obtain it and top up from the person they are attached to, and vice versa. These cords are established only with a prior contract before we incarnate, nevertheless this does not mean that they are always desirable; in fact, quite the contrary. For example, if one person is constantly drawing on the energies of the other, then the latter will feel drained and tired.

Sai Baba has realised how ubiquitous and detrimental these cords that tie us energetically and emotionally to others can be. In his attempt to combat this he has exten-sively trained a woman called Phyllis Crystal in how to cut those ties. The consequence is a best-selling book written by Phyllis and entitled *Cutting the Ties that Bind*. Taking Angelsword orally is tremendously effective in getting rid of the cords, but in Chironic healing the drops of Angelsword are applied topically on the feeling centre to achieve the same result. The feeling centre is approximately halfway between the navel and the base of the sternum—the ziphoid process.

Angelsword is incorporated in the Meditation Essence to provide psychic protection and clear spiritual communica-tion. As a spray it can be combined with Boab, Lichen and

Fringed Violet for clearing houses and spaces of negative energy, either from lost souls or darker energies.

A useful suggestion we have had from a spiritual healer is to apply Angelsword to the hands when working not on the physical body, but rather on the outer or subtle bodies.

Another aspect of Angelsword is that it helps you to access and retrieve gifts and skills which you have developed in former lifetimes. If you are working in the same field as one you have been in previously then this can be of great benefit, as you can draw on the deep ancient knowledge that you acquired earlier. Many healers, for example, have worked as healers lifetime after lifetime *and their current work would benefit greatly if they could access what they knew and used in the past.*

For anyone who doesn't feel comfortable with the concept of reincarnation, another way to interpret it is as a genetic memory being passed down through the generations. There could be, for example, healing knowledge which was gained by a great-great-great-grandmother and passed down generation after generation, but it has always stayed in the subconscious level and has never been accessed. I personally like Kahil Gibran's comments on reincarnation. 'Reincarnation? Of course it is a fact, but who cares about facts.'

Angelsword is a good example of how the majority of the more recently developed essences are working predominantly at a spiritual level, and a very deep one at that. This reflects the great shift in human consciousness and levels of awareness that is occurring at the moment. It is as if the essences coming down now have been held back and not made available until the time when we are ready and open to utilising their healing qualities. For centuries humanity at large has had an appreciation and awareness of how nature has been healing people on a physical level and to a lesser degree, with flower essences, on an emotional level. But nature has always been and is still very willing and capable of continuing this healing on a spiritual level as well. Also we find that as the needs of society change, new essences emerge to meet those needs while, at the same time, they work as catalysts to rapidly accelerate the evolution of human consciousness to a higher level.

I am now free of all negative energies which have ever been a part of me.
I now have clear communication with my Higher Self.

Negative condition

•

spiritual confusion

•

interference with true spiritual connection

•

spiritual gullibility

•

looking for answers outside of self

•

spiritually 'possessed'

Positive outcome

•

attaining spiritual truth and protection

•

access to gifts and knowledge from past lifetimes

•

repairs whole energy field

I now clearly and easily discern what is truth for me.
I am now cutting and releasing all draining cords attached to me from
  other people.

BOAB

(Adansonia gibbosa)

Yield to the current of life ... unencumbered by baggage—Anthony de Mello, in Unencumbered by Baggage

The Boab tree is found only in the north-west region of Western Australia, in the open sandy plains where there is good rainfall, and along rocky ridges, drainage lines and creeks. This tree belongs to the cotton or Bombacaceae family and the genus is named after the French botanist Michel Adanson (1727–1806). The large, swollen, smooth, grey trunk may attain a girth of up to 25 m but rarely exceeds 15 m in height. This large and spreading tree is deciduous during the dry season but just before the arrival of the wet season grows long alternate compound leaves. These are green above and paler and whitish below and have up to nine pointy, hairy, finger-like lobes. The flowering time is November through to February and the large fragrant flowers with their five fleshy petals are white to cream and have numerous lengthy stamens. The flowers are sized between 8 and 12 cm by 10 cm and may appear with, or just before, the new leaves during the early wet season. The large ovoid fruit can grow up to 25 cm by 20 cm and has numerous kidney-shaped seeds that are cased in a matrix of white pith within a brittle shell.

The main healing quality of Boab is to clear the negative patterns of the ancestors—the limiting, dysfunctional, emotional and mental beliefs and patterns that are invariably learnt and passed on from generation to generation. Boab can access and clear these core patterns and all the related ensuing beliefs.

Think of the worst aspects of your parents ... now I guarantee that you have those very same aspects to some degree,

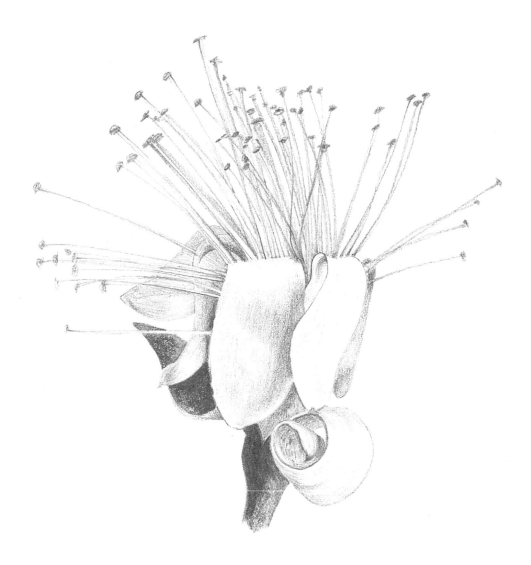

which is a very scary thought! We role-modelled our parents when we were young, and like all children, we assumed that they were perfect and God-like figures. It was only later when we were older and our cognitive ability much further developed that we realised that 'Dad is a bit neurotic—I don't want to develop some of his traits'. But by then it was too late. Boab breaks these family patterns and behavioural traits.

Sai Baba said that there were two crucial things that needed to happen for human consciousness to rise to a higher level and move into the new age. One of these was the need to release all the emotional baggage that we pick up from the family. This is exactly what Boab is all about.

Boab is helpful for people who have experienced abuse, persecution or prejudice. It is also for clearing the environment of negative energies. Boab offers us great strength and the opportunity to perceive our true spiritual essence, unencumbered by the layer upon layer of ancient and outmoded models of behaviour and thinking that are not what or who we really are.

For over two years I had been receiving a very similar message from several highly intuitive people about a large, candle-shaped white flower whose essence I would be making up in Western Australia. I was told this message in Australia, Europe and North America. I must admit to feeling a great deal of pressure to find and make this essence, especially as I had no plan or intention in the near future of going to Western Australia. Nor did I like the feeling of having something so seemingly predetermined thrust upon me. More importantly, I was concerned that I may not be able to fulfil the expectation of spirit guides who were passing this message on to me . . . if it really was from them!

It was in Darwin, while teaching in April 1993, that I saw my first Boab flower. I had been standing with a friend, Mark Skinner, in front of a Boab tree behind Darwin's GPO when I noticed a few very old and shrivelled up flowers at the base of the tree. On looking up, it was obvious that there were definitely no more flowers in the branches above. I lamented to Mark what a pity it was that we weren't able to see what the Boab flower looked like. We both scanned the tree again to see if there were a single bloom we hadn't previously detected. With a sigh I said: 'I would really love to see one.' Right then, with the words hardly out of my mouth, a perfect flower fell between us. We looked at each other incredulously and then, to cap it all off, I realised that this was the special white candle-like flower that I had been receiving information about. Then and there I decided to head off on an expedition to find a late flowering Boab, so we enlisted Julie Emery, a good mate and our workshop organiser for the Top End, together with her unique travelling van, and set out. Not surprisingly, for many years I had been strongly attracted to and fascinated by this amazing tree but I had never seen it in flower. What ensued was a fantastic week of tremendous fun and laughter, visiting many beautiful places . . . but no flowering Boabs. This was certainly not due to lack of effort on our part as I can remember on one dark moonless night driving through metre high grass in Julie's van with Mark and me hanging out of the windows, shining torches into every nearby Boab tree as we drove by. Mark and I decided at the end of that week to go back to the Kimberley later in the year when we knew the Boab would definitely be in flower.

In mid-December I travelled to Broome to first teach a workshop and then make the essence. It so happened that attending the workshop was a midwife who had worked with local Aboriginal communities. She told me how medical staff had great difficulty persuading the pregnant Aboriginal women to have their babies in a medical setting, how they would sneak out from these centres to give birth by themselves. The traditional birthing practice in this region, she explained, was for the tribe to give the woman Boab flowers if labour occurred during the flowering season. The woman would then go off, dig a hole and line it with the Boab flower. She would squat over the hole and deliver the baby into the cradle of flowers. So the baby's first contact in its life was the Boab. I realised just how intuitive these tribes were, because the healing quality of Boab is to break the negative family patterns that are passed down from generation to generation. What a wonderful headstart to give to a child by having it contact this healing energy of the Boab so early in its life.

The Doctrine of Signatures of the Boab tree is extremely interesting. It is quite common with this tree to have younger Boab trees growing around it in a circular pattern. These smaller trees are eventually engulfed by, and merge into, the older adult tree, once more pointing to the theme of family enmeshment which the Boab Essence addresses. In this particular case it is emphasising the insidious manner in which young children invariably become caught up in the long existing family patterns. Also, when the flower has withered, died and turned brown you will still see it being clasped tightly by the tree which seems to have a real reluc-tance to let anything go. No one can easily break free from and escape the behavioural traits that travel down the family tree. Interestingly, the Boab tree is also known as the bottle tree because it has a reservoir of fresh water stored in the trunk. Water, symbolically, is associated with the emotions, and the fact that this tree stores water is indicative of the deep emotions that the essence addresses. The creamy white flower with its tuberose-like scent is pollinated at night by moths. Night and darkness relate to the subconscious mind and Boab's healing sphere of action is very much directed to this area.

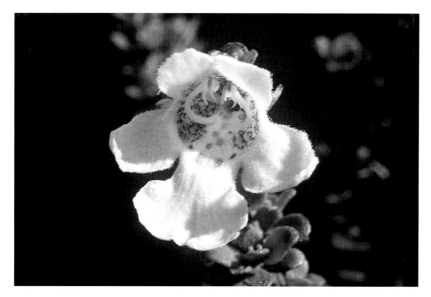

Alpine Mint Bush (*Prostanthera cuneata*). The healing qualities
of this essence include: revitalisation, joy and renewal.

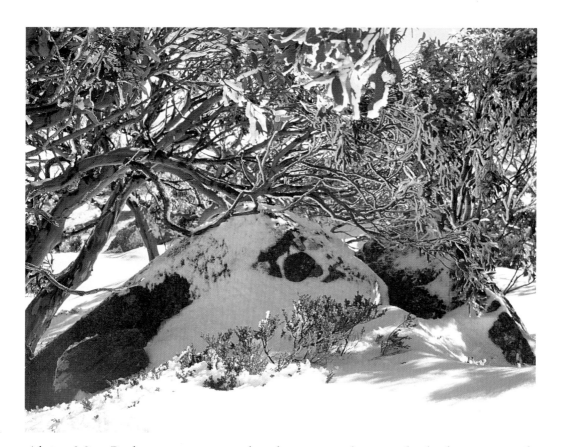

Alpine Mint Bush grows in exposed rocky sites in alpine and sub-alpine areas of
south eastern Australia and Tasmania.

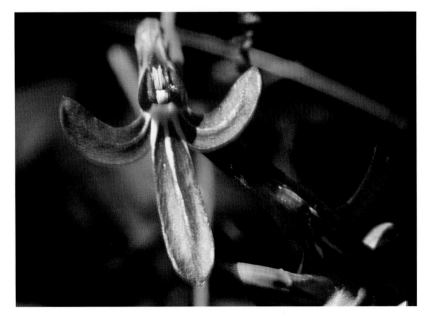

Angelsword (*Lobelia gibbosa*). The healing qualities of this essence include: attaining spiritual truth, protection and discernment as well as clear spiritual communication and release of negatively held psychic energies.

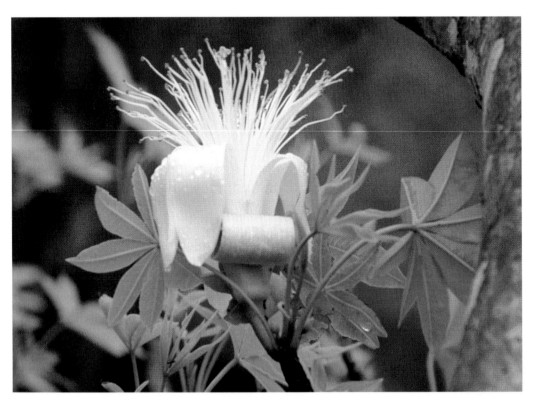

Boab (*Adansonia gibbosa*). The healing qualities of this essence include: engenders positive personal growth and also releases negative family behaviour and thought patterns that are passed down from generation to generation; heals effects of abuse and prejudice.

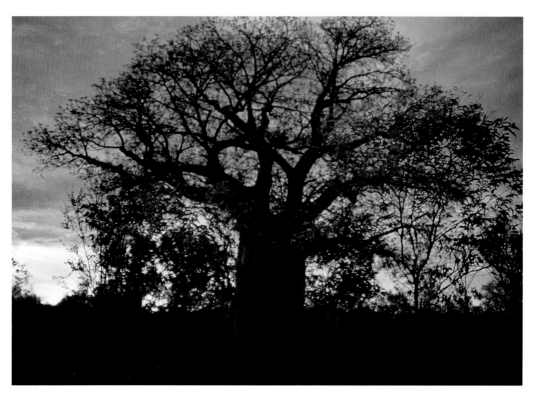

The Boab tree at sunset, in the Kimberley region of Western Australia.

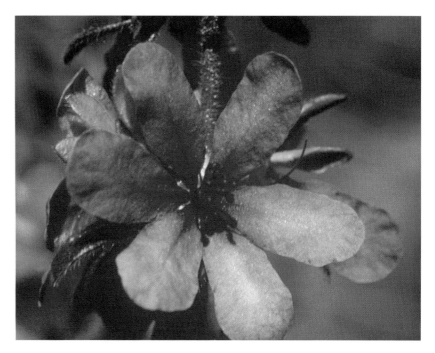

Dog Rose of the Wild Forces (*Bauera sessiliflora*). The healing qualities of this essence include: emotional balance; and calmness and centredness in times of inner and outer turmoil.

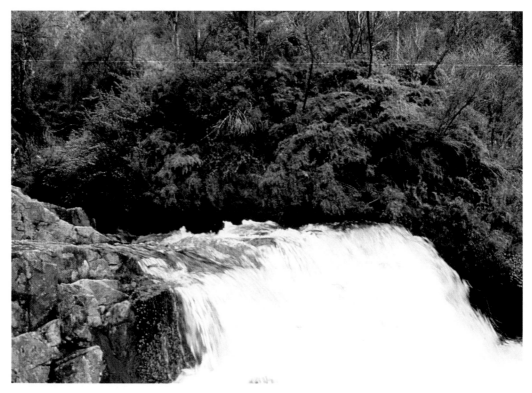

The Grampians, Victoria, Dog Rose of the Wild Forces country.

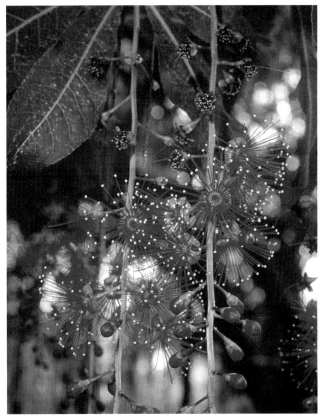

Freshwater Mangrove (*Barringtonia acutangula*). The healing qualities of this essence include: openness to new experiences, people and perceptual shifts, as well as healthy questioning of traditional standards and beliefs.

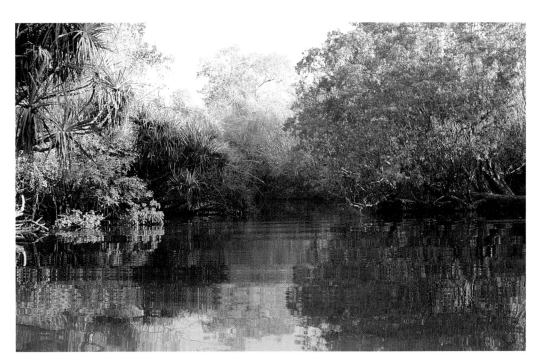

East Alligator River, Northern Territory, Freshwater Mangrove country. This short, robust, spreading tree can be found growing along the banks of fresh water creeks and rivers, and at the edges of billabongs and swampy areas, across the top end of Australia from the north west of Western Australia through to Cape York in Queensland.

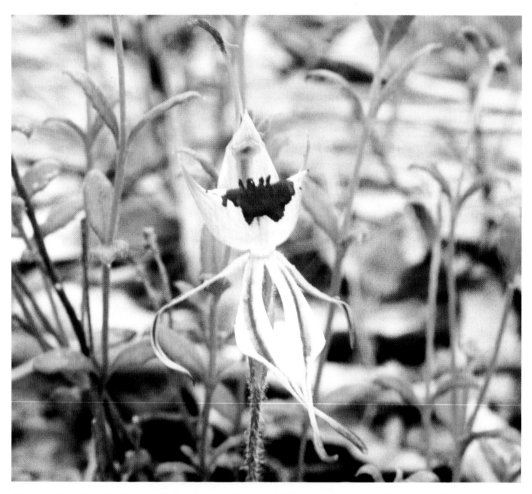

Green Spider Orchid (*Calandenia dilatata*). The healing qualities of this essence include: telepathic communication to other people, plants and animals; and the ability to withhold information until the timing is appropriate.

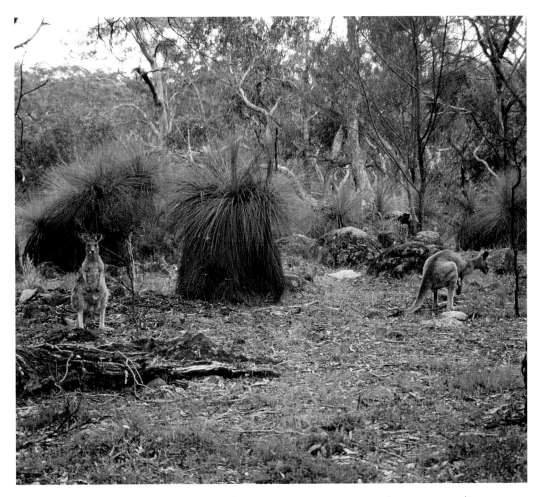

The Grampians, Victoria, Green Spider Orchid country. This perennial orchid is found widespread throughout all states of Australia in open forest and woodlands, though along the east coast it can also occur in open heathland.

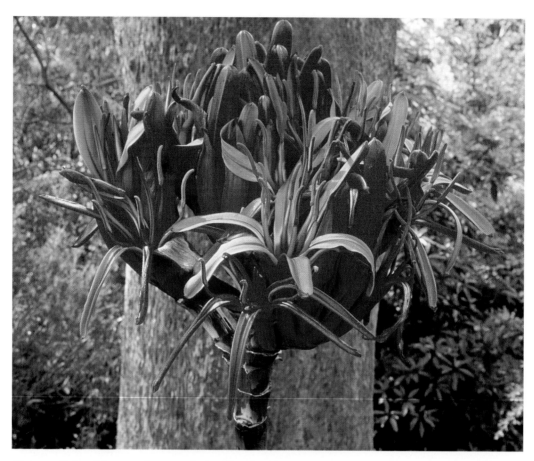

Gymea Lily (*Doryanthes excelsa*). The healing qualities of this essence include: courage to express your full power and who you really are; humility; allowing others to express themselves and contribute; awareness, appreciation and taking notice of others.

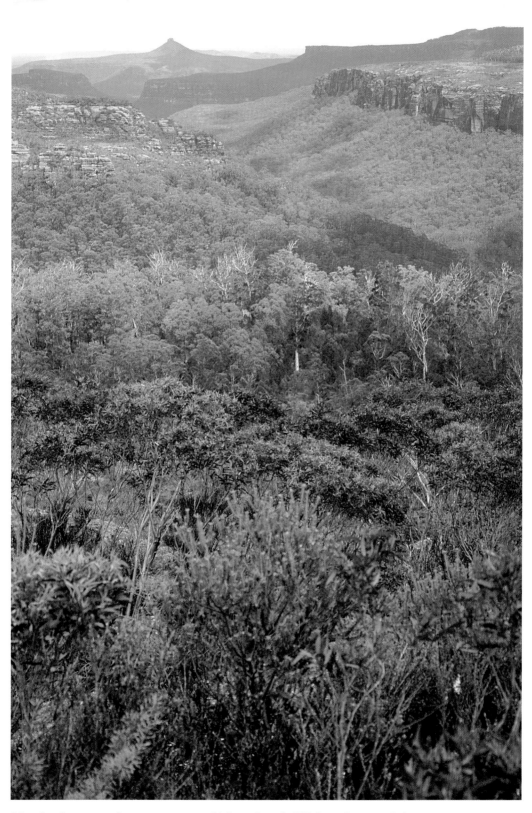

Hawkesbury sandstone region of New South Wales, Gymea Lily country.

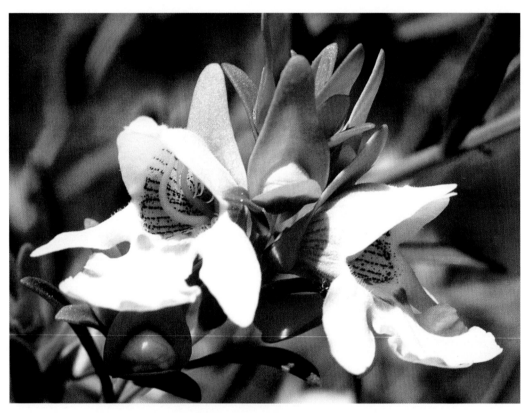

Mint Bush (*Prostanthera striatiflora*). The healing qualities of this essence include: smooth spiritual initiation; clarity; calmness; and ability to cope.

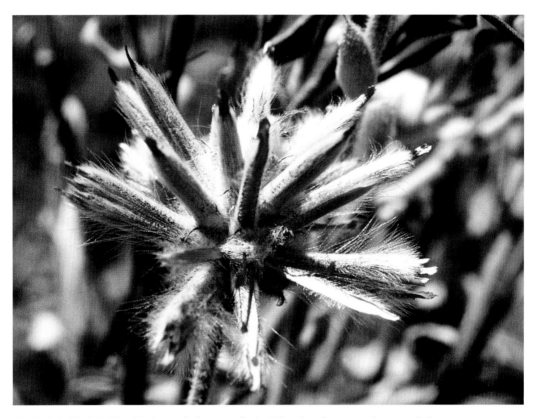

Pink Mulla Mulla (*Ptilotus helipteroides*). The healing qualities of this essence include: deep spiritual healing; and trusting and opening up.

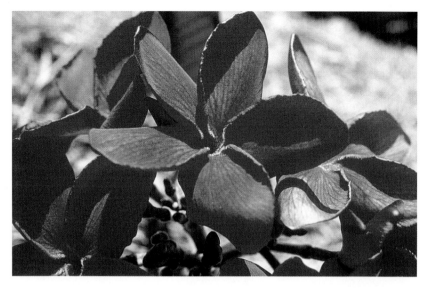

Red Suva Frangipani (*Plumeria rubra*). The healing qualities of this essence include: feeling calm and nurtured; and finding inner peace and strength to cope with relationship difficulties.

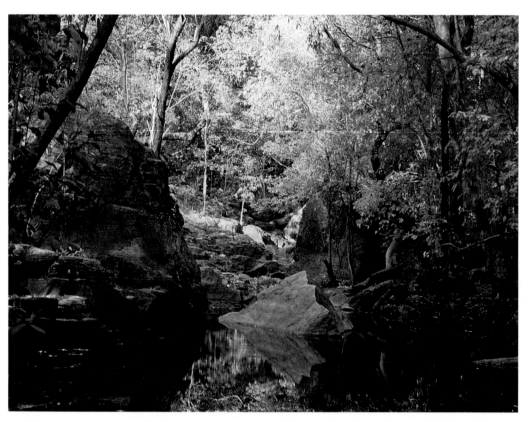

Kakadu, Northern Territory, Red Suva Frangipani country. This deep blood-red frangipani originated in Central America, and has now been introduced throughout Asia and the South Pacific region.

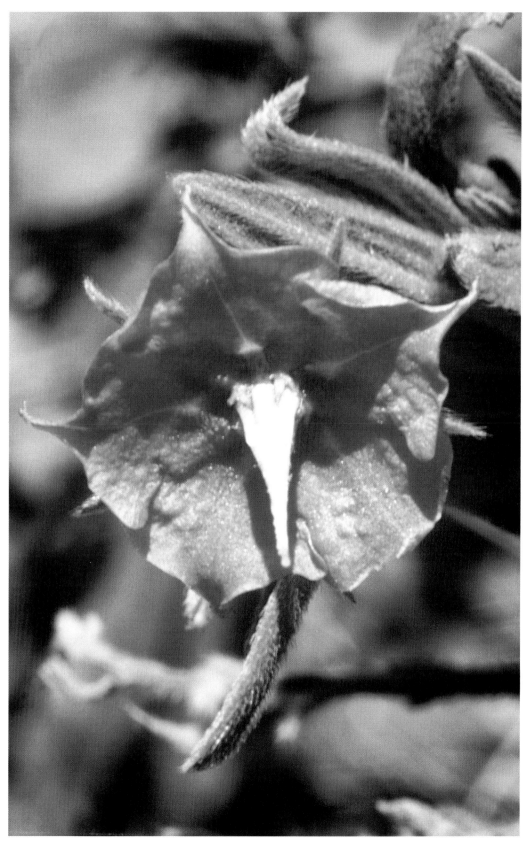

Rough Bluebell (*Trichodesma zeylanicum*). The healing qualities of this essence include: sensitivity, compassion and release of one's inherent love vibration.

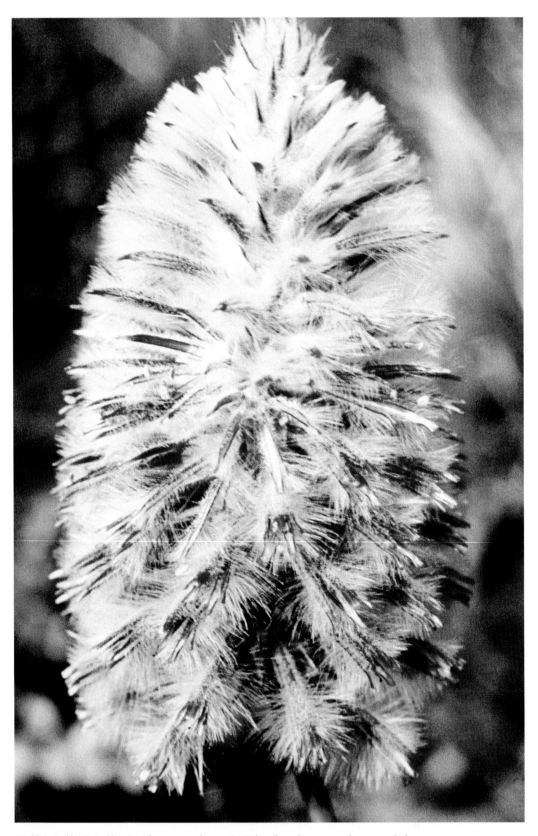

Tall Mulla Mulla (*Ptilotus exaltatus*). The healing qualities of this essence include: feeling relaxed and secure with other people; and encourages social interaction.

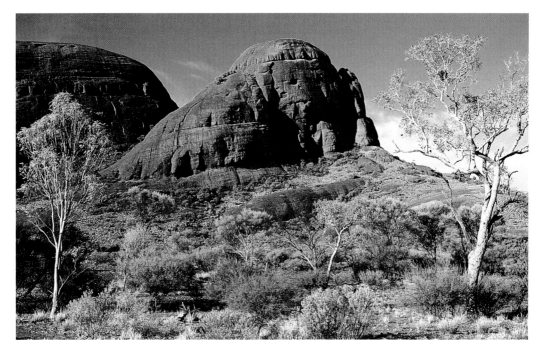

Katajuta (the Olgas), which many people believe to be not only the physical but also the spiritual centre of Australia. It is in this region that Mint Bush, Pink Mulla Mulla, Rough Bluebell and Tall Mulla Mulla flourish.

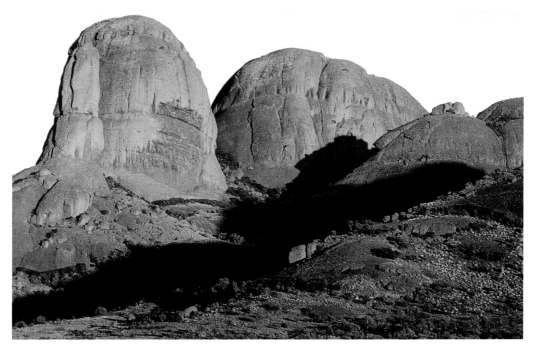

Katajuta at sunset, with the Landscape Angel of this region clearly visible amongst these magnificent red rock domes, where the energy is extremely powerful. Even on still days you can see the trees quivering and shaking with this energy. Each time I visit this magical part of the World, I attempt to explore a different area and I can spend all day out there in blissful solitude without seeing anyone—well, not anyone in a physical form anyway.

The sodium ring is a thick milky white ring that appears around the outside of the iris. It marks a hardening in the body, especially in the circulatory system, and is rarely seen in young people.

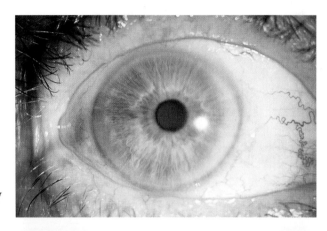

Lymphatic rosary. When the lymphatic system is becoming sluggish, white cottonball-like fluffs called 'tophi' will begin to occur in the outside of the iris.

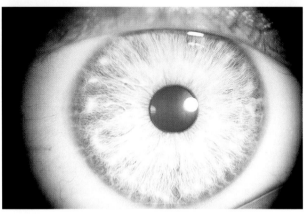

Nerve rings indicate stress and tension that is not being released from the body. They are found around the outside of the eye and are usually located in the zone of the iris corresponding to the neck and back although it is not uncommon to find them in the chest, solar plexus and head areas.

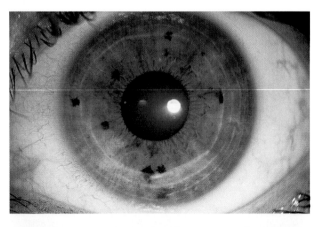

Toxic colon. In the iris, autotoxaemia will often show as a brown discolouration that often can be seen spreading out in the iris from the bowel region to other parts of the body.

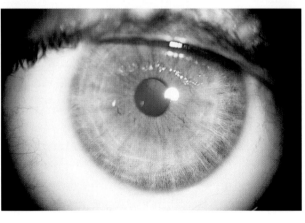

It has been indicated through channelling that the Boab tree is not originally of the earth but was given as a gift, in times past, from the star system Pleiades. The essence derived from the Boab is one of the most powerful healing forces with which I have ever worked.

Many cultures and their legends have likened the shape of the Boab tree to that of an upside-down tree with its head in the soil and its roots growing in the air. In Africa the Bushmen tell the story that God found his creation of the Baobab so ugly that he ripped it from the ground, and in his anger left it upside down. This seems to me a somewhat harsh description as the Australian Boab, which is closely related to the giant Baobab (or Boab) tree of Africa, is such a majestic and impressive tree. I much prefer the other comparison which claims it to be resembling a whale with its head stuck in the earth. In the North American Medicine Cards (tools of divination based on the insights and teachings of the North American Indians) the whale is connected to and represents the family. Boab is also all about the family. Whales swim around the earth in figure of eight movements and in some traditional cultures this is perceived to be a conscious action on the whale's part to balance the energies of the earth. In the human body the sacrum also creates a figure of eight movement. The sacrum's action pumps cerebro-spinal fluid all the way to the brain. Boab as an essence can be effectively used to correct cranio-sacral imbalances.

When Mark and I, along with another friend Tom Reeve, set out that morning I was quite content to drive along the Broome–Derby road—a trip of approximately two and a half hours—and wait for the appropriate Boab tree to call us over to it. It is a stunning drive, the whole flat landscape is dominated by these beautiful strong trees. By the end of the first hour we had passed many Boabs which I felt would have been perfect to make an essence from and I started to have the thought that we were getting closer and closer to Derby . . . and the prison tree. I quickly dismissed this thought, telling myself it definitely would not be the prison tree. By the time we were only half an hour from Derby I was still telling myself, a little bit more frequently than before, 'Surely it wouldn't be the prison tree.' And yes, the prison tree it was.

This tree, which is over 1200 years old, was used late last century to house chained prisoners (predominantly Aboriginal). They were locked up overnight inside the hollowed tree, awaiting their court appearance the next morning.

The advantage of working with this particular tree, which is very short and squat, was that we were easily able to climb it to reach the flowers. We didn't need to touch any of the ropes and pullies and rope-firing guns that Mark had brought along for the expedition. How we would get to the crown of the tree had certainly figured very high in our logistic discussions, because the tree has no branching before the crown. Just how did those Aborigines collect the flowers for the pregnant women in the tribe?

Initially, we spent quite some time just observing and taking in this special tree. And even though it was very different from all the other Boabs we had seen, its strength, presence and intensity were palpable. We were all very surprised to experience just how pure the energy among the branches and flowers above the rounded hollow trunk was, a sharp contrast to the heavy energy inside the tree and around it on ground level, which we felt was due to the purpose to which the prison tree had been put in the past. It seemed as if the top energy of the tree was working to balance the heavier energies surrounding the bottom half. Nevertheless, we were guided and spent quite some considerable time clearing this residual negativity both around and inside the tree.

The magic that occurs while making an essence was demonstrated to me once more when, towards the very end of the time the flowers needed to be in the bowl, we became increasingly aware and alarmed by the approach of massive dark menacing rain clouds which were rapidly blotting out the sky in a manner I had never seen before. There were only a few moments to go before the essence was ready and we were hoping that we would be given these few more minutes of sunlight, and we were. Just at that very moment of decanting the essence into the brandy we started to feel the first few large heavy raindrops falling on and around us. Within minutes we were scampering with all our equipment and Mother Tincture back to the safety of our four-wheel drive to avoid the torrential downpour, which didn't let up for the next four days. We ignored the official name of the cyclone and instead christened it Cyclone Boab!

Later that night, in meditation, I asked why it was that we had had to make the essence from the prison tree. The message came back that human consciousness has been in chains for thousands of years and that this is the essence to break those chains.

Considering the power and potency with which it can clear emotional, mental and behavioural patterns and the results that can arise from this clearing, I feel the Boab to be one of the most significant of all essences.

If there is one key major life scenario you keep repeating lifetime after lifetime you will invariably attract a family or cultural structure that will cause this pattern to be repeated. The Boab Essence will access and clear those core patterns and the connected beliefs and repetitive lifetime situations. A classic example of this is in certain trouble spots in the world such as in conflict-stricken Bosnia, where souls keep reincarnating lifetime after lifetime into basically the same tribal disputes or wars that have been going on for centuries.

The Hoffman Quadrinity Process, a ten day workshop that has been taught worldwide for over twenty years, has as its primary premise the belief that all human suffering stems from negative attitudes, feelings and behaviour. It is what Bob Hoffman calls 'the curse of humanity'. These patterns are unwittingly programmed onto children by each generation's parents who in turn were programmed by their parents before them. The Hoffman Process is designed to identify, trace to the source, then clear and replace the negative patterning. In Australia, the instructors spray Boab around the room during the workshop to speed up the process and facilitate even greater results. If you are already doing work on clearing negative patterns, then Boab will speed up this process.

Boab works on the spiritual level initially and then on the mental and emotional; it also has to do with clearing karma of past actions. If, in the past, an individual has acted in a detrimental way towards another then, when that injured person returns to earth in a new incarnation, they will carry with them a dark line of energy which is connected to the person who originally harmed them. This energy line will almost invariably bring them into contact with each other so as to commence the readdressing of the karma. The Boab will clear this negative/dark line of energy. Often if there are negative patterns operating between two people there can be lack of understanding at a conscious level as to why they are acting in a strange way towards each other. When that spiritual dark line is cleared so too is the confusion about understanding the other person's behaviour. Quite often they may have an insight regarding the situation or else have it revealed to them either through dream or in meditation. When taking Boab in particular, or Bush Essences generally, your dreams can be very revealing and insightful and it can be a good idea to make the time and effort to record them each morning.

There are no accidents on the earth plane nor can anyone hurt or kill another without there already being a contract or agreement between them. So even in a 'random' shooting where, on a physical level, the victim or victims had never had any contact with the shooter, on a karmic or spiritual level they certainly had. However, at this critical point in human history, we have far higher and more important opportunities and possibilities available to us than merely getting caught up in old karmic scores and scenarios. If we pursue this higher path then this can lead to us fulfilling our highest destinies. Once we stop being imprisoned by negative patterns, we can be open to far greater spiritual development, awareness and sensitivity.

The Boab Essence is also very powerful in helping people who are experiencing, or have experienced, abuse, persecution or prejudice. In most cases this, too, is a pattern that they have repeated many times in the past and are drawing to them again in this life.

When used as a spray in a misting bottle the Boab Essence is very good for clearing your space or environment of negativity that can arise from the thoughts and actions of people who are out of balance, or which stems from earth-bound spirits. Many of these lost souls have been around for a long time and the Boab will assist them to go towards the Light. However, the results will not be so effective if that energy is coming from a darker source. To counter this, add Angelsword to the spray. In fact many people also add Fringed Violet and Lichen to their spray. Boab is, however, my flower of choice to help move lost souls to the Light.

For over 200 years, homoeopathy has strongly asserted and worked on the premise that an individual's wellbeing and health disposition is, to a large extent, determined by the disease states from which his or her ancestors suffered. If, for example, syphilis had been present in the family tree, then future generations would be more prone to destructive illnesses of the tissues, such as heart disease and ulcers. But if gonorrhoea had been present then arthritis or conditions of excess growth, such as warts and tumours, would show up further down the family tree. These genetic tendencies to pass on disease predispositions are referred to as 'miasms'. The deeper-acting homoeopathic remedies have been shown to modify or clear these miasms. Boab also has that ability.

Many practitioners not only use Boab to clear emotional and mental traits but also prescribe Boab for illnesses which are genetic in nature. In many cases, where an illness passes through a family, it is a consequence of the children innocently and passively taking on the same behaviours and emotional responses as their parents and that had also led to the cause of the parents' or family's illness. There is no doubt, however, that some family illnesses are clearly of a genetic nature rather than being caused through a learnt emotional pattern. Boab, when used in these circumstances, is producing some very positive results, although it needs to be taken for longer than the normal one month period. This appears to be a very significant field of research for Boab.

Boab is a very important and incredibly powerful essence that brings about profound personal transformation; it also helps to bring about tremendous positive change on this planet by healing the collective consciousness.

I now release and clear all negative conditioning and family traits from my psyche.
I create my own reality which is now free of all persecution and abuse.
I now choose to fulfil my own destiny and not my family's.

Negative condition
taking on negative family thought patterns

•

repetition of past negative experiences

Positive outcome
releases past negative actions within families, abuse, prejudice

•

releases negative thought patterns

•

releases deep-held emotion

•

engenders positive personal growth

DOG ROSE OF THE WILD FORCES

(Bauera sessiliflora)

You cannot always control what goes on outside, but you can always control what goes on inside.—Wayne Dyer, in Everyday Wisdom

With its striking magenta flowers, this is the most flamboyant of the small *Bauera* genus and is endemic in many parts of the Grampians (in the Australian state of Victoria), where it is found chiefly in deep sandy gullies and along creek

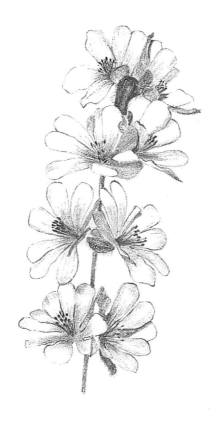

banks. It is also commonly named Grampians Bauera or Showy Dog Rose and belongs to the Saxifragaceae family. An evergreen shrub, it grows to a height of up to 2 m with a similar spread. It has a stout and erect stem with a compact, densely textured crown. The hairy leaves are trifoliate, sessile and opposite, being 3 cm long and occurring in whorls of six. Flowering time is in the spring from September to December, when the massed stalkless magenta flowers are produced along the stems towards the tips. The flowers are up to 2 cm long with six to twenty stamens. It is a sheer delight to come across the magenta splashes throughout the Grampians when Dog Rose of the Wild Forces is in bloom.

This plant belongs to the same genus as Dog Rose but is a different species. There is a fair degree of similarity between the two flowers: both usually have six brightly coloured magenta petals, although you can also have a colour which is lighter, pink or almost white, in the bloom of Dog Rose. With the latter, the flowers hang from the main stem on a thin tendril and have a bowed down, drooping appearance, whereas the flower of Dog Rose of the Wild Forces grows upright and is virtually attached directly on to the main stem. Its clearly visible stamens are black, as opposed to gold in the Dog Rose.

The Dog Rose of the Wild Forces Essence was made up from a plant that was dangling and quivering over surging white water just above Mackenzie Falls. Like Dog Rose, Dog Rose of the Wild Forces can usually be found growing around water.

There were some very harrowing aspects to the making of this essence, as I had to cautiously and often precariously inch along a narrow rock ledge next to the surging, swollen river over which the particular bush I was collecting from jutted out. The flowering stems of this bush were clearly seen to be shaking, as if trembling with fear, as the river roared past underneath. Less than a metre beyond this point the river cascaded over the sharp drop of the falls. I didn't even want to consider the consequences if I were to slip and be swept away.

After the flowers had been in the bowl for an hour, I came over to commence discarding them and start decanting the Mother Tincture, but my intuition was telling me strongly that it wasn't complete and that I should leave this final process till the following morning. Just as many years earlier, while making the Red Helmet Orchid in Western Australia, where I also had to leave that essence overnight, this one was left out under the full moon. Both the Red Helmet Orchid and the Dog Rose of the Wild Forces address some very yang behaviours and situations. It seems to me that by bringing the more nurturing lunar qualities into the essence-making process for both remedies, there occurs a softening of the harsher aspects of both.

Often found growing next to Dog Rose of the Wild Forces is a tall thick bracken that I had to clamber over so I could get close enough to photograph my flower. The bracken was so thick that I could actually lie on top of it and have my weight supported without falling through. From the Doctrine of Signatures' point of view this is like the safety net that the essence puts out to those people who need it, that stops them from plummeting to destruction. This essence gives tremendous support and helps an individual reach that point where they can serenely surrender and simply 'let go and let God'.

In Chinese medicine the element of water is represented

by the kidney meridian. The emotion associated with the kidney is that of fear, the main emotional state resolved by Dog Rose which addresses common and niggling minor fears, and anxiety. But as can be gleaned from the Doctrine of Signatures of Dog Rose of the Wild Forces—with the associated surging torrents of white water—this essence is involved with more intense, turbulent emotion. It is for a person's fear of losing control, when the emotions they are feeling within themselves or immediately around them are so intense that there is a sense of imminent loss of total control.

Dog Rose of the Wild Forces can be used when a person finds themselves in an environment which is an emotionally charged situation, where for example there may be hysteria all around them, such as in the case of an IRA bombing one year, during the peak Christmas shopping period at Harrods in London. Or in sporting arenas when some of the terraces have given way, or even the stampede to the exits in a crowded place or building at the time of a fire. In all these situations there is the very real possibility of being swept up into the cauldron of surrounding *external* turmoil and emotion.

The mourning that occurred in England at the death of Princess Diana, where the whole country was caught up in a shroud of shock and intense grief, was a situation where people were taken over by the intensity of their own *inner* feelings. Her death savagely rocked the psyche of England, a country and culture where, traditionally, deep emotional display is unusual, and even somewhat disapproved of. It was as if the floodgates holding back years, even generations, of suppressed emotions and denial of death, were suddenly opened and flowed out along with the grief. Dog Rose of the Wild Forces was dispensed frequently at this time.

On a higher level, Dog Rose of the Wild Forces helps to teach the necessity of gaining control over the emotions so that emotional intensity will not distort one's natural energies and balance.

Some people describe the feeling associated with the need for this essence as like being on a knife's edge. It is as if they were going to snap at any moment and either lose their temper, or lose complete control, and do something violent or destructive to themselves and/or to other people. Dog Rose of the Wild Forces is successfully used and should be thought of whenever anyone has the sense or feeling that they are going to lose it at any moment. Dog Rose of the Wild Forces, for this reason, is often added to Emergency Essence.

It can also relieve physical pain that has no obvious cause. Quite often the cause of this is an injury, a wound that was received in a past life. In many cases the current symptoms correspond to how they were killed previously. One of my patients presented with severe chest pain and shortness of breath. She had consulted numerous doctors and cardiologists, convinced that she had heart disease. Yet none of these medical practitioners could detect any abnormality or offer any explanation as to why she could be experiencing these symptoms. Using a technique known as age regression, I was able to lead her back to the earliest time that she had experienced chest pain. What surprised us both was how far back in time she went to find that memory, seeing herself in a Stone Age period, clothed in animal skins, screaming with terror as she was dragged from a cave and speared through the heart. She eventually reviewed seven other past lives in which she was mortally wounded by spears, arrows or bullets, each one passing through her heart in its own time slot. No wonder she was experiencing pain in her chest this time around. These regression sessions were so torrid that we were only able to deal with three episodes at a time, and as we released and cleared the cellular memory of each successive lifetime she would often be left sobbing almost hysterically. I have never experienced any patient having such a cathartic experience during age regression, and it certainly indicated the depth to which she had been traumatised, as well as the depth of healing she was now allowing herself. However, when we had finally worked back to present time, the severity and frequency of her symptoms had gradually abated and totally resolved after a course of Dog Rose of the Wild Forces, Fringed Violet—for the shock and trauma—and Sturt Desert Pea—for the deep hurt and pain. During the sessions, while she was still in past time, I was administering Dog Rose of the Wild Forces and sometimes Emergency Essence as well.

Ian Stevenson, from the University of Virginia, has done extensive research into the subject of reincarnation. In one study where he had access to the death certificates of the people his subjects claimed to be in their previous lifetimes, he was interested to see if there were any correlation between the manner in which they died and the markings found in the corresponding part of their body in this current life. Time after time he proved there was a correlation between the two. For instance, one subject in his perceived previous life had, according to medical records, died from a gunshot wound to the chest. Now, when a bullet enters the body the entry wound or opening is quite small; however, the hole made where the bullet leaves the body is much larger. In examining this particular person Stevenson noticed a small birth mark corresponding exactly to the point where the bullet had previously entered, and a much larger birth-mark again at the same point where the bullet had passed out through the back of his body. Stevenson's research and results are quite fascinating.

During a workshop I held in November 1997 one practitioner spoke of how he had found Dog Rose of the Wild Forces very good when working with Vietnam veterans.

> They are often very controlled, not losing their tempers— yet they just feel terrible inside. They have traumatic stress disorder and suffer multiple repressed feelings and problems which are coming up all the time. Having such good control, they are not expressing them, just holding them down. Taking Dog Rose of the Wild Forces helps them deal with their repressed feelings and allows these frustrations and horrors of their war experience to slowly dissipate, similar to a safety valve letting off steam and so preventing a meltdown or explosion.

Carolyn Jack, a metaphysical teacher from Calgary, Canada, has found a great need for, and subsequent benefit from, using Dog Rose of the Wild Forces with her students. Her course covers health and healing as well as spirituality, and attracts participants from a broad spectrum of the community, including many doctors. What she notices is that as her students are opened up to whole new paradigms of thinking, they often reach a stage where it feels as if their consciousness is expanding too quickly. They can often think they are going to go crazy and their mind will snap. This is the crucial point where she brings in this essence and describes the results as brilliant.

Another case history, involving Dog Rose of the Wild Forces, came from a therapist who wrote (in *The Essence*, Spring 1992):

> I would like to share with you an experience I have had with a single dose of the new Dog Rose of the Wild

Forces. I decided to try it when I was having a severely depressing, debilitating time. I cannot tell you how powerful its activity was. I had been unable to 'do' anything. I sat, as if held in my chair, weighted by no specific thing. I stayed with this state for perhaps an hour or so and finally in curiosity tried Dog Rose of the Wild Forces. One dose. For two minutes there was no response, then suddenly I felt as if my heart was ripping open. I shrieked in pain (not in a physical sense) but in the severity of the opening. I sobbed, allowing the intensity to come through me. The experience went on for fifteen to twenty minutes and was finally completed in a sigh of, 'What was that all about?' An incredible weight was lifted and I went about my business. As a therapist I was able to remain in the experience and watch what was occurring. This state or condition has not returned.

Earlier in this book, in the section on Alpine Mint Bush, I mentioned a doctor in England who was consulted by a patient who felt really furious with his wife and was worried that he might do her some serious harm. The case concluded the following way. Working intuitively, the doctor prescribed Dog Rose of the Wild Forces for his patient and suggested he take the drops regularly over the next several days. The fellow came back to see him three days later and said: 'It was really easy. I decided to forgive my wife this time.' He had calmed down and was now totally in control of his emotions.

As stated earlier, this remedy provides the safety net of being able to cope. There is the security that if you do go over the edge there is something to catch you instead of you plummeting to destruction down below.

I am now totally calm and serene.
I am in control of my life and actions.
I act always in the highest good for myself and others.

Negative condition

•

fear of loss of control

•

physical pain with no apparent cause

Positive outcome

•

emotional balance

•

calmness

•

sanity in times of turmoil

FRESHWATER MANGROVE

(Barringtonia acutangula)

*N*othing is either good or bad but thinking makes it so.—*Shakespeare*

This short, robust, spreading tree can be found growing along the banks of freshwater creeks and rivers, and at the edges of billabongs and swampy areas, during the rainy season. Freshwater Mangrove can attain a height of between 5 to 8 m and is usually multi-stemmed, with a dark grey, rough bark.

The leaves are up to 15 cm long and from 2.5 to 4.5 cm wide. They are distinctively crowded at the end of the branches. At any time of the year, but especially during 'The Wet'—November to March—small caterpillars, whose bodies are covered with stinging hairs, live on the underside of the leaves. One has to be careful to avoid these caterpillars as their hairs can easily penetrate human skin, producing an intense, irritating skin rash. The caterpillars are often called 'Itchy Grubs' and hence the reason for the *Barringtonia actuangula*'s lesser known common name of 'Itchy Tree'. The species name, 'acute angular', is derived from the Latin *acutus* which means sharp, and *angulus* meaning angled or cornered and refers to the fibrous four-angled fruit.

Freshwater Mangrove has a wide distribution across the top end of Australia, from the north-west of Western Australia through to Cape York in Queensland. Freshwater Mangrove is also found throughout South-East Asia and even as far north as India and Afghanistan.

When pounded, crushed and then placed in water, the bark and leaf of this tree release a substance that Aboriginal people use to temporarily stun fish, making them very easy to catch.

The main flowering time for Freshwater Mangrove is from July to September, although these attractive red blossoms can frequently be seen as late as February. The flowers, with

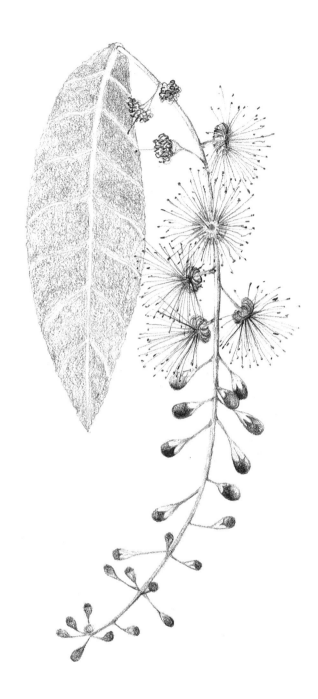

numerous stamens about 1 cm across, grow from a long, pendulous spike or raceme. The spikes can be up to 20 cm long and hang down from the branches. The buds furthest from the tip of the spike open first.

I had been aware of and interested in this flower since

1987, but I didn't make up its essence until September 1995, at the same billabong in the Top End where I had re-made Red Lily the previous year. Again, the making of an essence at this location wasn't without its difficulties. I needed to wade thigh deep in boggy, stagnant water, continually sinking further down into the muddy bottom while all the while keeping a wary eye out for crocodiles and, to a lesser extent, mosquitoes and leeches. In order to get out to the tree—I was by now almost waist deep—I started to place milk crates in front of me as stepping stones. As I disturbed the bed of sediment with each step, thick bubbles slowly rose around me releasing a foul sulphurous stench and making deep gurgling sounds as they reached the surface. In order to collect the flowers, and to take high quality photographs of them in good light, it was necessary to climb on to the tree, leaning against it and climbing up and over branches, continually trying to avoid the caterpillars. I think I was 'well looked after' that day as I clambered around this tree and prepared the essence, although at one point my hands did start to sting and itch and swell. I applied Emergency Essence every ten minutes and this was enough to quickly relieve the irritation, and I woke the next day with, thankfully, no ill effects . . . ah, the joys of making Flower Essences!

I was certainly glad I had my Emergency Essence with me that day as an Aboriginal man, with whom I had sailed down the East Alligator River, told me how he had just spent four days with his eyes puffed and swollen and almost totally closed as a result of inadvertently rubbing his eyes after merely touching the leaf of a Freshwater Mangrove!

The healing quality that the Freshwater Mangrove brings to humankind is the ability to release and heal mental prejudice. Often the seeds of this prejudice have been sown for a long time and in many cases it is generational. It is for the person who has already made up their mind about something or someone without ever having actually experienced them. One can see this, for example, in places of racial tension such as Northern Ireland where young Catholics are brought up from an early age hearing prejudice against Protestants from their parents, family and friends. All these seeds of intolerance have been sown generation after generation. Inevitably, because of the prejudices which have been conditioned into them, there arises a reference or filter through which they start to view and judge. Freshwater Mangrove would be a very useful remedy for the person growing up in this situation who has already, on a mental level, made up their mind about Protestants without having had much contact with them at all. Slender Rice Flower, on the other hand, would be prescribed for a person who has directly experienced, in a negative way, Protestant people, their culture or religion so that this has coloured their outlook.

Once you have a reference or expectation about someone it becomes quite easy to find things to reinforce your point of view. If you have repeatedly experienced your best friend being kind and considerate towards you, then you are likely to be accepting and forgiving of them if they are having a bad day and being really nasty to you. You know that their behaviour is not who they really are, it is just the circumstances or the way they happen to feel that day. However, if someone whom you have never met, although you have heard many negative things said about them by other people, starts behaving in exactly the same way as your friend, then almost undoubtedly your prejudice from those earlier references—other people's comments—will come through and you will find yourself judging and dismissing this person without giving them the benefit of the doubt.

Freshwater Mangrove was successfully prescribed by a practitioner for a colleague who was doing some research work but was having a lot of trouble finding the information, or even seeing it, because it wasn't appearing in the form in which he expected to find it. Expectations can be a dreadful curse! And very limiting. I was told of a spiritual group who were working with meditation on the chakras. One woman became very disheartened because none of her chakras were the beautiful colours that she had expected them to be. Yet throughout the whole meditation, she was aware of Jesus standing to her left, and she was still disappointed!

This essence is very beneficial in those situations where the heart is closed as a result of a mental prejudice. The Doctrine of Signatures in relation to the itching aspect of this tree is represented by the mental irritation that our prejudice can produce within us.

An example of such prejudice could be the reaction of the public in the United States to the trial of O. J. Simpson, who had been accused of the murder of his ex-wife. Everyone had already made up their mind about his guilt without having experienced the actual incident or before having heard the evidence presented at the trial. Another instance could be children who refuse to eat a certain food, saying that they don't like it, even though they have never tried it before.

Many prejudices are built because it is the culture's or society's belief that something *can't* be done. I know a man who successfully teleported his body from the United States to England, but at the last moment he started to doubt whether it was going to work and instead of 'landing' right inside the house as he had planned, he found himself stuck halfway through the ceiling of the loungeroom, with a number of broken ribs! This same man claims he knows of five other people in the world who have also teleported themselves from one country to another. It certainly sounds easier, and cheaper, than lining up at the check-in counter with all your luggage and then flying in a little metal box for hour after hour!

And I know of a man who, with some of my friends, was at a party in the Bay area of San Francisco, when suddenly he found his arm going through the wall right up to his shoulder. He didn't break the wall, his arm just passed through it. He was so shocked that he quickly pulled it right out again. There was a long stunned silence that followed: after all, in the paradigm of this man and his friends (and of ours), you are not supposed to be able to do that. They thought, 'Wow! This is a bit weird!' and wondered what they had been drinking! According to quantum physics it should be possible, theoretically, for this man to put his arm through the wall, but it is still very different from the reality we know and with which we are comfortable. After all, we have all had thousands of references that tell us that if we lean against a solid wall it will support us and not let us slip through it.

Back in 1954 two runners, Bannister and Landy, each broke the four minute mile in the same race. Prior to that race, everyone had said that it was physically impossible to break the four minute barrier. However, once it had been broken, almost immediately other athletes around the world started smashing the barrier too. Once people begin to believe that something can be done then it is only a matter of time until it is. It usually is an extraordinary, unique individual who is the first one to break through the old existing beliefs and barriers, taking whole cultures and societies with them to a new way of thinking.

When there is mass belief in society that something can't be done, then this gets so locked into our thinking that it becomes our reality. One of the important roles of Freshwater Mangrove is to open us up to an awareness that there are other ways of doing and perceiving which are different from what we have done before.

Our cultural beliefs about aging are that as we get older we will be less healthy, energetic and mentally sharp. Yet, after middle age we lose only 1% per annum from any of these areas. So the reality of aging does not have to be the grim experience that many people manifest for themselves because of their negative expectation.

Deepak Chopra often mentions in his lectures that we are surrounded and continually bombarded by billions of stimuli every second. It is physically impossible (or at least that is what we have been told!) to process such a volume of information. Consequently we usually only allow through our sensory filters those stimuli which reinforce our existing beliefs, blocking out all the rest.

The early Portuguese explorer, Magellan, recorded in his log book, hundreds of years ago, that when he sailed into Tierra del Fuego the native people were oblivious to his ship for the first three days after his arrival. This totally unfamiliar large object, anchored in the middle of their bay, was so different from their view of reality that it was invisible to them! Eventually a couple of the local people inadvertently crashed their canoe into the side of the ship. What a shock they must have received! Afterwards, as these wet and somewhat bewildered canoeists climbed on board, the ship suddenly became visible to the rest of the tribe.

It is well known, scientifically, that there are rod and cone cells in a cat's eyes which allow the animal to differentiate between horizontal and vertical lines. In his lectures Deepak Chopra has told of an experiment conducted at Harvard University, where one group of young kittens was put in a room where there were only vertical lines. After being there for an extended period of time it was observed that the kittens were unable to recognise any horizontal lines. The other control group of kittens was placed in a room with only horizontal lines and at the end of the same period they were unable to detect any vertical lines. So from that old adage 'if you don't use it you'll lose it' we could also extrapolate 'if you don't use it you can't see it'.

Freshwater Mangrove has the potential to allow us to fully experience and be open, on a heart level, to all the changes now occurring, and that undoubtedly will continue to rapidly accelerate over the next decade or so. At this present

Negative condition

•

heart closed due to expectations or prejudices which have been taught and not personally experienced

•

refusal to try new things for no good reason

Positive outcome

•

openness to new experiences, people and perceptual shifts

•

healthy questioning of traditional standards and beliefs

time there is a flood of new thoughts, ideas, experiences and evidence that drastically challenge, and are radically shaking our perception of, our world and reality. Who knows to what degree our sense of reality can be altered and, I dare say, enlarged and improved upon, if we can tear down some of our currently existing limiting filters. Freshwater Mangrove is a remedy that has the ability to do exactly this by opening us up to different paradigms and making visible the 'Magellan boats' of our future reality.

I now let go of expectations.
I never close my mind to something I have never experienced.
I am now open to new ways of perceiving.

GREEN SPIDER ORCHID

(Calandenia dilatata)

*L*earn to be silent.—*Pythagoras*

This perennial orchid is found widespread throughout all states of Australia in open forest and woodlands, although along the east coast Green Spider Orchid can also occur in open heathland. Generally it prefers sandy, gravelly or stony soils and clay loams and, like most native terrestrial orchids, is usually found in discrete patches. The slender flower stem can reach a height of 40 cm and bears one to two flowers. The solitary leaf is hairy, green and oblong to lanceolate and can be up to 12 cm by 18 mm.

The flower can be seen in the spring time, growing up to 10 cm across with elongated, slender sepals and petals. It is distinguished by long, yellowish-green comb-like fringes on either side of the blood red-stained recurved lip. The five spidery segments are all from between 3 to 5 cm in length and are also greenish-yellow, with a red central stripe.

This remedy was made up on the same trip as Dog Rose of the Wild Forces. Like the latter it too was prepared in the Grampians, or Gariwerd as the Aborigines refer to it, in central Victoria.

As I was driving out of the Grampians heading back to

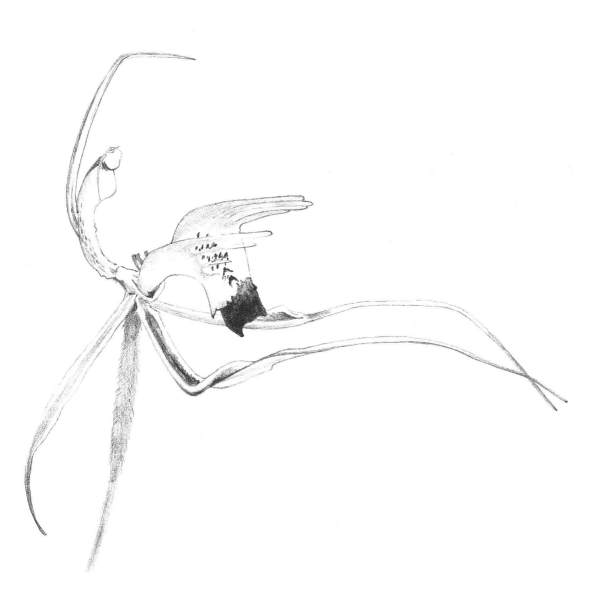

Melbourne, feeling very satisfied that I was leaving with the brand new Dog Rose of the Wild Forces Essence, I suddenly received a very strong message that I should do a U-turn and head off in the opposite direction. My curiosity aroused, I drove along on this new unplanned route for quite a few kilometres until, as a dirt road loomed up on my left, I received further instructions, this time to turn up that dirt road. After only a short distance, I had a very strong sense to stop driving, get out of the car and walk off into the bush, knowing that there was something very important to find there. One hundred metres or so later I found what was calling me—a colony of Green Spider Orchids. Initially I was aware of only one, but on looking more carefully I discovered there were close to twenty all around me.

These orchids were amazing to find and observe. They have an almost human-like appearance. It is easy to discern their 'arms', 'legs', 'torso', 'neck' and 'head' yet there is something alien about them: they look and feel as if they are not really of this planet. This impression is certainly reinforced by the antenna-like segment above the 'head' of the flower, which was shaking and vibrating, almost as if it were indeed very sensitive antenna through which the plant was communicating, sending out information of a very high and subtle nature. I certainly felt that the message that enabled me to find this flower had been sent out through the colony's antennae.

This essence can assist in working with telepathy between people. Not only can it help cut down the phone bill in talking to friends and family, it can also be very beneficial in communicating with deaf people and those with speech difficulties such as after a stroke, or between people from different countries where there is no common language.

Green Spider Orchid also helps one attune to, and be more receptive to, not only other people but also the plant and animal kingdoms. This remedy brings about a greater awareness of and communication with the spirit kingdom, especially with the nature spirits and devas of the flowers.

Green Spider Orchid Essence is very much aligned with higher teachings and philosophies as well as helping to provide deep spiritual insights. This remedy is excellent for those who are reaching out to new levels of awareness, and for those who are teaching spiritual matters and understandings. It helps them to fully comprehend that knowledge and then effectively impart it, not just verbally but also telepathically. Teachers taking this essence find that their spiritual message is conveyed on a much higher level than if they used words alone.

This essence creates within us a knowing of the appropriate timing of when to share new information and reveal our spiritual experiences and projects with others. Metaphysically, the energy behind a project can be dissipated if the people planning it discuss it widely before it is commenced or even fully manifested. Similarly, the potency and impact of a very powerful spiritual event experienced by an individual can be dispersed if it is shared and talked about with all and sundry. What's more, if the people with whom it is discussed are at a different level of awareness or development, then it will have far less meaning or value for them.

Green Spider Orchid helps an individual to keep information within. In its Doctrine of Signatures the flower appears like a sentinel, standing guard with its legs crossed, keeping its knowledge and information checked and withheld. The flower also has a prominent fringed tongue with large wine-red clubs, or calli, pivoted so that the slightest tapping of the stem will cause the tongue to vibrate rapidly, signifying the dichotomy between wanting to talk, but knowing it is best not to.

An interesting question for us all to consider is: 'Can I keep quiet when there is nothing to say?'. But it is not so much idle chit-chat for which this essence is used, rather it is for the awareness of knowing when to share knowledge or experiences of a slightly more profound nature. One of the reasons we include Green Spider Orchid in a mix that we spray around our workshop venues before the participants arrive is to help reinforce the discipline of silence that we ask of them when they first enter the room. I am frequently surprised by the difficulty people seem to have in being quiet and in their own space, even for the shortest periods of time!

Many personality types have great difficulty in not sharing their spiritual experiences and knowledge, and especially their projects. They have a strong desire to communicate something which they feel is very important or which has powerfully affected them. This can stem from a need for approval; looking and hoping for recognition and acceptance; wanting to show that they are really advancing or developing spiritually; or simply wanting to boast and hoping to impress. This remedy is very good for holding within new information until it has been assimilated and the energy around it built up, before that knowledge is shared— if it is appropriate to do so, as it may well be better just to keep the information to oneself.

Green Spider Orchid can release nightmares, terror and phobias arising from past lives. Many of the nightmares which beset young children are associated with past times, as they process a great deal of their former lives in their early years, especially the most recent life. If you observe the games or the toys with which a child likes to play you can usually pick up clues as to their major preoccupation or experiences from that last life. It can be very disconcerting for parents who advocate a peaceful and non-aggressive morality to find that their sons or daughters want toy guns or bows and arrows to play war games and kill people, or have a fascination with anything to do with war. Usually you will find that such a child has been a soldier in that past life.

Quite often it can be difficult to determine if a child's nightmare is due to something from a past life or from something in this one. An easy solution to this dilemma is to combine the Green Spider Orchid with Grey Spider Flower, as the latter is usually used for nightmares of a general nature.

A friend of mine suffered nightmares that were obviously stemming from past life experiences. Richard told me the amazing story of how every night, for a ten year period, he would go to sleep, dream all night of killing people in fights and battles and wake up in the morning feeling exhausted. He also said how in his dreams death wasn't quick and clean, as you see in the Hollywood movies, but rather brutal, gory and often slow. (Interestingly, this essence also addresses and clears the fear of blood.) Now in his early fifties, Richard has done a great deal of hypnotic regression to explore his past lives, and has discovered that this current life is the only one in which he lived past the age of thirty! Lifetime after lifetime he had been a soldier or warrior leading a very short and violent life. I get the feeling that Richard is a little disappointed and miffed that I hadn't made up Green Spider Orchid all those years earlier when he was having the nightmares.

Green Spider Orchid is for opening up the three higher chakras found above the crown. Red Lily and Kapok Bush also work on and balance these higher chakras.

At the time of making these two Gariwerd essences, Dog Rose of the Wild Forces and Green Spider Orchid, I received the message that both would stimulate rapid growth on the spiritual path. They heralded the fact that people were now ready to go to and work with higher energies, and the new levels of awareness with which these two essences were dealing. The next three essences that followed—Angelsword, Boab and Freshwater Mangrove—certainly reinforced and continued on this theme of speeding up the evolution of human consciousness.

Three years after that initial visit to the Grampians, I returned to take some new, and better, photographic shots for the then soon to be published *Flower Insight Cards*, as well as to replenish my supplies of Mother Tincture. My experience that trip confirmed once again just how much magic there is in working with the Bush Essences. After three days of blissful bushwalking in which I had made fresh supplies of Dog Rose of the Wild Forces, I hadn't sighted any Green Spider Orchids. Consequently, during my meditation on this third night, I asked to be shown, and received, very clear instructions as to where I could find Green Spider Orchid.

I was told to proceed 1.4 km up a specific dirt road and then after going 30 m into the bush I would find my Green Spider Orchid. The next morning in that exact location I found a Green Spider Orchid—very wilted, tattered, dusty and obviously at the very end of its flowering cycle. A good lesson was learnt by me on clarity: next time, I decided, I would have to ask for where I could find *lots* of Green Spider Orchids, all in perfect bloom. I also realised it is helpful to accurately record the location where I make up the more exotic flowers! For on my previous journey to this region I had stayed in a caravan park. Unfortunately, the caravan park, which was my reference point, had long gone by the time I returned on this trip.

I returned to Halls Gap, the main town in the Grampians, for dinner quite late on that fourth night as I spent a great afternoon after my lone flower discovery, rock climbing and meditating. When the third successive restaurant told me that its kitchen was closed, I began to feel somewhat frustrated but there was a strong sense that wherever I ended up for dinner that night, it would be perfect and I should simply trust. The fourth restaurant thankfully was open; what's more, they even served organic food, although they did not bother to mention this on their menu. At the restaurant I came across an old brochure promoting the Annual Wild Flower Exhibition, which had been held two months earlier, and listing the organiser and a contact telephone number for her. In my whole time in the Grampians I had not seen a similar brochure anywhere. The next morning I contacted this number only to find that the woman I wanted was in Melbourne for the week. Her husband wanted to know if there was any way he could help me. After explaining to him my desire to find Green Spider Orchid, he mentioned that he was the person in charge of putting together the Orchid display for the Exhibition. He had seen some flowering a few days earlier in an area and environment where I would not have looked. He generously offered to take me there that morning. Not only did Ken lead me to

Negative condition

·

nightmares and phobias from past life experiences

·

intense negative reactions to the sight of blood

Positive outcome

·

telepathic communication

·

ability to withold information until the timing is appropriate them, he also gave me some very beneficial photographic tips as well. The rest of the morning was blissfully spent crawling through the grassland, photographing, drawing and tuning in to Green Spider Orchid as well as making the essence. Another hard day in the office!

I now have greater communication with plants, animals and Spirit.
I now release all terrors and fears from my ancient past.
I now share, in perfect timing, what is appropriate.

GYMEA LILY

(Doryanthes excelsa)

Never be afraid to tread the path alone.
Know which is your path and follow it wherever it may lead you;
do not feel you have to follow in someone else's footsteps.—
Eileen Caddy, in Footprints on the Path

Arising from a large, bright green, thick rosette of sword-like leaves up to 1.5 m long, is a stiff, erect flowering stem 3 to 7 m tall. This stem bears a large, dense, spectacular head of fleshy, red, trumpet-shaped flowers. Gymea Lily's flower, which is borne in early spring, is colossal, frequently being over 40 cm wide, while the individual flowers, from the tightly clustered head, are each 6 cm long, and protected by bracts of a deeper red colour. Even the six long stamens, richly coated with their green pollen, stand upright, prominent and elevated, rising high above the petals.

A stunning member of the Agavaceae family, it is one of the most beautiful and striking flowering plants, and quite untypical of the other trees and shrubs that grow in its habitat all along the New South Wales coast north from Wollongong.

One and a half hour's drive north-west of Sydney, near an area known as Wiseman's Ferry, there is a magical location where Gymea Lilies are everywhere—it is like literally walking through a forest of them, of walking in a land of giants. It is such strong energy being with them all, and very uplifting. You just want to stand up straight and tall as you move among them.

The other common names associated with it bear witness to the extraordinary presence the Gymea Lily commands, as well as reflecting its size, appearance and distribution: Giant Lily, Flame Lily, Spear Lily and Illawarra Lily. Gymea was an Aboriginal name for this plant while the botanic name of its genus, *Doryanthes*, is a composite of two Greek words: *doratos*, meaning spear, and *anthos*, meaning flower. *Excelsa* is derived from the Latin *excelsus*, meaning high, lofty and exceptional.

Gymea Lily allows a person to draw from its powerful energy and attain the strength to be who they are, and do what they have to do. It enables them to achieve and fulfil their highest destiny, to find what gives them passion in their life and follow that passion, to do what really makes

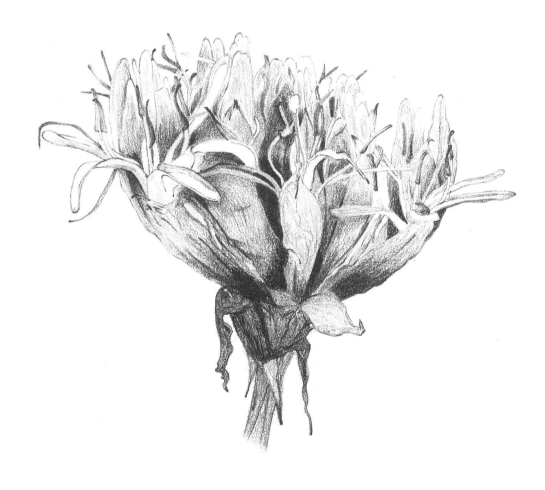

their heart sing. It is a remedy for those who are willing to lead an extraordinary life, flying high like an eagle, as opposed to living trapped, like the chicken in the chicken coop, in the numbing mediocrity and mindlessness of consensus reality.

It is very easy to allow your life to drift along in relative comfort and ease, with pleasurable distractions to fill your time, without ever questioning your own or society's views and beliefs. Yet so many of these beliefs, which form the foundation and structure of our society, are limiting and based on fear. They are programmed into us from an early age and are continually being reinforced through the media. People are encouraged to see themselves as victims, rather than empowered beings who are quite able to create their own reality within their lives.

However, there does seem to be a growing number of people all around the world who are searching for, creating and welcoming new challenges and opportunities that allow for their personal and spiritual growth and expansion. People whose focus is much more than that of merely the material and the physical, who pose questions such as: 'Why am I really here? What have I come to do?' and who then go on to base their lives and follow their dreams on the answers to such questions.

There are certainly not as many eagles as there are chickens and it can get a little lonely up there soaring on the thermals, although there is a much better view from the top. But it is not only the loneliness. Another problem is that the chickens know deep down that if they stay in the coop too long, they will lose the ability to fly and they can become envious of those beautiful birds flying high above.

If you are different from others in your views and beliefs or are very successful in your life, the Gymea Lily gives you the strength to stay in that position and not be affected or pulled down by any negative projections from those around you, or from those who may know of you. Gymea Lily helps you to stay so strong and focused on doing what you know you have to do with such single-minded purposefulness that you are not worried about what other people think of you or how they are judging you.

It can be a real threat to some people to see someone really succeeding because it focuses attention on what they are doing with their lives. Even though they may perceive their life to be nice and comfortable there still remains a niggling knowledge that there could be more than this, and that they ought to be asking questions about their own lives. But rather than do that there is often a tendency—and it is much easier—to try to pull the other person down or see them fail.

An aspect of the Doctrine of Signatures of the Gymea Lily flower is that it is so high it can't be clearly discerned from the ground; also, the flower is beyond the reach of, and out of touch with, those standing at the bottom.

In Australia we have what is known as the 'Tall Poppy Syndrome', something that stems back to this country's Anglo-Saxon origins. The syndrome describes the perverse pleasure, even celebration, our culture indulges in when a prominent or successful person appears to fall or fail. Success does not seem to be easily acknowledged, celebrated or even fully accepted in this culture, certainly in sharp contrast to a country like the United States.

As can be seen in its Doctrine of Signatures, the Gymea Lily is also beneficial for people whose personalities are very extrovert or for those who can be very dominating and charismatic, and used to getting their own way. These people are often natural leaders who find it quite easy to take control of a situation, and make split-second decisions. They do it so easily that they don't even think about it. They see what needs to be done, and instruct or order those around them to do it. Even if there is someone else in charge they will often automatically jump in and want to take over. It is not so much that they are trying to be bossy, it is just that they are used to doing it and they know they can make things work well. They are genuinely amazed when people get upset by them taking over. The Gymea Lily Essence tempers them somewhat, allowing them to consider if it is appropriate, or in fact necessary, for them to take charge. It also helps them to be a bit more aware of other people, not just riding roughshod over them, and to realise that these others have a real need to contribute in their own way, even if it is sometimes not very dynamic or efficient.

Erik Pelham offers an intriguing variation and addition to the more established understanding we have of the dominating personality aspect of Gymea Lily. I must confess I haven't worked with the remedy in this way nor do I have any case histories or feedback about it being used in this way, but I feel that it could offer a window to another dimension of this essence that, if researched and verified, could be very valuable. I offer Erik's Devic analysis to you in this context:

> Its purpose is to break down barriers of fear and trepidation that an individual has of powerful people, and help reconcile them to those who have power over them—if this is needed. Its most obvious use is breaking the fear and negativity that ordinary people have in dictatorships, and with those who wield power brutally and fearfully. This is a wide-ranging essence for alleviating fear and bringing reconciliation between an individual and anyone in power over them.
>
> The signature of this flower is of the fear inducing, menacing form that powerful people seem to have, which creates fear and trepidation of them in a person's mental perception of them. You can see this from the huge flower which has a rather weird and menacing form with its deep burgundy red flower parts and strange shapes within the flower—so often, those in authority of whom we are afraid, have this slightly menacing, larger than life quality in our perception.
>
> Gymea Lily has a very interesting dual action, as it transforms the negative thoughts one has about one's oppressor to positive ones *and* dissolves the fears that we hold of them as well. This is important because what keeps an oppressor carrying on oppressing people is the web of negative thoughts the people have of them. In other words, by thinking negatively about a ruler, and so defining them in a negative role, the people who think about them negatively actually keep them there in the role of oppressor. So, even if the Sadam Husseins of this world want to stop oppressing people, the sheer enormity of negative thoughts forms a huge sticky mire of negativity which holds him stuck in his ways, preventing him from changing. Thought is powerful, and these oppressors create their own prisons, but you must see that there is a responsibility on the oppressed for their own problem, as they are maintaining the problem through negative thought. By dissolving this negativity Gymea Lily makes it possible for an oppressor to really change—to be free from their self-made prison. By dissolving the blockage of fear we have about our oppressor, it makes love and reconciliation a possibility, leading to cooperation.

The difference between this quality of Gymea Lily, as portrayed by Erik, and that of Red Helmet Orchid, which is also about dealing with authoritarian figures, is that with the latter, people create their own problems by their rebellious challenging and attacking of those in authority; with Gymea Lily, however, they live in fear and trepidation of authority.

I made up this essence with my daughter Grace when she was only two years of age, around the Stanwell Tops area south of Sydney, near the Garden of Peace Sanctuary. A few years earlier, during a residential workshop there, the custodian of the Garden at the time implored me to make up Gymea Lily, a flower that she totally adored and which was prolific throughout the Sanctuary grounds. However the Gymea Lily wasn't calling out to me at that time and so I suggested maybe she should be the person to make the essence as she felt so strongly about it. Unfortunately, she passed over not long afterwards. Five years later, in the middle of a meditation, the Gymea Lily finally called out to me, saying that it was now the right time to make it up and that the place of choice was the Garden of Peace.

A few days after the meditation, I returned there, accompanied by Grace. As we were walking through the area I was surprised by how difficult it was to locate any of the plants in flower. So I told Grace that we would have to call out to it. Hand in hand, we continued our search, calling out 'Gymea Li-ly!!' as we went. It was a lovely time. Then, as we came up to a small ridge, she said excitedly: 'Daddy— it's over there!' We couldn't see beyond the ridge but as we clambered up it, we spotted a Gymea Lily in full flower immediately below. Grace made up her first flower essence that day. What a size flower to start with—it was nearly as big as she was! To make an essence from the whole flowering head would have required more a swimming pool than a bowl in which to float so we made the essence with a single floret from the head. Even then the very largest of my bowls just barely contained the flower.

While on the subject of young children, one of a newborn baby's very important early developmental needs is to receive the mirroring of total unconditional love from a nurturing person. If there is no one totally absorbed and besotted by the baby, looking into its eyes and sharing that love with it, then there will develop a deficit need from that stage of growth which will be very hard to redress in later stages. In adult life, such people may attempt to compensate by getting adoration from others. Being a rock star in front of 50,000 people could be an example of this. On a more ordinary note they will often have a desire to be noticed, to be the centre of attention or crave recognition. Gymea Lily addresses this attention-seeking behaviour and the constant need for status and glamour.

Astrologically, this essence correlates with the sun, and especially with Leo, with its emphasis on the sense of self, and of being seen and noticed. Gymea Lily can help to transmute into humility the excessive pride and arrogance that can often be found in an out-of-balance Leo.

Donna Cunningham, the internationally known American astrologer and flower essence practitioner, wrote to me telling how she gave this essence to one of her students whose:

> basic personality has contained strong aspects of condescension, spiritual arrogance, self-righteousness, and intolerance of 'double digit IQ's'. Although usually restricted to private thoughts, these characteristics do manage to seep through the seams. After the first five days it was noticed that her mind no longer occupied itself with those types of thoughts, which had been present in the personality since as early an age as ten months. At the time of this writing, after 14 days of the remedy, thoughts continue gentler and almost without judgment.

Leo rules the spine and this essence shows, once again, a correlation with this particular sun sign by the fact that it helps to align the spine. A number of osteopaths and chiropractors extensively use Gymea Lily for this reason and also because it is effective in working with problems in the bones and ligaments. Crowea, on the other hand, acts more on the muscles and tendons. In the ancient Chinese mystery schools, to break your word would lead to a breakage in one of your bones. Could there be any greater breaking of your word than to not honour your spiritual contract about what you agreed to achieve in this life, to fail to pursue your destiny with total commitment and passion?

I am now passionately following and fulfilling my life destiny.
I am now expressing strong leadership that acknowledges and utilises the help of others.
I am now expressing equally my power and humility.

Negative condition

- arrogance
- attention seeking
- craving status and glamour
- dominating and over-riding personality

Positive outcome

- humility
- allowing others to express themselves and contribute
- awareness, appreciation and taking notice of others
- reaching great heights

MINT BUSH

(Prostanthera striatiflora)

A *gem cannot be polished without friction.—Chinese* *proverb*

A native of New South Wales, Queensland, South Australia and Western Australia, Mint Bush can be found growing up to 3 m tall on ridges and rocky outcrops in the central parts of Australia, where it usually occurs as scattered plants and only occasionally forms rather dense communities. The stem of this evergreen shrub is erect, stiff and branching with a densely textured crown. The pale green leaves are 1 to 2 cm long, opposite, and ovate, and very aromatic, being rich in an essential oil containing antiseptic alpha-pinene and cineole.

This explains why many Aboriginal tribes and early European settlers used this plant either as a steam inhalation or as a wash for colds and influenzas. An ointment was traditionally prepared by mixing half a cup of leaves with one cup of animal fat, such as goanna or kangaroo, and heating them together to boiling point. When cooled, the mixture was applied topically for aches and pains, and the crusty sores of scabies.

These white 2 cm long flowers bloom prolifically in late winter, spring and early summer. In the majority of species of *Prostanthera*, which belongs to the Labiatae family, the flower tube is marked with dots or stripes which are regarded as a guide or landing strip for pollinating insects. But these markings are particularly prominent in the Mint Bush flower with its strong purple stripes in the throat and two golden yellow spots at the base. The corolla, or bell-shaped flower, ends in two lips, the top being notched and shorter than the lower one, which is three-lobed with a long central lobe, flanked by two shorter ones. Overall, the flower can seem like a small human figure with a hood or bonnet over its head.

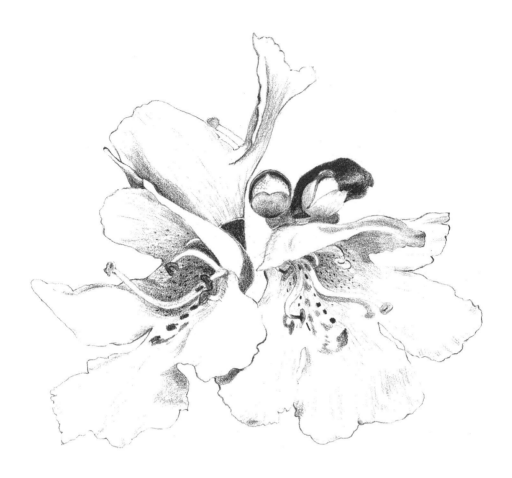

In 1989, I was given an understanding during meditation that if I were to go to Katajuta (the Olgas), in the Northern Territory, I would experience an important initiation. I was very excited by this. I hardly need any excuse, let alone a reason like this, to go back to this remarkable area, my beloved Katajuta. Ah! If only there were a surf beach there, it would be total bliss and my idea of heaven on earth! However my thoughts about the timing of this initiation were obviously very different from that of Spirit, as my intended trip to The Centre that year didn't eventuate: I was left stranded and frustrated in Sydney by floods and a prolonged airline strike. Anyway, the anticipation certainly made the trip the following year that much sweeter. I am not sure if I did actually receive an initiation then and there, for merely being at Katajuta is just so powerful, but it did trigger the beginning of a brand new phase in my life. As well, I left with a new essence—the Mint Bush—which, by coincidence, is all about helping a person cope and go through the intense experience of a spiritual initiation.

What that trip to Katajuta did do was herald and usher in the next twelve essences and a new phase of the Bush Essences. In their unique and powerful action, these new remedies reflected the spiritual emergence of both myself personally, and human consciousness and the planet, generally. Some initiation!

I had no intention of making any new remedies on that trip, Mint Bush in fact being the first new essence that I had made up in almost three years. At the very beginning of my work with the Bush Essences, I was told in meditation that there would be approximately fifty essences with which I would work. After the fiftieth essence, Yellow Cowslip Orchid, came through I was not led, nor did I receive any guidance, to prepare any other essences. I was quite open to doing more, but as the years went by I had basically become resigned to the fact that 'This is it' and that what would follow in my work would be to simply explore, research and go deeper with my understanding of each essence.

I made up the Mint Bush essence in the extremely sacred Valley of the Winds, which is one of the many places among these magnificent red rock domes where the energy is extremely powerful. Even on still days you can see the trees quivering and shaking with this energy. Traditionally Katajuta is a wandering place for men. I love going there, especially very early in the morning before the sun rises and while it is still dark, when I can literally have the place to myself. Each time I visit this magical part of the world, I attempt to explore a different area and I can spend all day out there in blissful solitude without seeing anyone—well, not anyone in a physical form anyway.

Even in spring, the sun can be quite hot and intense out in The Centre, and I am always very appreciative of coming across the very cooling and cleansing aroma that exudes from the Mint Bush, which is in sharp contrast to the dry arid heat of the area.

The morning I made this essence I was aware of the presence, on a spiritual plane, of twelve Aboriginal elders standing in a circle, surrounding me. They gave detailed instructions about making the essence, details of its properties and an understanding of both the plant and the Valley of the Winds. At one point I was being a little clumsy in my attempts to set up my tripod and photograph this flower, noisily stumbling over rocks and other plants, and I was sternly reprimanded by the elders. In no uncertain manner they let me know how very unimpressed they were with my trampling over this precious, sacrosanct spot, and that I should be far more respectful and careful.

Mint Bush is for the trials and tribulations that one goes through just prior to, or at the same time as, spiritual initiation. It is for the period when you feel you are being tested, often to your limits. There is the burning off of all the dross to allow you to emerge to a new spiritual level. Often at this time there is chaos and confusion—what is now currently referred to as 'perturbation'—and there can even be a sense of being in a void. Many people find their old beliefs and values obsolete, falling like crumbling stone pillars around them, crashing to the ground and smashing to smithereens. What also comes tumbling down, once these pillars have been removed, are the old structures that they have set up, and around which they have built their lives.

Mint Bush is fantastic when you find yourself in a period of perturbation, which can be likened to being in a washing machine where you are constantly going round and round in confusion and dilemma. An example could be in, say, a relationship: 'Should I stay in a relationship or should I leave?' You can see, and are weighing up, the pros and cons of all the options open to you, and you feel in turmoil. You just don't know which way to turn or how to act. Or alternatively, you can be in the same confusion and turmoil but with no sense of options. In both scenarios you get to the point where you feel as though you are going to crack up. You can't go on any more. There is not the total despair of the Waratah, but very much the feeling that everything is too difficult and too much to deal with and resolve. The nice thing about perturbation is that it does end, and with that ending comes clarity.

A few years ago, at the end of a teaching stint in Europe, I was intending to have a week's holiday in Amsterdam. Jim Wafer, a friend who had lived in that city for many years, had given me lots of addresses and phone numbers of interesting people who, Jim assured me, held the best parties in Amsterdam. I was looking forward to a wild and exciting week.

Jim, who is an amazing healer and masterful musician, had attached a long laser, with a site for a crystal to be placed in front of the laser, on to the top of his didgeridoo, giving it a bazooka-like appearance (he had previously been a paratrooper after all). He then would place a vial of a Bush Essence remedy in front of the laser and crystal, and also place a few drops of the remedy topically on specific points on a person. These might be acupressure points, the chakras or kinesiology test points for organs. As the person lay down he would place a Tibetan singing bowl over their heart or solar plexus, sometimes both, and then play the didgeridoo all around and over them, in his own unique style. Woahh!! So you had the essence being zapped into your body—and subtle bodies—with the extra addition of sound, crystal and laser.

However, once again, Spirit wasn't very interested in my intended travel plans. In between my English workshops, I was travelling along the St Michael's lay line doing earth healing work. When I was in Cornwall I met up with a Danish teacher who was taking a group of students from her Mystery School through England, also doing earth healing work.

When I arrived at my B&B after a long night of travelling, the owner asked if I were part of this woman's group. Apparently they had already gone out that evening to a nearby stone circle. I felt quite intrigued by them for some reason. The next morning I had hoped to leave early but I awoke feeling quite ill with food poisoning. When I finally made it down to the dining room, weakly sipping on a cup of peppermint tea, I noticed the group also at breakfast. I couldn't help but hear some of their conversation about their previous night's activity and meditations, and was quite fascinated.

Even though I tried to be inconspicuous and discreet, the group, especially their leader, would from time to time look over my way and start speaking Danish or German. I made two attempts to leave the house and get to my car but both times I fell asleep in front of the car! After waking up the second time, an English member of the group came over and started talking to me, inquiring what I did. She suggested that I might like to speak to their leader, Zana Ra.

Our first conversation together was innocent enough and she invited me to join them that evening for some earth healing meditation at another sacred site. At this next meeting, when alone together, she astounded me by telling me that they had been waiting for me and that I was two days late! She seemed a little annoyed by this. I had, in fact, taken two days out in Devon feeling as though I wanted some quiet R and R time, but I didn't know anyone else knew of my itinerary!

Zana Ra was a walk-in who was here on a two year assignment, just as the two previous walk-ins had been and who, like her, had shared that same physical body—although not all at once! When one left the next one would come in. Apart from her healing and teaching work, she was here to help counsel, train and prepare those individuals who were 'walking out' and moving to a new level of existence. Such people left their physical vehicle to be utilised by highly evolved spiritual beings like Zana Ra, beings who had specific and important roles to achieve but were way beyond, and in no need of, the normal third-dimensional life experience of being born into a young physical body. Not only was she to train the 'walk-outs' but also to train other walk-ins, helping them to understand how to maintain and balance their energies in a third-dimensional body. Adjusting to coping with a body, let alone with the third-dimensional life, is a difficult experience. She described the third dimension in quite derogatory terms, finding it difficult to be on a planet where the love vibration was so suppressed and denied.

At one point in England she said: 'I am being told that you have to come and spend a week with me in my centre.' So instead of raging in Amsterdam I had this quiet retreat in her spiritual centre—just the two of us for a week. No one else was around as the centre had closed for summer. It was one of the most remarkable and powerful times of my life. After my initial fears that she was going to tell me I was a 'walk-out' were allayed, I became like a sponge, intently absorbing every moment with her, every teaching, every new concept—and there were many. So many of my old beliefs disintegrated from my week with Zana Ra. At the same time I was also opened up to newer and greater realities; my understandings and awareness were broadened immensely to literally a much more universal spiritual view. This was a very positive Mint Bush experience on a grand scale.

I am now navigating my spiritual initiation with clarity and smoothness.
I am now letting go of all confusion and chaos in my life.
I am now lighting any darkness in my life with the dawning light of my new spiritual emergence.

Negative condition

·

perturbation

·

confusion

·

spiritual emergence

·

initial turmoil and void of spiritual initiation

Positive outcome

·

smooth spiritual initiation

·

clarity

·

calmness

·

ability to cope

PINK MULLA MULLA

(Ptilotus helipteroides)

*W*hen love beckons to you, follow him,
Though his ways are hard and steep.
And when his wings enfold you,
yield to him,
Though the sword hidden among his pinions may wound
you.—Kahlil Gibram, in The Prophet

Pink Mulla Mulla is an annual, ephemeral herb found in all states, except Tasmania, in the stony, dry interior country of outback Australia. Each bush comprises long erect branching flowering stems up to 50 cm tall and is sparsely covered with smallish, light green leaves, which are lanceolate. At the top of the stem is found a striking, purplish-pink, conical flowering head, about 2.2 × 1.5 cm, and comprising densely crowded blossoms, with a white tuft at the top. Each flower consists of five long, narrow, stiffened petals surrounding very prominent deep pink to magenta stamens, and covered on the outside with long fluffy hairs. The plant is in bloom through most of the year, although it is found less often in autumn. The small and inconspicuous fruit are enclosed by the base of the dead flower.

For many years I regarded the Pink Mulla Mulla as the 'black sheep' of the Bush Essence family. On a return trip to Katajuta (the Olgas) to replenish my Mulla Mulla (*Ptilotus atripicifolius*), I was shocked to find Pink Mulla Mulla growing all around it. When I had first made the Mulla Mulla, in Palm Valley, there was only the one obvious *Ptilotus* species. Now here I was suddenly confronted with the dilemma of what actually was the original species from which I had made the Mulla Mulla essence. My composure was certainly ruffled. The flowers of both plants looked quite similar, and quite a few years had elapsed since that earlier making.

After tuning into both plants, and desperately trying to recall the details of that earlier trip, I reached the stage where

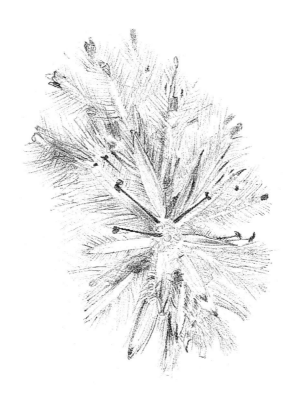

I was 95% sure which was which. However, there still remained that lingering doubt and so I decided I would make up what I later ascertained to be Pink Mulla Mulla— *Ptilotus helipteroides*—just in case. I reasoned that it would definitely be easier to have the essence already with me back in Sydney if later, through botanical research and extra tuning in, I decided that I had in fact mixed them up. So the Pink Mulla Mulla was birthed, so to speak, out of contingency factors rather than with the usual guidance and direction by which the other essences had come through.

Even when I was preparing the Pink Mulla Mulla Essence I didn't feel I was getting a full understanding of it, but was content to have it nevertheless. Botanically, there does seem to be quite some discrepancy between the various texts in regard to defining the different species, as well as agreeing on common names. Pink Mulla Mulla is frequently referred to as *Ptilotus exaltatus*, while I have often seen what I call Pink Mulla Mulla, *Ptilotus helipteroides*, labelled Tall Mulla Mulla. I must confess to having been guilty of perpetuating this confusion by, until recently, doing exactly the same thing in all our material—labels, promotional literature, insight cards and reference book! I am glad to be finally setting the record straight! Pink Mulla Mulla *is Ptilotus helipteroides.*

Quite a few people expressed interest in working with the Pink Mulla Mulla after they found out about it. So I decided to mention it in my newsletter, alongside the story and description of Tall Mulla Mulla, which was also prepared on that same trip. I did, however, honestly admit in *The Essence* newsletter of Autumn 1991 that 'its picture at this point is not particularly advanced but it will be interesting to observe, and will hopefully be filled in, by your observations and insights'. Possibly, because of the feeling of not having a total grasp of this essence, I rarely used it initially and didn't feel comfortable when people asked about it, even though the personality profile of Pink Mulla Mulla seemed to be clear enough.

Inspired by some great insights and results with this remedy by Ruth Toledo in Sao Paulo, Brazil, I made a special trip back to Katajuta to get to the bottom of this flower. This time, without that cloud of confusion hanging over it—or rather, over me?—I achieved what I felt to be both a thorough and satisfying experience and understanding of this essence. I felt greatly relieved to have all my 'flock' uniform and white once more!

The Pink Mulla Mulla is for those who have suffered a deep, ancient, spiritual wound, sometimes going back as far as their first incarnation, which has led to an old scar being left on their soul and psyche. The severe wound that often occurred as a result of such trauma is still carried in our psyches today, residing in the outermost level of our causal bodies. Consequently, we will put into place sabotages, at a very deep level, not at the psychological but at the causal body level, well hidden from our consciousness.

Being stored in the causal body means that neither the original experiences nor the sabotages will be perceived by most psychic healers and clairvoyants, who can usually only reach and read subtle bodies that are much closer to the physical. Kerrie Redgate with her spiritual astrology has, however, been able to pinpoint the earlier past life trauma and issues involved that create these sabotages. She cites an example in *The Essence* (Summer 1993): 'it may have been a traumatic experience when engaged in pioneering work that established authority figures of the day did not approve. All sorts of nasties befell those of us who dared to think differently in centuries past.' In the article Kerrie put forward the view that as a result of such a death experience and ensuing suffering undergone, a false concept about life may have been formed and as a consequence sabotage patterns are created. Kerrie has found only two modalities that can shift blocks or sabotages at the causal level, one being Spiritual Healing and the other Flower Essences, but only those essences released since 1977, the year when the comet/planetoid Chiron was discovered.

Kerrie goes on to say that 'the higher self resonates at the causal level, or the outermost of the rim of the aura'. She describes how the task of the higher self is to help you reach your chosen destiny. Yet sometimes those deep sabotages, as a result of old wounds on the psyche, can trigger within us an intense fear about ever again totally committing to and following our spiritual path or destiny because of this dread that those earlier traumas would be repeated. (Kerrie's forthcoming book *Astrology's Seventh Veil* will greatly expand on this theme.)

It should be noted that Pink Mulla Mulla has the ability to go right out to these causal bodies and heal that original trauma. According to research in Richard Gerber's book *Vibrational Medicine*, of the three most widespread forms of vibrational medicine—homoeopathy, gem elixirs and flower essences—it is the flower essences that work at such a high level. They have the ability to work right out to the outer subtle bodies, whereas homoeopathic remedies generally are restricted to the nervous system and chakras while gem elixirs operate about halfway in between.

I am often asked my opinion of homoeopathic radionic copies of the Bush Essences. Well, given that the Bush Essences work at this deeper level, as mentioned by Gerber, and that they are self-adjusting without side effects, why would you want to make the homoeopathic copy? What is the advantage? Also you introduce the possibility of aggravations when they are made homoeopathically and, even more importantly, you lose the devic and nature spirit connection from the remedy when it is made from a radionic card. In my opinion and experience, the resulting radionic remedy is only a pale imitation of the original flower essence.

In the Doctrine of Signatures of Pink Mulla Mulla it is easy to discern the human figure, its head, arms and legs, and from the centre of its solar plexus, cording back to that early experience, are the prominent stamens emanating from the very central core of the plant. The stamens are like cords that connect our current life back to the ancient traumas.

The Pink Mulla Mulla pulls out these cords, helping to disconnect the earlier trauma and any resulting sabotage patterns.

On an emotional level, Pink Mulla Mulla is for those who put prickles out to keep people away. These people tend to be quite isolated and loners by choice. They have often felt wronged or hurt or, they believe, have been treated unjustly in the past, which has affected them deeply. This impinges on their attitude to those around them and can make them suspicious of people and people's motives. They are often on guard against being hurt again and they may protect themselves by saying hurtful things to others. What they say to those around them doesn't always reflect what they really feel, it is merely a way of keeping people at a safe distance, for they have a fear of opening up and being hurt or abused. Southern Cross is more for people who act as victims, who blame others for their circumstances rather than taking responsibility for them, and often feel that life is not fair to them, whereas the Pink Mulla Mulla is more for protection against the possibility of being hurt or taken advantage of again. The Pink Mulla Mulla allows these people to trust, open up and interact more freely.

In transpersonal psychology a number of psychotherapists have been working with the Pink Mulla Mulla, claiming it to be one of the most important of the Bush Essences. They find that it assists clients in their process of breakthrough with tremendous efficiency and speed whenever there is resistance to change. They claim that previously this resistance had been extremely difficult to work with, because the origin of it goes back such a long way that the patient is unaware of it. The client may even feel that the therapist is attacking them when trying to bring this out into the open. One such psychotherapist, Janos Varga, has written (in *The Essence*, Summer 1991) that the Pink Mulla Mulla 'facilitates break-throughs, assisting people to overcome their resistances very, very quickly. The remedy provides recognition and understanding of where the resistances lie and once this understanding comes the energy which has been invested in resisting can then be used as a source of raw material to use in the process of self transformation'. Somatic psychotherapists, who also incorporate bodywork, report that as well as the obvious positive effectiveness of the remedy on the emotional and spiritual levels, this remedy will also correct long-term physical stiffness. This stiffness, the therapists

Negative condition

•

deep ancient wound on the psyche

•

an outer guarded and prickly persona to prevent being hurt

•

keeps people at a distance

Positive outcome

•

deep spiritual healing

•

trusting and opening up

feel, stems from and is a direct consequence of any resistance the client has in effecting profound change.

While still on the theme of physical conditions treated by the Pink Mulla Mulla, Erik Pelham claims the remedy works on the spleen and liver and is able to successfully treat haemolytic jaundice. This results when the red blood cells are more fragile than normal and are rapidly destroyed by the spleen, leading to anaemia. Erik believes that this unpleasant disease results from disregarding our Higher Will, being idle and neglecting our true path. This toxic condition in the Will creates blockages in the physical body in the area of the spleen and liver which then cause the haemolytic jaundice. The Pink Mulla Mulla, he states, works by initially vibrating the causal body to a higher rate of vibration so that this type of toxicity in the Will is dissolved and cleansed while, at the same time, dissipating physical blockages in the spleen and liver. The Pink Mulla Mulla, by cleansing and purifying the Higher Will, gives it great impetus not to get side-tracked by unimportant issues again.

I am now passionately and fearlessly following my spiritual path.
I am now trusting and opening up to myself and others.
I now know myself to be, and live my life, as a radiant being of light.

RED SUVA FRANGIPANI

(Plumeria rubra)

Earth has no sorrow that heaven cannot heal.—Thomas Moore, in Susan Hayward (ed.), A Guide for the Advanced Soul

The essence of this deep blood-red frangipani was made on the coast near Darwin in the Northern Territory in 1990. It is not a native of Australia, having its origins in Central America, although it has now been introduced throughout Asia and the South Pacific region. The Plumerias are a member of the Apocynaceae family which also includes many other delightfully scented plants, including the Oleanders, Allamanders and the Star Jasmin. There are over

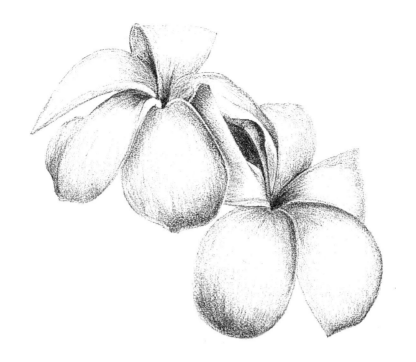

2000 species in this family, which is widespread in tropical and subtropical regions throughout the world. All its members have a milky white latex and the five lobes of the corolla are convoluted and twisted in the bud. There are seven distinct species in this genus which was named after Charles Plumier (1646–1706), the French botanist who, under royal charter, made three expeditions to the Caribbean area.

There seem to be two quite distinct explanations of how this frangipani acquired its common name. French settlers in the Caribbean termed the thick white latex of the cut tree *frangipanier*, French for coagulated milk. The second, and by far more interesting explanation, starts back in the sixteenth century in Italy when an Italian nobleman produced an exceptionally popular and tantalising perfume by combining together a number of volatile oils. This perfume, named after its inventor and used for scenting gloves, was quite famous throughout Europe for centuries afterwards. The early white settlers in the Caribbean instantly recognised the scent of the Plumerias to be almost identical to this perfume. The Italian inventor's name? Marquis Frangipani!

Red Suva Frangipani is a deciduous tree that grows to a height of 6 m with a spread of half that. The grey, stout, erect and branching stem carries these intensely coloured, beautiful, five-petalled, spicy fragrant flowers most of the year. They occur in terminal clusters and create a striking contrast to the long, leathery, elliptical dark green leaves that can grow to a length of 30 cm.

This species is unusual in that it does not have the sweet aromatic quality of other frangipanis, but rather a balmy, musky odour that reminded me of the cooking smells wafting from the dimly lit Nepalese and Tibetan huts that greet and entice you as you walk past at night. The tactile sensation on touching the Red Suva petals is one of a cool, thin, fine-cut velvet.

In the Yucatan of Mexico the juice of the plant is reportedly used to treat skin and venereal diseases, while in India the bark is known as a powerful anti-herpetic and is used as a cure for gonorrhoea or venereal sores, as it is in Puerto Rico and Indonesia. The heated leaves are topically applied as a poultice to reduce swellings, while the flower buds act as a febrifuge, lowering fevers, and are taken with betel leaves. The sap, too, is widely used internally as a purgative and is topically painted over an area where there is local inflammation.

Plumerias are one of the most loved of all flowers in tropical countries and held in high esteem, as evidenced by the number of countries making their greeting leis from these flowers. The tree symbolises immortality to many Muslims and Buddhists due to its extraordinary ability to continue to survive and produce leaves long after it has been raised from the soil. This is why it is frequently planted near temples and cemeteries. The Hindus regularly worship and make offerings to the Gods with these flowers. In Asia and the sub-continent a common name for the Plumeria is Temple Tree or Pergoda Tree.

This essence addresses the great emotional intensity, difficulty and hardship that people can go through when a relationship is ending, close to ending or going through a very 'rocky' period.

I have never had a more intense, passionate, healing experience with Nature as I had in making the Red Suva essence. I had been strongly drawn to this plant the night before a Darwin Australian Bush Flower Essence workshop, as I wandered around in the Botanic Gardens where a great deal of the workshop was to be taught outdoors over the next two days. Whenever I found myself in the vicinity of the Red Suva, it seemed to be always enticing me.

Throughout my time in Darwin I was going through tremendous turmoil and emotional upheaval. During the part in the workshop where everyone tunes into and draws a flower that has attracted them, I headed straight to my Red Suva and sat in the shade underneath it. The tree had a distinct heart shape formed by its branches and stem. A little while later, when meditating at the base of the tree, I was told to stand up and go up to the flowers. Immediately on doing so I felt tremendous ease and calm descend over me, it was as if I were bathed with the energy of these flowers. During my whole time with this tree I felt very loved and nurtured and released a great deal of the sadness I was feeling.

It was an incredibly healing time there, so much so that I wanted to stay with that tree for the rest of the workshop and found it very difficult to tear myself away.

Finally, as I was walking away, I noticed that another person from the workshop was also tuning into and drawing this plant, but from afar. I wanted to go over and tell her what I had been experiencing with the Red Suva but in the end decided against it, not wanting to disturb her or influence her own unique experience and rapport with this tree. However, she called over to me, telling me how she had been observing and drawing my interaction with the Red Suva. She also mentioned how she had felt that there was a lot of sadness with me when I had been sitting under the frangipani. Then she went on and described how she had seen the aura of the Red Suva come from its flowers, travel down and gently wrap and weave itself around my chest and heart chakra. It then lifted me up from its base, where I was sitting, to the flowers above where this pink and purple energy band totally encased me in a cocoon of pink light, which was doubly thick around my heart area.

Soon after, I asked permission to make up the essence of the Red Suva with all the workshop participants and was told that this essence was a personal gift to me from the plant kingdom to help me through my own personal dilemma. So it was with great reverence and gratitude that I made up my Red Suva. It is always quite amazing to me how and when the essences choose to come through and manifest. While the flowers were 'brewing' in the bowl we moved off, taking the workshop to a different part of the Gardens. When we returned to decant we found, lying neatly next to the bowl on the ground, a small branch half a metre in size. No one else had been near the spot because a couple of the people in the group had been keeping their eye on the area. 'Just another part of the gift', the plant kingdom told me.

I prefer to make the Bush Essences out in the bush in wilderness areas, and not from cultivated plants, because I know that the life force has to be very strong for a plant to survive in the wild without any human help or intervention. And it is not in my lifestyle or inclination to be a gardener and tend the plants. I am much happier going out and finding them where they naturally grow. However, I took both my gifts home—the essence of this Red Suva and my small branch. The latter I lavished with tender loving care and to this day it is still strong and healthy, possibly the only plant that has come under my care that I can make that claim about.

Red Suva is one of the most popular and widely prescribed of the Bush Essences. From talking to people from many different countries over these last few years, I believe there are not many relationships that haven't been tested very deeply as we come to the end of this very intense and, as the Chinese say, interesting age. We are currently in the middle of tremendous change and there is a need for so many things, including relationships, to be sorted out and resolved or completed. We are seeing, frequently, long-term and seemingly very stable relationships suddenly transformed and, often, come to an end.

Many relationships have the litmus test put on them if one person is changing and growing rapidly. Are both partners able to grow at the same pace, and in the same direction, and if not, is the relationship able to accommodate this?

There are many karmic completions between people that need to be made before we complete this present time cycle. The lessons to be learnt and the reasons behind a relationship these days can be, and are frequently, resolved in a much shorter period of time without the necessity of being within the framework of a long-lasting relationship. Spirit will then see to it that the partners are removed from one another and lead off in their new directions. The structure and values of the old society, where staying in a relationship, no matter what, was so important, are rapidly falling away. The old society is being replaced by one where the spiritual needs of the individual and society are of paramount importance and the structure within which this can occur is being set.

Negative condition

•

initial grief, sadness and upset of either a relationship at rock bottom or of the death of a loved one

•

emotional upheaval, turmoil and rawness

Positive outcome

•

feeling calm and nurtured

•

inner peace and strength to cope

The Red Suva Frangipani is for when there is a lot of difficulty, emotional rawness and intensity in a relationship. It is as if this essence creates a time out of the heat of the situation, out of the firing line, and then provides soothing, nurturing and large doses of tender loving care to help the person cope. One doesn't need to wait until a relationship has ended before considering taking this essence: it can be used at any time when a relationship is going through a very rough patch.

Physically, this remedy calms the overwrought nerves, the lungs where grief is stored, and the stomach or solar plexus which is also highly affected by what is being experienced.

As well as for relationship difficulties, Red Suva can also be taken for the enormous initial pain and sadness of the loss of a loved one. Emergency Essence is very appropriate for the shock and trauma, especially if the death is unexpected. Red Suva can even be added in with the Emergency Essence at this time. Sturt Desert Pea, too, is often combined with the Red Suva, although the former is really more for dealing with grief and sadness after the event. Whereas this remedy is for when one is right in the middle of the experience—in that acute crisis, and feeling greatly disturbed— not suicidal and despairing as in the case of Waratah, but just very torn apart by the event or situation.

A number of years after having first made this essence, I was walking through the Botanic Gardens in Singapore when I came across a section entirely devoted to Plumerias which included my Red Suva, and I was extremely excited to find printed on a little tin plaque embedded into the trunk that its common name was Bleeding Heart.

I am now full of inner peace and serenity.
I am never given anything in life I can't cope with.
I now have peace and harmony in my life and my relationships.

ROUGH BLUEBELL

(Trichodesma zeylanicum)

*H*e who focuses on only his own needs often doesn't end up with very much.—*Anonymous*

Rough Bluebell is an evergreen shrub that grows to a height of 1 m with a spread of 1.5 m. It is found in the tropic and subtropic areas of South-East Asia, India and Africa and in all states of Australia, except Tasmania and Victoria. Although seldom abundant, it can be found in a wide range of habitats but mainly in the open woodlands, sparse savanna woodlands, and grasslands extending to the dry central regions. It belongs to the Boraginaceae family that also contains Forget-Me-Nots, Comfrey and Borage.

The erect and branching stem, with its open textured crown, has a dense covering of stiff hairs, which can often be sharp. The leaves are lanceolate, up to 10 cm long, with the lower ones being opposite on the main stem, while the upper leaves, near the flower, are alternate. The deep blue, five-petalled flower has a central, white, spear-like projection where the stamens surround the style. The flowers are borne in clusters at the ends of the branches throughout the year, but more profusely during spring.

Initially, because I was unable to find very much information about this plant and no mention of a common name, I christened it 'Blue Spikey', for obvious reasons. But it never felt totally right and eventually I came across an old botanic text which listed it as Rough Bluebell. I found this to be very interesting, for both Rough Bluebell and Bluebell were made in Katajuta (the Olgas). Not only that, they both act primarily on the heart chakra, whereas Bluebell is all about opening the heart and expressing deep suppressed emotion. The healing quality of Rough Bluebell is for helping a person fully express the love vibration innate within them, and for showing them how to love and to see their potential.

No matter how dark the path a person is treading, or no

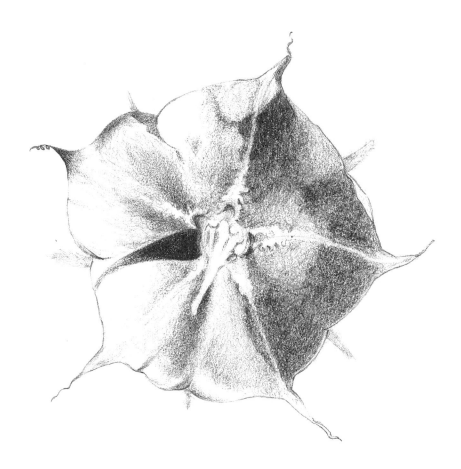

matter what their choices and actions, they can never totally suppress or destroy the spark of love and light within them. The Rough Bluebell helps to ignite this spark and unlock it from deep in their psyche, bringing it to a conscious awareness.

In the Doctrine of Signatures, you can see the central spike piercing through the darkness, or negativity, to bring through the Light. It resembles the lance used by St George in the slaying of the dragon. The latter symbolically represents evil or darkness, and also our shadow, which is really only a reflection of the areas in our life we have yet to integrate with love. Evil, in the religious sense, is nothing more than the absence of love.

The Archangel Michael is often described as having a blue flaming sword that he clasps as he charges to fight the evil forces of darkness. In Tibetan mythology, the Bodhisattva Manjushri is also depicted as carrying a blue flaming sword, which he uses to cut through ignorance and bring about a sense of oneness. A Bodhisattva is an enlightened being who chooses to return and stay on earth to help alleviate suffering till everyone is enlightened. It is impossible to attain enlightenment until one experiences the merging into the Universal Love of oneness.

Rough Bluebell is an excellent remedy for anyone to use as it helps to get them in touch with, and express, unconditional love; however, many people back away from taking this essence because they connect it with some of the more vicious and callous aspects of human behaviour and, subconsciously, don't want to associate themselves with such behaviour.

Certainly, Rough Bluebell has had some very profound results when used with people who have committed horrendous or incredibly malicious and violent crimes against others. These are not the type of people who would usually drop in off the street to see a practitioner for help. They are usually found in the underworld or locked deep in the criminal system. These people are manipulative and non-feeling with an impersonal way of behaving. Medical practitioners and psychiatrists admit that people with such a condition or disorder are untreatable, and that they have nothing which can alter the psychotic behaviour of people who commit such hideous acts—acts that they know will be destructive and hurtful to others yet which they coldheartedly and deliberately commit anyway, without any remorse, sometimes even with pleasure. A superb characterisation of this psychotic personality type was brilliantly portrayed in the movie *The Silence of the Lambs*. Anthony Hopkins, playing the role of Hannibal Lector, the former psychiatrist with the strange eating habits (!), uttered this remarkable line to end a telephone call, and the movie: 'I can't talk any more . . . I am having an old friend for dinner'!!

At the Bush Essences we have received exciting feedback from a psychotherapist working with this type of person in the New South Wales prison system. Using the Rough Bluebell, he has achieved remarkable breakthroughs and shifts with over twenty prisoners. In *The Essence* (Summer 1991) he wrote: 'Rough Bluebell acts as a "can opener" allowing the prisoner to become aware of their cool anger, cool resentment, cool cruelty and cool feeling to others. With Rough Bluebell they begin to open up quickly to their shortcomings and to their way of coming around to change.'

Rita Carter in her book *Mapping The Mind* discusses how

two areas of the brain have been found to be dysfunctional in antisocial people. One, the amygdala, found in the unconscious brain, generates feelings of alarm and emotion. The other, the frontal lobe, gives us control over our impulses. In normal people the amygdala is triggered by anything with emotional significance, especially signs of emotions in others: a baby's cry or a glare from someone. Alarm signals from amygdala activate initially our 'fight or flight' response in the hypothalamus, another part of the brain. The alarm signals then reach and trigger the frontal cortex and what we sense as emotion. However a psychopath's brain will fail to respond to a potential emotional stimulus. Either the amygdala doesn't respond or the signal from the amygdala doesn't reach the cortex. A normal person will feel uncomfortable hurting another person because the amygdala responds to others' pain or hurt so it acts to curb selfishness. Psychopaths aren't inhibited in the same way by their feelings. Usually it's only the awareness that hurting another may be detrimental to themselves legally or otherwise, that stops them.

The frontal lobe in healthy people has a control mechanism sufficient to stop impulsiveness, but in others the frontal lobe isn't sufficient to negate the spontaneous compulsive desires or urges.

Frontal lobe and amygdala dysfunction may bring about shocking, callous, cruel and immoral behaviour. Possibly what Rough Blue Bell is doing on a physiological level—the measurable 'tip of the iceberg'—is stimulating the frontal lobe or turning down activity in the amygdala. Maybe brain-mapping by functional imaging will be able to show this.

This essence is also for people who are manipulative and who use people, either subtly or openly. They put themselves and their own desires first, even if such behaviour is likely to bring about pain and suffering for others.

Rough Bluebell differs from Kangaroo Paw in that the latter is for those who hurt, or ignore the needs of, others, but this comes about through them being so self-centred that they are totally unaware of how their behaviour is affecting others. With Kangaroo Paw there is not the deliberate intent that there is with Rough Bluebell.

This essence can be for those who play the role of the martyr and like to have others obligated to them. Mostly, they do not care about the needs of others, but only themselves. They want love and affection but are not too concerned about, or have difficulty, giving it back.

In Indian herbal medicine this plant was used to cure mad dog bites, as one of the treatments for snake bites, and for warding off scorpions. Some very interesting symbolism is contained in these three! In Arnhem Land, this plant is used as a bush tobacco while in Australian Aboriginal medicine, the boiled plant is applied topically to treat skin sores and lesions.

Interestingly, as a Flower Essence Rough Bluebell has a very powerful action to release toxins from the skin and body, and can be employed both topically and internally at the same time. To enhance this cleansing effect, after each dose of the remedy you may wish to do the following:

With the breath held, imagine the skin opening. Release the breath and imagine the pores opening. Then breathe in the colour blue through the pores of the skin. Breathe out the colour, which is perceived . . . whatever colour that may be. Continue with this process until the awareness comes that the colour blue is being breathed out.

Skin breathing works on releasing toxins on the etheric and astral levels, as well as the physical. This remedy would be beneficial added to a bath and then bathed in, following this colour visualisation.

Rough Bluebell has also been used to heal severe itches and irritations. The excessive consumption of animal protein, especially red meat, can produce a build-up of toxins and fat in the physical body. The normal organs of elimination can't effectively cope with all these damaging substances and so the skin, often unsuccessfully, attempts to eliminate them through its pores. It has been suggested that this essence be used specifically to cleanse the tissues of the skin of these unhealthy deposits.

Recently, I finally came across another common name for this plant—the Camel Bush. I must admit that at first I was at quite a loss to connect this name to the healing properties of the plant. Yet almost invariably the historical use or naming of a plant reveals a particular side of its essence quality; there are no accidents. Then, at one of my work-shops, after mentioning the dilemma I was having with this other, new, common name, someone told me how camel drivers, approximately every six months, strip off their clothes and throw them at the feet of their camels. These clothes are then trampled upon, ripped and chomped into tiny shreds. Straight afterwards the camels become quite placid again—well, at least for a few months. The camels thereby take out in one intense, violent burst the pent-up

Negative condition

•

deliberately hurtful, manipulative, exploitative or malicious

Positive outcome

•

compassion

•

release of one's inherent love vibration

•

sensitivity

irritations, resentment and anger that have been slowly building up towards their drivers. If only these drivers knew about Flower Essences their wardrobe expenses could be reduced dramatically!

I am now fully expressing the love within me.
I am now acting with compassion and sensitivity.
I can now give and receive love in honest and direct ways.

TALL MULLA MULLA

(Ptilotus exaltatus)

To avoid criticism or conflict, do nothing, say nothing and therefore be nothing.—Ian White

Worldwide there are over 900 species and sixty-five genera belonging to the Amaranthaceae family, of which 131 species are found in Australia. Tall Mulla Mulla, of the genus Ptilotus, is one of the species more frequently found here in this country. This essence was made up in the Olgas, or Katajuta, which many people believe to be not only the physical but also the spiritual centre of Australia.

All of the three Mulla Mullas with which I work prefer the stony soils of the dry inland parts of the continent where they become a feature of the landscape after rainfall.

The Tall Mulla Mulla plant and flower aptly deserve the species name, *exaltatus*, which in Latin means tall; it has been recorded growing as high as 1.5 m, although it is usually found at around 80 cm or less. The erect sturdy stem can be branched or simple and is hairless. The large, fleshy and pointed, light grey-green leaves of this perennial are much larger at the base of the plant than on the stem and are a welcome addition to salads. These leaves grow up to 20 cm by 7 cm and are alternate and either obovate or oblong lanceolate in shape.

The magnificent, purplish-pink, conical, cylindrical flower heads of the Tall Mulla Mulla occur in spring and early summer, growing up to 20 cm long and 4.5 cm wide. The individual flowers of the spike are densely covered with

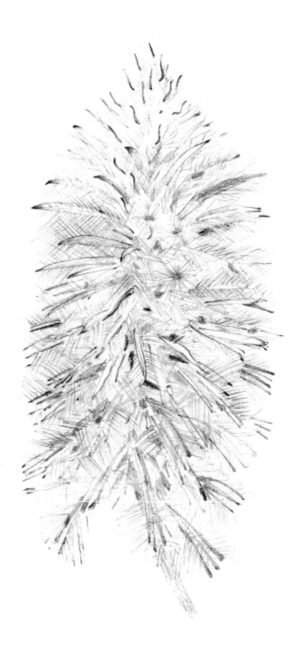

long, silky hairs and the stamens are crimson. The colourful, flowering spikes have a feathery, soft appearance and create a fantastic desert scene when you have a large patch of these glorious flowers yielding, in wave-like motions, to the wind.

This is a strong feature of the plant's Doctrine of Signatures, for the Tall Mulla Mulla person is definitely someone who bends a lot with the wind. They will often go to any length to keep the peace even if it means agreeing to, or saying things, they don't believe. They frequently act as pleasers and say what they think people want to hear. When they are with people they have a strong desire to create, and for there to be, harmony, and as soon as they can they will try to slip away. They just like things to go nice and smoothly with others and have a definite dislike of, and aversion to, conflict, disharmony and especially confrontation. The dread of these things occurring is so strong that they basically prefer to be away from people and by themselves. They are very comfortable in their own company and enjoy being alone where they know their own environment and can easily keep it peaceful and conflict free.

So, like Pink Mulla Mulla people, Tall Mulla Mulla people are loners by choice but there is not the aloofness or 'prickliness' about them that is found in the former. They simply want to live without scenes and fuss, believing that it is almost impossible to have a nice quiet time if you are among people. For, if you have a group of people together, they want this and they want that and there is conflict and it is all so horrible! They don't enjoy circulating with people as it feels too uncomfortable, troublesome and unsafe and, as a consequence, they miss out on the emotional growth that interaction with others can bring. Nor do they breathe in deeply of life, for they prefer holding on to the familiar rather than being open to the new.

On a physical level this remedy is specific to difficulties with circulation and the breath. Tall Mulla Mulla aids blood flow to the extremeties, therefore being very good for conditions such as cold hands and feet, varicose veins and alopecia. Getting better blood, oxygen and nutrient supply to the scalp can be of great benefit in stopping, correcting, and even reversing baldness in men and also hair loss, that is not of a hormonal cause, in women. This essence will help to re-oxygenate the tissues and cells of the body.

Tall Mulla Mulla is one of the first Bush Essences I think of when treating asthma. Other essences to consider along with Tall Mulla Mulla for this condition are: Crowea—for muscle spasm and bronchiole constriction; Flannel Flower—for establishing strong, healthy boundaries and overcoming emotional smothering; Sturt Desert Pea—for grief and sadness, which are the major emotions that affect the lungs; and the combination of Fringed Violet, Bush Iris and Dagger Hakea. Fringed Violet works to decrease the body's reaction and sensitivity to environmental irritants such as pollens, dust and dust mites, and chemical pollution. It is a great irony that, at the end of the last century and early in this one, English people were sent to Australia in the belief that the climate would be very beneficial to their health and they would have the opportunity to have their asthma healed. Yet our air-borne pollen levels are so high and of such a nature that Australia has a disproportionately high number of asthmatics. Bush Iris works very powerfully on the lymphatic system, clearing excessive mucus and toxins from the sinuses, throat and lungs, while Dagger Hakea, by working on and releasing the annoyances and resentments we feel towards others, stops us externalising these irritations, and makes us manifest them as allergic reactions to the foods that we eat or the air that we breathe. Emergency Essence should always be thought of when dealing with an acute episode of asthma, although I would suggest adding Tall Mulla Mulla to the bottle and having it on hand in case of an acute attack.

Although many people have successfully overcome asthma simply by using Tall Mulla Mulla alone, it is always wise to consider that, in working with any physical imbalance, one should ideally be knowing, assessing and treating the whole person and the unique soul journey of their life.

If I were seeing ten different patients I am sure that they would all receive Tall Mulla Mulla; however, it is most likely that each one would have their own very different selection of essences that would either be combined with or given separately to the Tall Mulla Mulla, during their treatment. This is because their ten individual life experiences and personalities are always going to be different.

However, the fact that they all have the same disease and somewhat similar symptoms suggests that they would share some common beliefs, attitudes, emotional responses or aspects of personality. All illness is a tap on the shoulder and an indicator that something is out of balance on an emotional or spiritual level, or about your lifestyle. The location of the illness in your body is the clue behind the tap, indicating the area of your life that is crying out to be addressed.

There are many cultures around the world which have been aware for thousands of years of the correlation between symptoms in specific parts of the body and the emotional states and predispositions that cause them. Anger, jealousy and resentment, for example, will produce gall bladder and liver problems, while fear and anxiety will create problems in the kidney and bladder. The emotional trigger for the lungs is, as previously discussed, grief and sadness.

The following is a devic analysis of Tall Mulla Mulla by Erik Pelham reprinted here in its entirety because it offers an original and somewhat different hypothesis to a possible cause of respiratory disease. It also offers another explanation as to how Tall Mulla Mulla has a very specific action on the breath.

This essence works on the Causal and Physical bodies only. It works on the Causal body by enhancing it to overcome disharmony, and it removes blockages from the Physical body.

Tall Mulla Mulla is a clearing essence for disharmony and dissipation of our Higher Will, and a whole host of respiratory problems associated with that. It is a reconnecting remedy with our Higher Will, when events come along which make us blocked, uncertain and unclear within the working of our Willpower. There are many reasons why this happens, but it often connects with recurrences of past events resurfacing in our lives, in which we had been blocked, unhappy and confused. It has a very important action in clearing breathing problems, and removing energy blockages in our respiratory tracts also. These kinds of blockages occur when disharmony grows in our Will centres, so the clearing of this disharmony of Will in our Causal bodies will alleviate physical respiratory problems through the dual action of this essence.

By harmonising the Causal body, any confusion as to what we should do in our lives becomes cleared, so any dissipation of our precious life force on negative or wrong application of our personal energy is curtailed. By dissolving energy blockages in the respiratory tract in the physical level, the entire respiratory processes are toned, healed and harmonised, making breathing deep, regular and healthy again.

Tall Mulla Mulla is excellent for use in regression work, where there is a need to clear blockages connected with past events and their effects. It is also excellent at alleviating a whole range of respiratory problems and diseases, such as asthma, sinus problems, etc., where they are connected with blocked or disharmonious effects from past events or confusion in the present within our will centres.

Negative condition

•

ill at ease

•

sometimes fearful of circulating and mixing with others

•

loner

•

distressed by and avoids confrontation

Positive outcome

•

feeling relaxed and secure with other people

•

encourages social interaction and room for discussion

This is a good example of how a range of physical problems connect with a particular type of problem in a Higher Body.

I am at ease and enjoy being with people.
I now breathe in deeply of life and life's experiences.

Update of
First Fifty
—Essences—

Since the publication of my book *Australian Bush Flower Essences* in 1991, there have been some very exciting new information, insights and revelations discovered about the original fifty remedies. This is certainly not surprising, as I have always contended that, when the essences first came through, they could be likened to a raw diamond; that as people worked, and became familiar, with them, we would be able to see their different facets which would become more polished and clear as time went on.

With She Oak, for example, my original information and understanding of this essence was that it was for infertility. Then, over a period of some months, we had quite a number of patients being sent over to my clinic to get this remedy by a Sydney gynaecologist who had realised that the She Oak had a balancing effect on a woman's hormonal and reproductive systems. A year or so later, while running a workshop in Tasmania, the practitioners there were quite surprised by the fact that I wasn't aware of how this essence was specific in its action for correcting fluid retention associated with menstruation.

It is for this reason that we are always encouraging workshop participants, practitioners or anyone using the Bush Essences to let us know about any interesting insights or case histories they have experienced. We are incredibly appreciative when anyone takes the trouble to do so.

Such information is well noted, recorded and filed and, via our news-letter, communicated worldwide to the members of the Australian Bush Flower Essence Society.

One of the very rewarding things about teaching the Bush Essence workshops all around the world is the opportunity to collect and collate data on the remedies, and discuss it at first-hand with the individuals doing research into or having the insights about them.

As the demand has increased for both the Bush Essences and my work-shops on them, I have spent progressively more and more time overseas. This has necessitated the relinquishing of my naturopathic practice, which for sixteen years had been a very rewarding and fulfilling part of my life. So for the last four years I have rarely been treating any patients which, although depriving me of direct observation and case histories of the essences, has allowed me the opportunity to train thousands of people, from medical specialists to teenagers, in the use of the Bush Essences. At the same time it has enabled me to gather new information on the remedies from all around the world, and to open up some unique research projects centred on the Bush Essences.

The following is a brief summary of some of those new insights and awarenesses that have arisen since the first book. You will note that with some essences in this chapter there is little or no text and this is because the picture of this essence has not changed to any great degree.

Banksia Robur (*Banksia robur*), sometimes called Swamp Banksia, is the first essence to be thought of in treating ME or chronic fatigue.

Bauhinia (*Lysiphyllum cunninghamii*) corrects the ileocecal valve. Most chiropractors conservatively estimate that six out of ten people have problems with their ileocecal valve. This valve separates the small and large intestines. It keeps the chyme in the small intestine up until suf-ficient processing on, and absorption of nutrients from it, has occurred for the remainder to be released into the large intestine, where more water will be absorbed from it and different bacteria will work on it until it is excreted as faeces. The pH of the small intestine is alkaline, while that of the large intestine is acid. Problems with the ileocecal valve can lead to: the valve jamming and subsequent fermentation of the contents in the small intestine; the valve opening too soon and the body being deprived of nutrients; or the valve being leaky and there being back flow from the large intestine, with its different pH and bacteria, into the small intestine. This, by far, represents the biggest threat to one's health and wellbeing. Symptoms arising from such problems of the ileocecal are neck pain, bloating, abdominal disten-sion, headaches and malaise. (In a recent workshop in Switzerland I was discussing Bauhinia's role in working on and correcting the ileo-cecal valve when I was told that Casper Bauhin, a Swiss physician who lived from 1560 to 1624, was the person who discovered the ileocecal valve! Was the plant named after him? Ah, the magic of the essences and synchronicity …)

Billy Goat Plum (*Planchonea careya*) also addresses shame and embarrassment. It allows one to have awareness of sexuality on a spiritual and emotional level, not just the physical. It has produced very good results when used topically for acne.

Black-eyed Susan (*Tetratheca ericifolia*): as this is one of my major constitutional remedies, I had already used it frequently and came to understand this essence quite fully before writing the last book! However, one area in which it is being used very successfully and frequently is in attention deficit disorder (ADD).

Bluebell (*Wahlenbergia* species) has a sphere of action on the veins as well as the heart.

Boronia (*Boronia ledifolia*) essence is now being successfully utilised to enhance one's ability to maintain intense focus during creative visualisation or in guided meditation.

Bottlebrush (*Callistemon linearis*): you no longer have to be concerned about giving this to a child under twelve, as it can now be given to anyone at any age. There have been tremendous shifts in consciousness and spiritual awareness in the last ten years and as a consequence that original information no longer holds. In terms of bonding, not only does this help the mother bond to the child, it also works the other way around in that it can help clear any difficulties the child has in bonding back to the mother. Bottlebrush can also be used for pain relief. Some people even add it to Emergency Essence for this reason. Physically its major action is on the large intestine. It has a very tonifying and balancing effect on most disorders associated with this organ, such as irritable bowel syndrome. In addition it has a very definite draining and cleansing effect on the large intestine and helps to really open this vital channel of elimination.

Bush Fuchsia (*Epacris longiflora*): what I have noticed is that not only are we evolving but also the flowers and the essences are. I originally made this essence up in 1986, but during a residential four day workshop in 1996 we made up Bush Fuchsia as a group. I was quite surprised to find that its qualities had recently changed. Rather than just helping you listen to your own intuition, Bush Fuchsia was now able to assist you in listening to and being in tune with the rhythms of the earth and to have a sense of what nature is telling you. The animals tune into this so well. One of the most accurate ways to predict volcano activity is not from all the high-tech sensing equipment but observation of well documented animal behaviour which precedes a major quake. What I found interesting as well was that it wasn't only the essences made up that year that had these new qualities but also that the original Mother Tincture had now evolved in the bottle and was addressing those very same qualities as well! Bush Fuchsia not only helps greatly with speech by improving the tone, timbre, inflection and melody of the voice, but it also works at the point where sound is received—the ears. It is very effective in treating chronic ear infections (what in Australia is known as glue ear). It is also used to successfully treat the following conditions: tinnitus; vertigo; travel sickness; and sense of balance. Bush Fuchsia has been found to be one of the most effective treatments in resetting the thermostat of the hypothalamus which can be seriously thrown out of balance from the prolonged use, over six months, of the contraceptive pill and hormone replacement therapy (HRT). As well as integrating the left and right hemispheres of the brain, it also balances the front and back hemispheres of the brain—which helps to explain why it is so effective with learning problems and dyslexia. It should also be thought of in helping to re-establish the correct neurological connections in the brain after trauma such as a fall or a stroke (cardiovascular accident) or in conditions such as epilepsy and dyslexia.

Bush Gardenia (*Gardenia megasperma*) essence will help a person to be aware if their intended communication is being perceived in the manner they originally intended. One older man, on returning home from work, used to give his wife what he perceived as an affectionate pat on the bottom. To him it was expressing his affection to her, yet he was totally oblivious to the fact that she used to find it quite annoying and irritating. So with the Bush Gardenia he became more receptive to how his communication was being received.

Bush Iris (*Patersonia longifolia*): many years ago, in the Australian Bush Flower Essence Newsletter, I wrote how Fringed Violet and Dagger Hakea were wonderful in treating hay fever or sinus conditions. Afterwards I received feedback from a number of people, saying if you added Bush Iris to this formula the results were even better. I was at a loss to explain how Bush Iris was working for these conditions. It led me to quite a lot of research, with the end result being that I realised Bush Iris has an extremely powerful action on the lymphatic system in the body. For most people, the lymphatic system is a great mystery. They have little clue as to what it does or how much lymph they have. We have, in fact, over 5 L of lymph coursing through our body. The lymphatic system serves to help digest fats; boost and support the immune system; and, most importantly it helps to cleanse and detoxify the body. The heart pumps the blood, but the lymph requires muscular contraction to move it. Diets high in fats, especially from dairy products, together with a sedentary lifestyle, are a wonderful recipe for a clogged lymphatic system, where basically the body is swimming in a cesspool of its own waste. Bush Iris can be thought of in treating the following types of symptoms, which all stem from a sluggish lymphatic system: oedema (Bush Iris is in Travel Essence, so to combat swollen feet at the end of a long flight, massage some

Travel Essence into the feet an hour before arriving and a few times a day after the flight); elephantitis; acne, excema and other skin rashes; body odour; and chronic illnesses generally. Through its regulatory action on the pineal, Bush Iris helps balance one's body clock, so it is of great assistance to shift workers and to negate the effects of jetlag. The American space agency NASA claims that for every two hours of time difference between your departure and destination points, it takes a day for your body clock to readjust. So if you are flying from LA to Sydney where there is a time difference of up to nineteen hours, depending on daylight saving, theoretically it would take ten days for the body clock to readjust after arriving, and then another ten days on returning home! I have flown from Sydney to London, where there is an eleven hour time difference, arrived on the Friday and taught a Bush Essence Workshop on the Saturday and Sunday. This would have been impossible without Bush Iris and the Travel Essence. Bush Iris has also been very effective in treating seasonal affect disorder (SAD) where, during the long northern winters in places such as Scandinavia and Alaska, the lack of light exposure on the pineal, or third eye, slows down one's body clock and, in some individuals, produces depression over time. Bush Iris helps activate and balance the higher chakras.

Crowea (*Crowea saligna*) has a very specific action on the stomach whereby it regulates the amount of hydrochloric acid being produced. If there is too much (a common cause of gastric ulcers), it will lower it while, if there is too little hydrochloric acid in the stomach (the person digests their food through fermentation in this situation and consequently doesn't effectively digest, and later absorb, nutrients from their food), Crowea will raise it to a sufficient level for good digestion. Some people can develop allergies to certain foods because their digestion is so poor that the protein molecules are not being broken down, and further along the digestive tract, the body perceives these large protein molecules to be a foreign substance and sets up its defences to protect against them. If these same protein molecules consistently come down undigested, the body can over time develop a memory for these substances as being foreign so that whenever they are encountered the body can release a full-blown allergic reaction to it.

  Crowea has a very beneficial action on not only the muscles but also on the tendons and is wonderful in treating sports injuries. It is also very good especially in helping a woman go from stage one to stage two in labour, as the uterus is a muscle. In breathing problems Crowea assists the diaphragm which is a muscle too. In asthma it helps the diaphragm and also helps to release constricted and spasmed bronchials and intercostal chest muscles.

Dagger Hakea (*Hakea teretifolia*) is a major component of a formula I call the Detox Essence. It is included in the formula because it has a draining and stimulating effect on the liver, one of the major channels of elimination in the body. In treating allergies one should always consider this Essence as in many cases the cause can be attributed, at least to some extent, to the individual not being able to resolve annoyance, irritation or resentment they feel towards another, which then becomes internalised so that they start to become annoyed and irritated by the food or environmental factors such as pollens.

Dog Rose (*Bauera rubioides*) essence is included in the Detox Essence as well because it has a draining and stimulating effect on the kidneys. However, this remedy also works on the spleen which, in traditional Chinese medicine (TCM) helps people to absorb the spiritual essence of their food, which is then taken to the pineal or third eye to assist their spiritual awareness and understanding. Consequently, for a powerful digestive combination, Dog Rose can be combined with Crowea, Paw Paw and Peach-flowered Tea-tree.

Five Corners (*Styphelia triflora*): in my practice I always made a point of finding out the reason a person came in to consult with me and, whether it be to lose weight or gain weight or create a happy and loving relationship, or even to be self-employed, I would muscle test them while they stated their goal out loud. In many cases their arm would go weak while stating what it was they wanted to achieve. Consciously they obviously wanted to achieve their goal, but subconsciously they had a sabotage to achieving it. Almost invariably, the bottom line of these sabotage programs was that they didn't love themselves enough or felt they didn't deserve to have what they wanted. This is where Five Corners would come in because it would clear this lack of self-worth and self-love to the point where their sabotage program would no longer operate. On a physical level many acupuncturists give their clients this essence before a treatment as it helps the energy flow of the meridians.

Flannel Flower (*Actinotus helianthi*): whenever treating women who have experienced physical or sexual abuse I now always add Flannel Flower to the combination of Wisteria and Fringed Violet, and the results have been even better. This essence is very good for helping a person to establish healthy boundaries with others, whether that be of a physical or emotional nature. Some people without boundaries would find it hard to open up to one person but at the same time, keep others at a comfortable distance. They either keep everyone at bay or else everyone could just literally walk all over them and they would have great difficulty in saying 'no'. Flannel Flower has a very special balancing action on the testes.

Fringed Violet (*Thysanotus tuberosus*) works hand in hand with Angelsword, both found in the Meditation Essence. Fringed Violet heals any break or hole in the aura while the Angelsword releases any energies or entities that entered while the aura was wide open. Fringed Violet didn't have the ability to release these energies or entities in itself. It must be emphasised that by taking Fringed Violet alone to repair the aura you won't entrap any such entities or energies within. It can be combined with Red Lily to reduce the effect of engine vibration when flying. Such vibration can weaken the endocrine, immune, nervous and lymphatic systems.

Grey Spider Flower (*Grevillia buxifolia*): when a person is experiencing terror, their astral body is usually fully or partly disconnected from their physical body, and this is why some people experience the inability to move, or feel frozen. Grey Spider Flower will reconnect the astral to the physical.

Hibbertia (*Hibbertia pendunculata*) essence regulates and balances the parathyroid glands, two pairs of small glands located near or attached to the thyroid glands. Their secretion, parathyroid hormone, controls the metabolism of calcium and phosphorus in the body. Hibbertia can be thought of when there are problems of rigidity in the body, especially in the bones, and even when there is a softening of the bones.

Illawarra Flame Tree (*Brachychiton acerifolius*) and **Isopogon** (*Isopogon anethifolius*): the knowledge about these has not changed to any great degree.

Jacaranda (*Jacaranda mimosaefolia*): the underlying reason why some people can be so scattered and are always asking others' opinions is they have a fear of responsibility and of making mistakes or the wrong choice or even simply just a fear of making decisions. The scattered energy of Jacaranda also manifests in a condition known as hiatus hernia or gastric reflux, where gastric juices escape from the stomach and travel back up the oesophagus, creating much discomfort. It's as if the acid doesn't know where to go. Jacaranda is very effective in addressing this problem.

Kangaroo Paw (*Anigozanthos manglesii*): the knowledge about this essence has not changed to any great degree.

Kapok Bush (*Cochlospermum fraseri*) remedy along with Red Lily and Green Spider Orchid works to open and harmonise the immediate three chakras above the crown.

Little Flannel Flower (*Actinotus minor*), **Macrocarpa** (*Eucalyptus macrocarpa*) and **Mountain Devil** (*Lambertia formosa*): the knowledge about these essences has not changed to any great degree.

Mulla Mulla (*Ptilotus atripicifolius*): over the last twelve years, this remedy has brought about tremendous healing for thousands of people suffering from many conditions. A common theme it addresses is always heat or fire. Whenever there is any burning sensation anywhere in the body, think of Mulla Mulla, whether it be vaginitis, eczema or menopausal hot flushes. It works very well to lower fevers. Children commonly get fevers when they are sick: their life force is so high they are able to quickly burn up the toxins. Many children, however, are very scared when they have a fever because they are not used to them and can even feel they might literally burn up. Mulla Mulla not only lowers the fever, it also eases their fear around the fever. The fear robs the body of oxygen and makes it harder to control the fever. We have had numerous case histories where Mulla Mulla has been used with people suffering from third-degree burns—including my daughter when she was five years old—and subsequently have not needed the skin grafts which were originally planned. Even for first and second-degree burns, Mulla Mulla will ease the pain almost straight away and in most cases there won't even be any marking on the skin the next day, even when there has been scalding with boiling water. We have three separate case histories of people who had gone to the casualty department of their local hospital after accidents to determine if they had broken any bones. In all three cases they each took a dose of Mulla Mulla immediately prior to their X-rays and, much to the astonishment of the radiographers and other hospital staff, they were unable to obtain an X-ray. Each person was put on three different machines! Normally after taking Mulla Mulla one would be able to get an X-ray but wouldn't be left absorbing as much of the radiation. It is for this reason that we have included Mulla Mulla in the Travel Essence for, when you are flying at 12,000 m above the ground, you are absorbing a great deal of radiation. I have come across varying estimates from radiographers that equate the amount of radiation absorbed on an around the world trip as being equal to as much as forty chest X-rays. Mulla Mulla also helps release static electricity that you absorb while flying, especially at take-off. It results in a decrease of potassium, oxygen and water in the cells of the body. Also, if anyone is undergoing radiation therapy for cancer, they would do well to consider taking Mulla Mulla immediately beforehand as well as morning and night during the course of treatment. Numerous case histories have clearly indicated that Mulla Mulla reduces the amount of burning these patients suffer and that they recover much more quickly. Mulla Mulla greatly reduces the amount of emotional trauma associated with this treatment, and also allows a person to be able to tolerate higher levels of radiation so that the treatment can be more effective.

Old Man Banksia (*Banksia serrata*): the knowledge about this essence has not changed to any great degree.

Paw Paw (*Carica papaya*): applying this essence topically on the lung acupuncture points has proved to heal or, at the very least, reduce the symptoms of malaria. This technique was developed and extensively utilised in the late 1980s by Mary Jane Russell, a kinesiologist, in the Solomon Islands, where this disease was rife, even to the point that some of the local people chose not to go out of their huts at night for fear of the mosquitoes and the disease they carry.

Peach-flowered Tea-tree (*Leptospermum squarrosum*): as mentioned in my earlier book, this remedy balances the pancreas. Since that publication we have had a number of case histories where insulin dependent diabetics taking this remedy, in consultation with their medical doctor, have been able to come off all medication. In fact two women who had both been taking insulin injections for over fifteen years were able to come off all insulin within a month of being on Peach-flowered Tea-tree—and with neither needing to ever go back onto insulin again!

Philotheca (*Philotheca salsolifolia*): there has been some recent reporting of Philotheca, like Bush Iris, having a very strong action on the lymphatic system. Though there have not been enough substantial case histories and testimonials to totally endorse this finding, I offer it to you so that we may have some more research conducted.

Red Grevillea (*Grevillea speciosa*): we have included Red Grevillea in the Heartsong Combination because of its special healing capability on the temporomandibular joint (TMJ). This joint is exceedingly rich in nerve endings. If one's TMJ is out of alignment, not only may there be pain, discomfort and cracking in the joint, not to mention difficulty in opening the mouth wide, but also it is highly likely that there will be considerable emotional mood swings and imbalance. Red Grevillea, like Bauhinia, also has a balancing action on the ileocecal valve.

Red Helmet Orchid (*Corybas dilatatus*): not only does this essence help men bond to their children but it also assists children in their bonding to their father. It serves to help an individual to work through and resolve issues with their father even if they themselves are quite old or even if their father has passed over.

Red Lily (*Nelumbo nucifera*): this essence works to open both the crown chakra and the higher chakras above the crown. The earlier differentiation between Sundew and this essence was that the former was for individuals under the age of 28 whilst Red Lily was for those over 28. This however no longer applies. Anyone at any age can take either of these essences. The main distinguishing feature between these two essences is that Red Lily helps one to be very grounded and balanced while pursuing one's spiritual practice, whereas Sundew is more for being grounded and paying attention to detail in day-to-day activity or at any time when there is a lack of consciousness, whether arising from anaesthetic, drugs, alcohol or severe trauma. Red Lily Combination with Fringed Violet helps negate the effect of engine vibration when flying.

She Oak (*Casuarina glauca*): in hospitals in Brazil and Switzerland She Oak is successfully being used as an alternative to hormone replacement therapy—without the increased risk of breast and cervical cancer or of elevating cholesterol levels. Because of She Oak's hydrating action it maintains moist vaginal secretions so that sex does not become painful, while at the same time slowing the aging process by keeping all the cells hydrated. Its balancing effect on the ovaries enables the individual to maintain a high enough oestrogen level so that osteoporosis is not an issue. To find a woman's ideal dosage prescription of this essence for menopause can involve some degree of trial and error. As an initial starting point I recommend taking She Oak for a month, then taking a two-week break and then taking the essence again for a month. This is then followed by a month's break and then taking the essence for two weeks followed by a six-week break and once more taking the remedy for two weeks. Ideally a woman only needs to take the She Oak two weeks every two months. Some women however have found they need to take the remedy more frequently to have the desired result. Some in fact have found they need to take the remedy on a daily basis. One very pleasing and exciting comment that has come from a number of women is that not only have they greatly benefited from this essence in terms of relieving and allaying the more common consequences of menopause but they have commented how they feel far more feminine within themselves. We have included She Oak in the Travel Essence for not only alleviating symptoms of dehydration, common in air travel, but also for counteracting the effect pressurised cabins have on a woman's hormonal balance. It is very common for female flight attendants to suffer from mid-cycle bleeding and to have difficulty in conceiving whilst regularly flying, even up to a year after they stop flying.

Silver Princess (*Eucalyptus caesia*) will reset your inner gyro system for latitudinal or north/south air travel.

Slender Rice Flower (*Pimelea linifolia*): any cut, whether it be from an accident or surgical incision, that is deep enough to require stitches, will frequently impede the flow of energy along any meridian line that it crosses. This remedy, when used either internally or topically along the scar, reintegrates that scar so that the energy can once again flow along the meridian. Retained in the scar tissue is also the emotion the person was feeling or experiencing at the time of the accident or surgery. Slender Rice Flower will also work to release both the embedded emotion as well as to heal the physical wound.

Southern Cross (*Xanthosia rotundifolia*): the knowledge about this essence has not changed to any great degree.

Spinifex (*Triodia* species) treats any bacterial infections in the lungs. This remedy can also be considered if there has been damage to nerve endings anywhere in the body.

Sturt Desert Pea (*Clianthus formosus*) can be used for any lung or breathing difficulties, such as bronchitis, as grief and sadness primarily affect the lungs.

Sturt Desert Rose (*Gossypium sturtianum*): the knowledge about this essence has not changed to any great degree.

Sundew (*Drosera spathulata*): anyone at any age can take Sundew. This remedy addresses day-to-day vagueness and lack of attention to detail whilst the Red Lily enables one to be very focused and grounded while pursuing one's spiritual practice. Sundew will reset your inner gyro system for longitudinal or east/west air travel.

Sunshine Wattle (*Acacia terminalis*): this remedy combines wonderfully with Bush Iris when treating seasonal affect disorder (SAD).

Tall Yellow Top (*Senecio magnificus*): there have been some very excellent results achieved with treating depression with this essence. It is normally the first essence I would think of for this condition, followed closely by Waratah and then Kapok. Some people experience chronic neck pain at the level of the second or third vertebra. In many cases the cause of this is what is referred to as dural torque—whereby the dura matter, the outer connective sheath of the spine, is twisted as a result of structural imbalance in the lower spine or pelvis. As a consequence the rest of the spine compensates for this, but at the level of the higher cervical vertebrae there is nowhere to pass the compensation to and these vertebrae are often pulled out of alignment. Not only does this produce neck problems but gives rise to what appears to be one leg longer than the other when they are measured against each other, with the person lying down. In actual fact there is no difference in the length of the legs, just the rotation of the pelvis giving this illusion, though the person will take a longer step with the leg that appears to be longer and this will affect the gait. Tall Yellow Top effectively corrects dural torque and all its associated complications.

Turkey Bush (*Calytrix exstipulata*): the knowledge about this essence has not changed to any great degree.

Waratah (*Telopea speciosissima*) is being used, with fantastic results, in Brazilian hospitals by cardiologists when treating ventricular failure and mitral valve insufficiency in particular, and heart imbalances generally. Waratah when used to treat glaucoma not only halts this condition but can reverse it as well, something that allopathic medication rarely achieves. Waratah has also been used in hospitals to overcome transplant rejection. This essence should also be thought of, along with Tall Yellow Top, whenever treating depression.

Wedding Bush (*Ricinocarpus pinifolius*): not only did the early white settlers use this flower in their wedding ceremonies but also the Aborigines. Whenever a man and a woman from one tribe in the south west of New South Wales wished to wed each other, they would exchange Wedding Bush flowers. I was told that later if one or both got 'tired' of one another then they only had to give their partner some Wedding Bush flowers a second time and it was all over! Interestingly at one residential workshop someone commented how the scent of Wedding Bush was just like marzipan—a major ingredient of the icing on the traditional wedding cake!

Wild Potato Bush (*Solanum quadriloculatum*): this essence is the crucial ingredient in our new combination remedy called Detox Essence. Wild

Potato Bush is able to mobilise heavy metals, especially lead, as well as many other toxic substances, out of the cells of the body where they are usually stored. The rest of the Detox Essence works to optimise the body's eliminative channels so that the heavy metals and other toxins can be flushed out of the body.

Wisteria (*Wisteria sinensis*): as well as working to bring about an enjoyment of sex and ease of sexual intimacy for women, this essence will also allow a woman to be open to and enjoy her sensuality.

Yellow Cowslip Orchid (*Caladenia flava*): in my last book I mentioned how this essence balances the pituitary gland and since that time, there have been case histories sent into us reporting how pituitary tumours have been healed using this remedy.

Combination
—Essences—

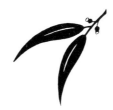

The following sixteen combinations are all derived from the sixty-two individual Australian Bush Flower Essences. Each combination addresses a specific theme whereby the different essences contained within it work on different aspects of that particular theme. All of these combinations, with the exception of Detox Essence and Radiation Essence, are available in our retail range. The combinations are as follows.

Abund Essence

This combination is made from the essences of Bluebell, Boab, Five Corners, Philotheca, Southern Cross and Sunshine Wattle. It aids in releasing negative beliefs, family patterns, sabotage and fear of lack. In so doing it allows you to be open to fully receiving great riches on all levels, not just financial ones.

Adol Essence

This combination is made from the essences of Billy Goat Plum, Boab, Bottlebrush, Dagger Hakea, Five Corners, Flannel Flower, Kangaroo Paw, Red Helmet Orchid, Southern Cross, Sunshine Wattle and Tall Yellow Top. It addresses the major issues teenagers commonly experience. It enhances acceptance of self, communication, social skills, harmony in relationships, maturity, emotional stability and optimism.

Cognis Essence

This powerful combination of essences is unsurpassed for bringing about mental clarity, recall and focus, and for enhancing all learning skills and abilities. It comprises Bush Fuchsia, Isopogon, Paw Paw and Sundew.

Confid Essence

This combination of Dog Rose, Five Corners, Southern Cross and Sturt Desert Rose brings out our true inherent positive qualities of self-esteem and confidence. It allows us to feel comfortable around other people and resolves negative subconscious beliefs we may hold about ourselves, as well as any guilt we may harbour from past actions. This combination also helps us take full responsibility for the situations and events that occur in our lives and realise that we have the ability and power not only to change those events, but also to create those that we want.

Detox Essence

This combination is for cleansing and detoxifying the body. It contains Bottlebrush, Bush Iris, Dagger Hakea, Dog Rose and Wild Potato Bush. The latter works to release heavy metals, especially lead, from the tissues in the body where they are stored, and it will also help to mobilise chemical toxins and poisons. The other four essences help to stimulate the body's major eliminative channels—namely the colon, lymphatic system, liver and kidneys—so that, once released, the heavy metals and other toxins can be effectively eliminated and flushed out of the body.

Dynamis Essence

This combination brings about abundant energy, vitality, enthusiasm and joy for life. This is achieved by balancing and stimulating the major glands associated with energy: the thyroid with Old Man Banksia and the adrenals with Macrocarpa. Also in this essence are Crowea, which balances the organs and muscles, Banksia Robur, for temporary loss of drive and enthusiasm, and Wild Potato Bush, for vitality.

Emergency Essence

The Emergency Essence is a combination of Crowea, Fringed Violet, Grey Spider Flower, Sundew and Waratah and should be thought of for any physical or emotional upset. It has a calming effect on the mind, body and emotions during minor and major crises. It will quickly ease fear, panic, severe mental or physical stress, nervous tension and pain. If a person needs specialised medical help, this essence will provide comfort until treatment is available. The wide variety of uses for this combination ranges from pre-examination nerves to gross physical injury. You can administer this remedy every 10–15 minutes if necessary, until the person feels better. It can also be mixed into a cream.

Femin Essence

This combination is made from the essences of Billy Goat Plum, Bottle-brush, Crowea, Mulla Mulla, Old Man Banksia, Peach-flowered Tea-tree and She Oak. It harmonises any imbalance a woman may experience from her first menstruation through to, and after, menopause, so it addresses such problems as period pain, premenstrual syndrome (PMS), infertility, irregular menstruation, candida, hot flushes, as well as offering a safe and effective alternative to hormone replacement therapy (HRT). It allows a woman to discover and feel good about her own body and beauty.

Heartsong Essence

This combination is made from the essences of Bush Fuchsia, Turkey Bush, Red Grevillea, Crowea and Flannel Flower. It frees your voice, improving tone, timbre and melody, and opens your heart. It inspires creative and emotional expression in a gentle and calm way and gives courage and clarity in public speaking and singing while, at the same time, correcting any blocks in the temporomandibular joint (TMJ) so that you can open your mouth wide.

Meditation Essence

This combination is made from the essences of Angelsword, Bush Fuchsia, Bush Iris, Fringed Violet and Red Lily. This is a wonderful combination to awaken one's spirituality. It allows one to go deeper into any religious or spiritual practice. It also enhances access to the Higher Self while providing psychic protection and healing of the aura. This is highly recommended for anyone practising meditation.

Radiation Essence

This combination is made up of Bush Fuchsia, Crowea, Fringed Violet, Mulla Mulla, Paw Paw and Waratah. The Radiation Essence can be used to negate or reduce earth radiation, found where lay lines cross, or in houses under which underground streams run; electrical radiation emitted by meter boxes, overhead power lines, fluorescent lights and electrical equipment, especially televisions; solar radiation, such as bad sunburn; and radiation therapy used to treat cancer. With radiation therapy, this combination helps the normal, healthy cells withstand the radiation and recover after therapy. It would also be useful against nuclear radiation. In all these situations, the combination stops the storage of radiation in the body and helps to emit the radiation already stored, and to keep the body's energies intact and the neurological systems functioning normally.

Relationship Essence

The essences of the flowers of Bluebell, Boab, Bush Gardenia, Dagger Hakea, Flannel Flower, Mint Bush and Red Suva Frangipani help enhance the quality of all relationships, especially intimate ones. This combination clears and releases resentment, blocked emotions and the confusion, emotional pain and turmoil of a rocky relationship. It helps one verbalise, express feelings and improve communication. This essence breaks the early family conditioning and patterns which affect us in our current adult relationships. For intimate relationships, a perfect remedy to follow this combination is Sexuality Essence.

Sexuality Essence

This combination is made from the essences of Billy Goat Plum, Bush Gardenia, Flannel Flower, Fringed Violet and Wisteria. This is helpful for releasing shame and the effects of sexual abuse. It allows you to feel comfortable with and to fully accept your body. It enables you to be open to sensuality and touch and to enjoy physical and emotional intimacy. Sexuality Essence renews passion and interest in relationships.

Solaris Essence

Solaris Essence is made only from the flowers of the Mulla Mulla plant which is found in the desert of Central Australia, the hottest part of the continent. It is an essential first aid remedy, greatly relieving the fear and distress associated with fire, heat and sun. Solaris is excellent for healing and easing the pain of all types and degrees of burns. It also significantly reduces the amount of radiation one absorbs from X-rays and the sun.

Transition Essence

This combination is made from the essences of Autumn Leaves, Bauhinia, Bottlebrush, Bush Iris and Lichen. It eases the fear of death as well as helps one to come to terms with it. This combination allows one to easily and gently pass over with calmness, dignity and serenity.

Travel Essence

This combination is made from the essences of Banksia Robur, Bottlebrush, Bush Fuchsia, Bush Iris, Crowea, Fringed Violet, Macrocarpa, Mulla Mulla, Paw Paw, She Oak and Sundew. The use of this essence is beneficial for the distress associated with all forms of travel, although it particularly addresses the problems encountered with jet travel. It enables a person to arrive at their destination feeling balanced and ready to go.

Companion —Essences—

I have called Autumn Leaves, Green Essence and Lichen 'companion essences' because, even though they were prepared by the Sunshine Method similar to how I prepare all sixty-two of the Australian Bush Flower Essences, they were not derived from flowers. These companion essences do, however, work in a very similar fashion to the Bush Essences.

Autumn Leaves

Autumn Leaves allows one to hear, see and feel communication from the other side and be open to that guidance and communication. It also further emphasises the sense of letting go and moving on in a very profound way. The leaves themselves were collected from a sacred area in (surprise, surprise) autumn, at the exact moment of their release from the trees. The essence was made only from these leaves.

The work of Elizabeth Kubler-Ross and other workers in this field of death and dying all note how common and important it is for the one passing over to be aware that help and guidance are around, especially the presence of loved ones who have already died. This essence will ease the transition of the passing over from the physical plane to the spiritual world.

Green Essence

Green Essence is made from the stems and leaves of traditional fresh green herbs, using the same method we use to make flower essences. It is used to clean the system of yeast, mould and parasites. It should be taken orally for a two-week period, five drops five minutes before meals, three times a day. Topically Green Essence can be used to treat skin problems such as eczema, psoriasis or fungal infections. Place seven drops of Green Essence in a dessert bowl of water, splash on the affected area and allow to dry. Do this morning and night for two weeks. You will need to make a fresh batch at least every two days. *Do not use Green Essence externally at the same time as it is taken internally,* as the reaction can be too strong: the skin may peel.

If you are using Green Essence to treat candida, the following regime is recommended. Both Green Essence and Peach-flowered Tea-tree are to be taken for two weeks, the former before meals three times a day. For the next two-week period take a combination of Bottlebrush, Peach-flowered Tea-tree and Spinifex morning and night. Then take the Peach-flowered Tea-tree again for a further two weeks morning and night.

At the beginning of the process take for one month a good brand of acidophilus and bifidus powder which should have been refrigerated prior to purchase and certainly after opening. During this time avoid sugary and yeasty foods such as alcohol, vinegars, Vegemite, yeasted bread, etc.

You can douche if necessary morning and night for two weeks with

Green Essence. To make it, place seven drops of Green Essence in a bowl of water. After you have completed two weeks of douching, take Green Essence internally for two or four weeks. Alternatively Green Essence can be taken before commencing the two weeks of douching. *Never use Green Essence orally and topically at the same time.*

Lichen Essence

Lichen helps an individual to be aware of, look for and go to the Light at the moment of physical death. The alternative to the soul going through to the Light is to stay earthbound in the astral plane—what we commonly refer to as 'ghosts'. There is a great deal of darkness operating on the astral plane and it is certainly a level through which the soul would be well advised to move quickly.

A violent or sudden death can also result in the increased likelihood of the Spirit staying earthbound; the spraying of Lichen would be of great benefit for those souls. Even in cases where there is an unexpected sudden death—for example, a car accident—the individual who dies in such an experience was fully aware at the level of their Higher Self of what was about to happen and that they were going to pass over. Two weeks before such an event the etheric body starts to disengage and unravel from the physical body. Lichen assists the etheric and the physical bodies to separate to prepare for passing over.

A person who suicides usually has to spend a certain period of time on the astral as a karmic penalty before going through to the Light. In this situation the spraying of Lichen from an atomiser will assist that soul to deal with existing on the astral and, in many cases, speeds up the time required before he or she goes through to the Light.

Transition Essence, which contains Lichen, was originally designed to help people in passing over, but can also be taken by anyone going through major changes in their life, such as moving house or changing career. In this circumstance their etheric body would definitely not separate from their physical body!

Emotional Patterns and Balance in Pregnancy and —Labour—

In the fifth century BC, Plato said, 'the cure of the part should not be attempted without treatment of the whole. No attempt should be made to cure the body without the soul and, if the head and the body are to be healthy, you must begin by curing the mind ... for this is the great error of our day in the treatment of the human body, that physicians first separate the soul from the body.'

This chapter is intended as a brief overview of the Australian Bush Flower Essences and their potential for bringing about a happy, healthy pregnancy and labour. In particular I look at predominant emotional patterns that can hinder this and how specific essences can be used: leading up to conception; during the pregnancy itself; the labour; and the initial bonding period afterwards. Like Plato, I believe that thoughts are creative and, whether they are negative or positive, they influence a person's emotional state which in turn affects their physical body.

The Australian Bush Flower Essences are the perfect remedies to prescribe during pregnancy because they are safe for the unborn foetus and have a harmonising and balancing effect on the mother, always only bringing her back to her own equilibrium. They are ideal also because many women embark upon childbirth with inadequate emotional preparation and support for the enormous physical and emotional changes happening to them. Flower Essences are and can be in the front line of action prescribed by supporting health practitioners and childbirth educators.

Having a baby is a normal event in life; it is not an illness. As it requires a co-ordination of mind and body, the mental attitude of the woman and her sense of calmness and security is crucial if she is to give birth with ease, joy and spontaneity. Ideally, it is an experience with which she will cope and deal very satisfactorily, with pride and joy, and one from which she will emerge as a more complete person, who will be free to express all the love and nurturing that this new soul requires from her.

Birth is shaped by a woman's integration of a number of factors: expectations and fears about the labour; her relationship with both her body and her partner; feelings about, and acceptance of becoming a mother; as well as other deep hopes and fears.

Pregnancy can bring up a multitude of feelings and memories, some good, some not so good. Certainly it is a wonderful time for releasing a lot of negative beliefs and attitudes so that in your new role as a parent you project less negativity on to your child.

Infertility and She Oak

However, before discussing the Bush Essences relating to pregnancy, I'd like to mention briefly a closely related field—infertility and the role of She Oak. Twenty-five per cent of infertility is of unknown cause. This together with the success rate in IVF and GIFT programs being less than 15%, not to mention the amount of financial and emotional stress and disappointment associated with these treatments, makes it worthwhile to look at some of the emotional factors which may be influencing or creating infertility.

To start with, a young girl can grow up with a belief that motherhood is very hard and unrewarding, something which she may have picked up from her own parents, especially her mother. Such an attitude could hamper her ability to conceive. One client didn't want to conceive on a subconscious level because of a trauma she had experienced in a past life, where, as a mother, she had to mercifully kill her four young children in order to save them from a brutal death at the hands of a neighbouring marauding tribe. The agony of this event left such a deep scar on her psyche that she did not ever again want to be a mother or in such a position of responsibility. She Oak will usually successfully address infertility stemming from such deep emotional causes.

From a naturopathic point of view, dehydration of the uterus is a common cause of infertility. She Oak is also a tissue rehydrator and will correct this problem while at the same time helping to bring about hormonal balance in the woman, regulating her cycle and her oestrogen/progesterone levels—all of which greatly enhances her fertility and ability to conceive. Many practitioners, including myself, working with She Oak alone have over a 75% success rate in treating infertility; one medical doctor of my acquaintance has enjoyed over a 90% success rate in her Sydney practice!

Pregnancy and Birth

Once conception has occurred, the actual confirmation of pregnancy can come as a great shock, even for people who have been desperately trying to conceive. The remedy Fringed Violet is specific in dealing with shock.

If the pregnancy was unplanned or unwanted by one or both the parents yet it is still going ahead, rejection of the child may be an issue here, especially if a termination has been considered or even attempted. Perhaps the parents want their child to be of a particular sex. The baby, if it is not of the desired sex, picks up the feelings of rejection instantly. Some breech and overdue babies reflect this rejection, by not wanting to be born, so to speak. Numerous studies (such as in T. Verney's *Secret Life of the Unborn Child*) and regression work have shown that the child does pick up on the parents' feelings, right from the earliest stages of the pregnancy, and can carry these feelings throughout the rest of their lives.

Tall Yellow Top addresses feelings of abandonment and isolation, while Illawarra Flame Tree is for rejection. Both are extremely beneficial in cases like this. The latter essence is also for feeling overwhelmed by responsibility, a reaction people can experience when contemplating parenthood and the commitment it requires.

Another common cause for a baby to be breech is fear, as if the woman were holding the child close to her heart for fear of letting it go. Fear is common during pregnancy—fear of the labour, fear of the pain, perhaps a fear that her body won't return to its pre-pregnancy shape or that she won't be able to breastfeed. Sometimes the fears can be vague and nebulous. Dog Rose is the remedy for fear and helps to bring about a sense of confidence and courage. Fear is a major contributing factor in morning sickness, and for this reason Dog Rose can be added to a mix containing Crowea and Paw Paw—to help digestion; Dagger Hakea to help the liver detoxify the extra hormones and any other toxicity in the body; and She Oak to help regulate hormonal balance.

If the woman is experiencing a great deal of fear, the child will pick up on this. In fact any major upset the mother experiences leads to a release of catecholamines. When produced, they cross the placental barrier, going straight to the baby where, according to Verney, they create fear and anxiety in the baby.

Another consequence of fear, especially during labour, is that it leads to a construction and a tightening of many muscles, including the pelvic ones, which can in turn lead to a longer labour with more complications. With fear think of Dog Rose. Yet if there is terror, the remedy to be thought of is Grey Spider Flower, which is one of five remedies in a combination called Emergency Essence, the others being Waratah, Crowea, Fringed Violet and Sundew. The Emergency Essence can be used for any emotional or physical trauma and it is of particular value during the labour itself. It helps the woman to continue in spite of over-whelming feelings of not being able to, perhaps because of fatigue or pain, or because she is disassociated and cut off from what her body is doing. During labour Macrocarpa can be used to increase stamina and endurance and alleviate any physical exhaustion. To help a woman to move from first to second stage in labour, a combination of Bauhinia, Bottlebrush and Crowea can be used. Bauhinia is for embracing change, Bottlebrush for facilitating the transition and letting go of the previous stage, while Crowea works directly on the uterus, which is a muscle.

Emergency Essence is wonderful for providing pain relief during the birth and is also very good in dealing with any birth trauma, shock or medical intervention, such as surgery or the use of forceps, that may occur. It can certainly be used for any unusual complication. It is very calming for the woman and for others around her too.

Verney's studies have shown that many people convicted of violent crimes have all had in common extraordinarily traumatic births, which suggests that birth is an event that powerfully imprints itself on an indi-vidual's personality. When a birthing woman is feeling very fearful or extremely stressed, her body responds by releasing adrenocortiecotropic hormone (ACTH) and other stress hormones. These hormones affect the child as they flood into his or her system. It has been shown that ACTH has the exact opposite effect of oxytocin, in that it helps retain memory, whereas most children don't have a memory of their birth because of the high levels of oxytocin with its amnesiac-like effect. ACTH inhibits that function of the oxytocin and hence many young newborns remem-ber and retain the experiences of their birth if it was traumatic. They have a memory of what to them was a very disturbing and stressful event. The Emergency Essence will help these children with processing, dealing with and coming to terms with any such trauma.

One of the other remedies from the Emergency Essence—Fringed Violet—has an ability to heal and protect a person's aura, to give psychic protection and decrease a person's susceptibility to the influences of other people or of unpleasant experiences. Many pregnant women in their last trimester have used this essence to protect themselves from the negative experience of having women, whom they have never met before, come up to them in the street and tell them unsolicited stories of horrendous birth experiences. A lot of these pregnant women find that after taking Fringed Violet they no longer encounter such women—nor their stories.

Some cultures suggest that the newborn should not be taken outside the house for six weeks, because his aura is too open and he needs this time for the development of his own psychic protection and emotional wellbeing.

Fringed Violet, rubbed topically in the sign of the cross over the baby's soft spot, the anterior fontanelle, will close off the aura and bring about that very same protection, and as a consequence the child can be taken outside much earlier.

Frequently it has been observed that babies in their first week often have a daily outburst of crying for no apparent reason at a time that corresponds with the exact time of their birth. One theory put forward by Michel Odent claims that this is the baby reliving and thereby processing the actual birth experience. If this seems to be the case, Fringed Violet is quite helpful for the child.

If the baby is born 'floppy'—that is, very slow and sluggish—Emergency Essence can bring the baby's soul down into her little body very quickly. This 'floppy state' is commonly due to the mother smoking tobacco, either actively or passively, while the baby was in the womb, or to any medical drugs used during the birth. In such cases, it is the action of Sundew in the Emergency Essence that brings the child 'back into the body', grounding her and putting her in the here and now. At this point, the other most important thing to bring the soul back in is the love the parents have for the child. Also, if the mother has haemorrhaged or had a really hard time during the labour then Emergency Essence will work swiftly and effectively, helping her to stay fully present in her body.

There is a very strong argument in favour of immediately applying Boab to the mother's breast for the newborn to suckle on straight after the birth, as this essence helps to prevent any negative emotional pattern being transferred across from the parents or from their family tree down to the child.

Pregnancy can be a time when a woman has a greater need for communication and increased sharing with her partner. To help with any difficulty the male has in the area of emotional communication, the remedy Flannel Flower would be of great assistance. It will help him to develop trust, and let out and express his feelings. Some people, have difficulty in showing their love. The partner may feel resentment towards the child because he feels she has taken over the role that he used to have with his lover before the child's birth. He feels more a sense of jealousy, like the sibling rivalry which occurs with other young children. The remedy Mountain Devil would be appropriate in these cases.

While some women can feel increased self-esteem at the changes in their body, others can feel resentful that they are losing their shape. There can even be resentment, that is deeply held in, towards the baby, who they feel is preventing them from experiencing freedom, independence, leisure, and so on. A woman may feel that her whole being has been changed and affected by this baby and she can't do what she wants anymore. Perhaps the resentment is directed towards a partner for not doing more or for doing things that displease. The remedy Dagger Hakea helps with these feelings of resentment and bitterness and also helps us to remember that all feelings are appropriate and valid, and that we have a choice in the way we respond to these feelings.

It is not uncommon for the woman to experience much grief during pregnancy, and many women report crying without knowing why. Grief and letting go is a large component to any major life change and if a woman allows herself to fully enter into this process she will emerge transformed; if her partner is also willing to go through his own process, then their relationship is likely to be transformed. Sturt Desert Pea is the essence specific for grief.

A woman may worry that her partner will no longer have any physical desire for her because of her change in body shape; she may fear the loss of her lover. If we look underneath this fear there may be lack of confidence about what is happening to her body. For this the remedy Five Corners is excellent. To me it is the most important of all the remedies because it helps a person develop a sense of self-love and self-confidence. It does this by bringing about confidence in the body. This is an especially important quality during pregnancy and in facing labour, the confidence and knowledge that the body is doing exactly what it has been programmed to do, and has been doing, and will continue to keep doing, as long as there is a minimum of intervention (except in emergencies) and natural medicines are used as much as possible.

Five Corners is one of the Flower Essences in another combination called Confid Essence. For the same reasons regarding the need to feel confident in the body mentioned earlier, this combination is ideal for pregnancy. It also comprises Dog Rose for fear and Southern Cross which is for taking responsibility, and not being a victim. This is often necessary for the woman to help her to not be a victim, perhaps of a medical system, or of her situation, whatever that may be. The last essence in the combination is Sturt Desert Rose which is for guilt and following her own morality. A woman during labour or about to give birth needs to feel free to follow her instincts, she needs to feel she can do whatever she wants, especially during labour: if she wants to howl and scream or send someone away from her because she cannot tolerate them, she has a right to do this without feeling guilty.

Another remedy, Bush Fuchsia, is also for helping a person to trust and follow their intuition and instincts. No person knows better than the mother what to do for a child, yet there are often times, especially early on with a first-time mother, when she will not trust her intuition and instead will be influenced by books or other women. There will be a sense of what she should do, but she is not trusting her knowing. The Bush Fuchsia is a remedy to help bring through that intuition and also the ability to trust it. It is a very important remedy because it makes a woman confident in what she is doing, gives her greater self-esteem, and allows her a more satisfying experience as a mother.

There is another remedy called Wild Potato Bush, which is made up in the deserts of Central Australia. It can be used near the end of a pregnancy for any frustration a woman may be feeling due to physical restriction and limitation, such as feeling big and cumbersome, and not being able to sleep comfortably or move freely. It addresses all these feelings of being burdened by the physical. For the unborn child, it will also greatly help with his physical restrictions within the womb before birth, and with his frustration due to his lack of control of his own body after the birth. It also addresses the frustration the spiritual being experiences of suddenly finding themselves crammed into a non-responsive, tiny body in a third-dimensional reality. By rubbing Wild Potato Bush on her belly, the mother will allow both herself and her baby to experience the benefit of this essence.

Towards the end of a pregnancy, many women become impatient and want the birth over and done with, perhaps because of this feeling of being burdened. A remedy called Black-eyed Susan can be given to women who become too impatient. There is a wonderful old expression: 'Nature is hurried at our peril'. Perhaps both the mother and the obstetrician could be given this remedy!

The ability of a woman to feel comfortable and to enjoy her sexuality and be orgasmic can make it easier for her to surrender into the energy of labour. Yet for some women pregnancy brings up a lot of feelings and memories of any previous sexual trauma, assault or incest. Current surveys suggest that up to 70% of women encounter some form of sexual abuse or assault during their lives. This can quite obviously affect their attitude towards sex, and their own expression of their sexuality.

When combined together, the remedies Fringed Violet, Flannel Flower and Wisteria are specific for helping a woman who has experienced such sexual abuse. Fringed Violet deals with the shock; Flannel Flower helps re-establish ease with physical touch and intimacy; and Wisteria brings the ability to relax and feel comfortable with her sexuality and her lovemaking. Even if the woman has not experienced any sexual abuse, Wisteria can be useful in strengthening her connection to her feminine sexual energies and sensuality. Labour is a powerful sexual landmark in a woman's life. This remedy will also encourage spontaneous, affectionate and gentle lovemaking during pregnancy which can help a woman to relax and enjoy herself. It can only lead to the baby picking up feelings which will lead to a healthy attitude towards sex later in his life.

The combination of Fringed Violet, Flannel Flower and Wisteria can also be useful if the woman feels traumatised after the birth experience, especially if there was medical intervention with surgery or if forceps were used. Wisteria can also be used for women who feel apprehensive, perhaps after an epesiotomy, or for those who just feel that resuming sex could be quite painful and so they are unable to relax.

While anticipating the actual labour, if feelings of revulsion come up regarding the body, a sense of feeling dirty or unclean, Billy Goat Plum is for feelings of self-disgust about bodily functions, especially related to sex and the genitals. A woman or her partner can feel very uncomfortable about the amount of blood, faeces and other body fluids which are a common and normal part of labour. The woman may find the idea of breastfeeding repugnant—usually if she hasn't been breastfed herself—or even that she really dislikes how her body looks, pre or post labour. Billy Goat Plum helps a person to accept her body and its functions.

Pregnancy is a time of change for a woman and her partner, and it affects every aspect of their lives. The Flower Essence Bottlebrush is for major change, whether that be of a physical nature—such as becoming pregnant, lactating or menopause—or a situational one, such as moving house, changing jobs, etc. Moving house to accommodate a growing family, especially towards the end of pregnancy, is extremely traumatic for a woman and can influence her to such a degree that bonding is affected.

Parenthood and Bonding

Bottlebrush is the remedy for helping the woman bond to her child, for it is well known that the bonding, the nurturing and the acceptance of the pregnancy leads to a physically healthy and emotionally stable baby. If a child is removed from the mother because of health reasons and put in a humidicrib for more than six hours before it has a chance to go on the mother's breast, then frequently there will be a difficulty in the bonding between the mother and the child. Some women have told me that it took years to re-establish the same level of bonding which they had enjoyed with their other children who had gone straight on to the breast.

Bottlebrush doesn't help the man bond to his child, but a remedy called Red Helmet does. This essence is for the male who is so preoccupied with his business, sport or other activities that he misses the connection to his child and her development. Red Helmet helps a man to be aware of and to spend more time with his child, thereby establishing a healthy, strong bonding with her. It is just as important for the child to bond with her father as it is for her to bond with her mother.

The Little Flannel Flower addresses the child in us all. It is also a good remedy for all parents, especially older ones—helping them to be light and spontaneous, to lose some of their inhibitions and become playful, because it is through play that children and adults learn.

On the subject of love, the Chinese have a saying: 'Children bring certain sorrow and uncertain joy'. Parents can certainly experience deep sadness and sorrow if there are complications in the pregnancy or if there is a miscarriage, stillbirth or cot death. As well as Emergency Essence for the initial shock, there is also Sturt Desert Pea for the deep hurt and sorrow. The Bush Essences can be of great assistance to parents who are grieving. The other phases of grief, apart from the numb shock and sadness, are guilt and anger, which are addressed by Sturt Desert Rose and Mountain Devil, respectively.

Pregnancy, birth and parenthood are powerful physical, emotional, mental and spiritual experiences. The physical and mental sides are well covered by the high standards of health care and information, both medical and naturopathic, available in this country. These days, there is the best potential for both mother and baby to be delivered in fine health; however, as is too often the case, the emotional and spiritual aspects are dealt with all too briefly and inadequately. If we continue to ignore these aspects we lose our very humanity and our ability to grow as human beings through these experiences which are truly mysterious, mystical, awe inspiring and humbling at the same time. Sexuality and birth ensures the continuation of our race, however there is also the opportunity for the quality of these experiences to continue to add richness and growth to our lives.

Goal Setting and Goal —Achieving—

'**Y**ou are the gifts of the Gods. You create your reality according to your beliefs. Yours is the creative energy that makes your world.' Those are the thoughts of Seth as revealed in Jane Roberts's book *The Nature of Personal Reality*, while Buddha had these words to say on manifestation: 'What we are today comes from our thoughts of yesterday and our present thoughts build our life of tomorrow. Our life is the creation of our mind.' Interesting views, both indicating the importance of our thoughts and especially the relevance of having goals in our lives, for without them, our lives will meander along, devoid of any clear direction, and without us having as much control over our destinies as we would like. In this chapter I will be looking at various Bush Essences and how they can greatly enhance the process of individuals determining and achieving their goals.

> If any one thing can be conceived or pondered it exists,
> For whatever is dreamed or imagined is already in the realm of existence.
> That is how all of creation came into existence (Ramtha)

Our goals usually stem from the very deep point of our being, which is known as the higher self, the part that knows our overall life plan and what is in our best interests, not only for ourselves but also for all those people who will be affected directly or indirectly by our goals. Quite often our goals seem clear to us but the overall impact of them is often far greater and way beyond what we could possibly imagine. However, it is enough for us to only have an understanding of the end point of our goal without having to know the full picture. An appropriate analogy is the bee doing its morning rounds, collecting nectar. The bee does not set out with the thought of pollinating the flowers in order to guarantee the continuation of the different plant species; rather its job is to collect nectar to be used in the beehive. In doing this it is fulfilling a role that leads to a far greater outcome. This is also one of the reasons why it is important and beneficial to have goals. It helps to fulfil both our personal as well as the planetary destiny.

If you are intending to do a goal setting session I would recommend that before focusing on future goals you take some time, even an hour or two, to review the previous year and allow all the fantastic and wonderful moments that you experienced to come flooding back to you. Let them come one after another. Go through the last year month by month so you don't miss anything. This will really help you to get into an unlifted peak and motivated space to plan for and see yourself achieving new goals. A dose of Isopogon taken before such an exercise will help you more easily recall those great moments. Reflect also on things that you didn't enjoy in the last year and, which is the whole point of this particular exercise, what you learned from it. What new decisions or realisations did you make or come to as a consequence? This will further enhance your goal-setting ability, motivation and success.

It is of the utmost importance to understand that, for any goal to be achieved, initially it has to be known and then seen on an internal or mental level. Before establishing that inner view, a few essences could be considered to easily allow and create that mental insight or concept of the goal.

Sundew aids one's ability to be creative and imaginative. It could be used by an individual who, while in a daydream state, and with their spiritual doorway open, gets a great idea but who then ignores or forgets it and so the idea is lost and not put into practice. As Henry David Thoreau said: 'If you have built castles in the air, your work need not be lost; that is where they should be. Now put the foundations under them!' Sundew can be used to ground and make the idea practical, while still retaining the image from that intuitive moment. Of course, after having the insight or the sense of the possibility of the goal, take the time to write it down. This tends to earth it and helps to bring it into reality and give it greater power. Sundew also eliminates procrastination and provides the attention to detail necessary for committing it to paper.

Your goals can easily arise when you are in an intuitive or dream state. The remedy Bush Fuchsia greatly enhances your intuitive awareness and abilities, while also helping and increasing your communication in the dream state and the recall of any dreams on awakening.

Being still and quiet and listening to your inner guidance brings you to an increased awareness of, and movement towards your goal. Black-eyed Susan is the remedy if you are a very busy and active person who is always on the go. It allows you to slow down and find your reflective, inner space where you can both become aware of your goal and, at the same time, realise the strategies and the best way to achieve that goal. Silver Princess can be thought of at times when you have no clear sense of life direction. It helps activate a sense of what the next major goal is to be. By following that goal, your life once again will be on track and this is one of the mechanisms by which Silver Princess enables you to be aware of and to pursue your life purpose.

Boronia is an essence whose key function is to greatly improve and deepen creative visualisation, so you can focus on and see the desired outcome.

Once you can see yourself in, or doing the completed goal then get excited by it. Allow yourself to totally feel what it would be like having achieved your goal. The more intense your emotions are the easier it will be to manifest what it is you're desiring. I would advise you however to take a moment to decide beforehand whether or not the thing you wish to manifest is in your highest good. Manifesting something you don't need can take a lot of energy. Energy that may serve you better if directed elsewhere.

The remedy Boronia works very powerfully on the mental body, allowing you access to the power of your consciousness in a very positive way. It is particularly beneficial to kinaesthetic or auditory people who tend to perceive primarily in a non-visual way.

> The mind is the limit. As long as the mind can envision the fact that you can do something, you can do it—as long as you believe one hundred per cent. It's all mind over matter. (Arnold Schwarzenegger)

Our minds are exceptionally powerful. I often reflect on the story of a recently graduated German medical student travelling through Russia between the World Wars. Being broke, his preferred mode of travel was hopping on freight cars and travelling for free. On one particular journey Hans hopped into a freight car, pulled the door closed and, to his concern, it locked. What was of greater worry to him, however, was the realisation that he had jumped into a refrigerated van. His desperate banging on the door to attract the attention of the guards and have it opened before the train took off was to no avail. Realising that he had before him a twelve hour journey without stops, Hans knew he would not survive the trip. He had only a small amount of food and a pen and paper to write letters. He decided that to make the best out of this dreadful situation he could, at least as a legacy, record the various stages of hypothermia (freezing to death). When the train arrived at its final destination the officials who opened the freight car found three things: Hans's frozen body; his notes describing all the stages of hypothermia that he had experienced, up until he lost consciousness; and finally they realised that the refrigeration was switched off! Yet for Hans, believing that he would freeze was enough for his body to go through the various stages of hypothermia and die. If we can harness that same amount of power and certainty from our minds and use it in areas where we choose to channel it positively, then that potential is awesome.

Once having achieved a sense and vision of the goal, there are a number of Bush Essences which will help take that goal to the next stage, where you now start to take practical action to implement it. You can feel overwhelmed by having a head full of ideas. Paw Paw is a good remedy for this and also if you feel overcome by the amount of information you are receiving, or by the number of steps you need to take to reach your goals. You can also help overcome this dilemma by breaking down the goal with the aid of a PERT Chart (PERT means 'Project Evaluation Review Technique'). This technique is widely used in the academic, corporate and government sectors. PERT allows you to turn conceptual ideas into physical road maps whereby a vision or a goal can be systematically worked backwards to its beginning in small logical steps. This method has proven to be highly effective in reaching a goal efficiently and successfully.

Kapok Bush is for any of you who, at this point of commencing the goal, gives up and does not even bother attempting to begin bringing about the goal because you feel it is too hard and difficult. This remedy assists you to be able to establish and see all the smaller steps that need to be done and followed, so that the final outcome can be easily achieved. Your focus becomes not merely the overwhelming goal but also the easily obtained journey along the way. So in working with any goal, especially if you are working with a PERT chart, Kapok Bush is a great essence to help facilitate the sense of what the next step is. For example, if your goal were to plan a memorable dinner party, you would start at the very last step of that goal—that is, the guests leaving at the end of the night—and then focus on what happens immediately before they leave, which might be cleaning up. Then look to the step immediately before cleaning up which might be clearing the table. Without going too far into PERT charts, one can then assign roles—for example, who will be doing the walking out the door or who will be doing the cleaning up, how much time each activity will take. Your goals can be well planned using this method.

However, regardless of the method used, one of the most important elements of bringing about the successful completion of your goal, is to see yourself, in your mind, acting out and doing the goal; to feel—and this is what many people fail to do—what it is like being and doing the things that you want to achieve, to really give yourself the 'juice' of them.

You may also want to communicate with and inspire those people who will be directly involved with the goal, and enlist the support of colleagues or friends along the way. However, discussing a project with everyone before it is actually started tends to dissipate the energy of it. It is a very important metaphysical teaching that the more people talk about something before it is started, the more the energy of it will be lost. Green Spider Orchid is invaluable in enabling people to keep their goals to themselves, rather than leaking out the energy of the goal by talking to all and sundry about it before they have even commenced it. This Essence helps you to keep your goals and ideas within and share them only when the timing is right.

Illawarra Flame Tree is for when you know the goal but fear the responsibility of it, while Sunshine Wattle can be utilised to create a sense of optimism and hope when contemplating and commencing the goal, and to realise that any mistakes or struggle in the past need not be repeated or expected again, for what you focus on you move towards and create. Southern Cross empowers you to realise you can create and take charge of what you want rather than merely hoping it may happen.

As Goethe understood centuries ago: 'Concerning all acts of initiative (and creation), there is one elementary truth, the ignorance of which kills countless ideas and splendid plans; that the moment one definitely commits oneself, then Providence moves too' (*Faust*).

It is necessary to make the goal tangible, attainable and measurable so that you can know when the goal has been reached. Put a time deadline on your goal for even greater focus, clarity and certainty. Also review your goal, and your actions to bring it about, as frequently as possible. The more often the better. Probably the next step is to make a commitment and develop a burning desire to bring that goal about. Of course the essence for commitment is Wedding Bush. This remedy gives the ability to hang in there with the goal and to be single-mindedly committed in pursuing it.

Once you have decided on the goal and committed yourself to it, Five Corners is a valuable remedy to consider. Many people have subconsciously sabotaged the achievement of their goals and from clinical research that I have carried out, in 95% of cases, Five Corners will clear such sabotage. I detect the sabotage by asking my client to state their goal out aloud and then I muscle test them using kinesiology, checking that their conscious and subconscious commitment and desire for the goal are in alignment and free of sabotage. If not, it is sufficient to take Five Corners for only one or two weeks to clear any sabotage. The bottom line behind most sabotages is that the person does not feel worthy enough to deserve what it is they want.

Five Corners floods the psyche with a self-love and self-worth. Even without muscle testing, if you have a goal, it is good to have Five Corners either individually or in combination with some other essence, just to make sure there is no sabotage program going on.

Five Corners is an excellent remedy for those who don't start a project or goal, not because of their fear of failure, but because of the fear of revealing themselves to be inadequate in the process of attaining the goal. This sense of inadequacy is often shame-based and derived from early shaming or blaming from early childhood.

A step in the wrong direction is better than staying on the spot all your life,
Once you're moving forward you can correct your course as you go,
Your automatic guidance system cannot guide you when you're standing still. (Maxwell Maltz)

The step after creating a positive mental attitude and clearing the sabotage might be the simple act of starting on the path towards your goals. Here there are two remedies which can be helpful. Hibbertia is for those who feel that they need to read a few more books, do a few more workshops or study a little bit more before they are ready to do it. As Krishnamurti succinctly put it: 'This is your life and nobody is going to teach you, no book, no guru. Learn from yourself, not from books. It is an endless thing and when you learn about yourself from yourself, out of that learning wisdom comes.' Sometimes we focus too much on the outcome rather than realising the process of attaining the goal is a journey within itself. For that matter, the Hibbertia person tends to be a bit inflexible for many goals.

There needs to be adjustment and flexibility. The *Apollo* spaceship that took Neil Armstrong to the moon was on course for only 3% of its journey; there was continual correction to keep it on course. This applies very much to our goals. To reach a goal we should be flexible, willing to learn and be able to see patterns that we have repeated previously in order to make corrections and change. Isopogon is helpful in letting us see the similar patterns in our behaviour and thus helps us not to repeat the same mistakes.

Procrastination, another aspect of starting, can be addressed with Sundew, which can be used to cut through procrastination and take that first practical step to bring the goal about. Legion are the goals that lie fallow in the field of life because that first step was put off and never taken. One has to act straight away while still enthused, inspired, 'juiced up' and excited by the goal. For as the old Dutch proverb proclaims: 'He who is outside the door has already a good part of his journey behind him.'

Personal motivator Tony Robbins in his seminars emphasises the importance of never leaving the site of setting a goal without doing something towards attaining it, suggesting you do two simple actions and one that is done immediately that will initiate the goal into physical commencement.

Once action has been commenced on the goal, the following Bush Essences will help a person to stay focused on and follow through with the goal until completion. Peach-flowered Tea-tree is for anyone who begins to easily feel bored once the project is going along nicely and the initial challenges have been surmounted, or for those who start off enthusiastically but later lose interest. Jacaranda can be used by those who are scattered and easily distracted from the goal, starting the next project before they have completed the previous one.

The final stage is attaining the goal and locking in that success which will give the motivation for wanting to achieve other goals. We can do this by celebrating and acknowledging ourselves for achieving our goals and be open to any praise and acknowledgment from others. Philotheca is for those who have trouble letting in acknowledgment, whether from self or others, after having achieved their goal.

Finally, Silver Princess is for helping people find a new direction once they have achieved a major goal. When people focus on an important goal they often ignore the day-to-day aspects of life, so that when they achieve the aim they are left feeling very flat with a sense of 'Well so what! Is that all there is?' As Michelle Demonier poignantly writes: 'The great and glorious masterpiece of life is to know your purpose.' The essence for that is again Silver Princess and, although it may not give your whole life purpose in one vision, it will certainly help when you are at the crossroads and not quite sure of the next step to take. To finish, a quote from Stuart Wilde, that tends to say it all:

If you move towards your goals expressing all your power, opportunity will find you as a result.

—Iridology—

If there is one area of naturopathy that never fails to interest and fascinate it is, without doubt, iridology. There are many signs in the iris, the coloured part of the eye that signals and indicates someone's state of health and wellbeing. In this chapter I want to feature four such commonly found markings, ones that can be readily observed in a person's eye simply by looking, without the need of any extra equipment. I will discuss what these markings indicate and which Australian Bush Flower Essences would be the most appropriate for the health conditions they underlie.

Iridology is a wonderful system and a useful tool for analysis. Every part in the body has a corresponding zone in the iris (see Iridology chart). The top of the body corresponds to the top of the iris as the lower part of the body does to the lower part of the iris. For example, the zone for the leg, feet and toes is found in the bottom of the iris. The outermost part of the body—the skin—has a corresponding zone in the outer part of the iris, while the innermost part of the iris around the pupil indicates the area of the innermost part of the body, namely the digestive system. The left iris reveals the left side of the body, the right iris the right side of the body. Through the study of iridology we can gain an insight into not only the physical strengths and weaknesses of the body, but also the emotional balance of the individual.

The iris is very rich in nerve endings and is on the information highway between the brain and all other parts of the body. So if you are walking along the beach and stub your toe the message goes up the various nerves from the toe to the brain. The brain deciphers and interprets the message and responds accordingly. In this case the response would be to say 'Ouch', withdraw the toe and hop up and down. That message of trauma going from the toe to the brain branches at the ganglia in the neck and is diverted to the iris. If there were serious damage to the toe,

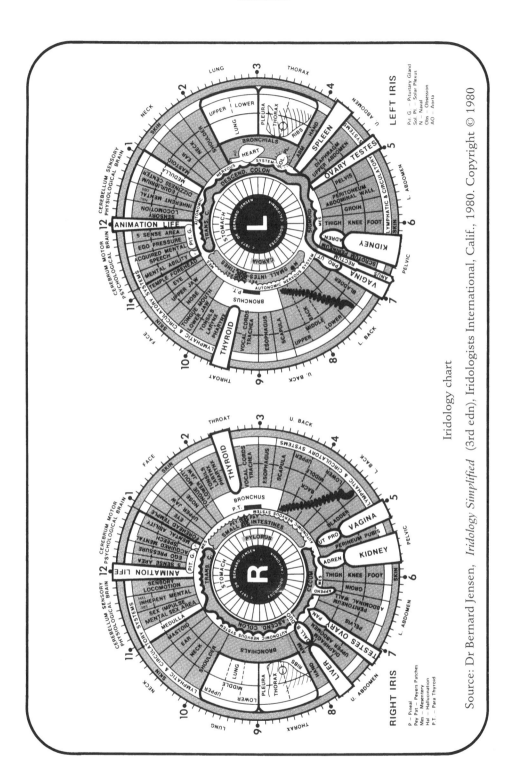

Iridology chart

Source: Dr Bernard Jensen, *Iridology Simplified* (3rd edn), Iridologists International, Calif., 1980. Copyright © 1980

a mark would appear in the toe zone of the iris and that mark would register on the top layer of the iris. There are, in fact, four layers of the iris and if the injury to the toe did not heal quickly and became degenerative, that mark would work its way down through to the second, third and eventually fourth layer of the iris. If an iridologist looked at a mark or almond-shaped lesion in an iris, he or she could determine the level of healing going on in that zone by the depth of the mark or lesion. Acute bronchitis would show as a white acute mark in the lung area of the iris. If the condition became more chronic, this would be revealed in the deterioration of the iris around the bronchial area. Theoretically, as the lung healed, you would notice healing marks occurring over that lesion.

However, I did not find this to be a very accurate assessment of the healing process and, on many occasions in my clinic, a recovery of health and healing was not indicated by the iris. I personally found kinesiology a far more efficient way to assess the current state of health of an individual. I find the benefit with iridology lies in it being able to reveal potentially weak physical and emotional areas before they later manifest as a symptom or problem.

Like the Flower Essences, iridology has a long history, with records of its use going back many thousands of years to ancient Chinese and Egyptian medical records.

In this chapter I want to present four markings, starting from the outside of the eye and working inwards, and the corresponding essences to be considered if you see these markings. Travelling on public transport or parties may never be the same again!!

Sodium Ring

The sodium ring is a thick milky white ring that appears around the outside of the iris (please refer to the photograph in the colour pages of this book). This is rarely seen in young people. It marks a hardening in the body, especially in the circulatory system. People with this marking are more prone to a hardening of the arteries and veins and to the eventual blocking of blood and oxygen to the heart and the brain (what is commonly known as a heart attack or a stroke respectively), where the blood vessels become so rigid that they lose their flexibility and burst in the brain (what we call a stroke). Basically, as the blood vessels close up or occlude, less blood and hence less oxygen can get to the head and brain so all the mental functions are impaired. When there is increased mental or physical exertion, the heart has to pump very hard to get extra blood and oxygen to the tissues through the narrow, more rigid blood vessels. In a healthy state the blood vessel is flexible and can easily expand to accommodate the extra surge of blood. The resistance caused by the plaque and calcium-encased arteries and veins creates much stress for the heart, not to mention the veins and arteries themselves.

If this ring only occurs on the top of the iris, it represents a medical condition termed arcus senilis. People who have this marking are commonly noted to have a poor memory.

Some of the Bush Essences used to address the problems associated with a sodium ring are: Tall Mulla Mulla, which is an excellent essence for improving circulation; and Isopogon, which assists memory and helps to optimally access the memory bank when there is decreased blood and oxygen supply. Emotionally, Hibbertia can be thought of for mental rigidity because a rigid mind usually precedes a rigid body—or rigid blood vessels. Bluebell is another essence to consider for the emotional cause of this problem. It helps people who are blocked off from their emotions to open their hearts and express love and joy. Blocked and held-in emotions are a common trigger for hardening the blood vessels. Flannel Flower to help express feelings and Little Flannel Flower to be light, playful and open to joy would certainly be very useful essences to consider in this condition. Those born under the astrological sign of Leo also seem to be very prone to heart-related conditions so Gymea Lily could also be thought of.

The sodium ring basically shows that the body is calcifying: there is hardening occurring in the body. This can also be an indication of arthritis and again the essences already discussed could be thought of, as well as Dagger Hakea and Sturt Desert Pea. Holding in resentment and sadness are two of the most common ways to block the flow of love and joy in your body, and take away its flexibility and lead to hardening. I have noticed that many people who have strokes usually, at some very deep level, do not want to be on the planet any more—they want to leave. You may think of Waratah and Kapok Bush: the former for suicidal feelings or any subconscious death wish and the latter for giving up.

Lymphatic Rosary

The lymphatic system is one of the greatest kept secrets of the body. There is more lymph (in fact over 5 L) than there is blood in the body. The heart pumps the blood while muscular contraction pumps the lymph. There are three major functions of lymph in the body:

- the transportation and breakdown of fats;
- the transportation of white blood cells, enhancing the immune system; and
- the purification and detoxification of all cells in the body.

The area in the iris related to the lymphatic system is just within the outer border of the iris (please refer to the photograph of the lymphatic rosary in the colour pages of this book). Blue-eyed people are more prone to having problems with their lymphatic system, while brown-eyed people usually have more problems with their intestinal organs. There are only two basic colours in the iris—blue and brown. If you have green eyes they are simply blue with a yellow overlay. The yellow indicates the kidney, so the old romantic Irish notion of a green-eyed Colleen is really a woman with kidney problems—not quite the same! The pigments for brown in the iris are not available until a child is between three and six months old. Some parents with knowledge of iridology panic when their blue-eyed young babies suddenly go brown-eyed, fearing that suddenly their children are being clogged with toxic waste from their bowels.

When the lymphatic system is becoming sluggish, white cotton ball-like fluffs called tophi occur in the outside of the iris. They are most commonly seen in the lung and bronchial areas which, if we were to see the iris as a clock divided into twelve segments, would be at 3 o'clock and 9 o'clock, respectively. Another common area for them to be seen is in the throat and sinus area which can be found at either 2 o'clock or 10 o'clock, depending on whether you are looking at the left or right eye. As well as indicating congested lymph, white tophi appearing in this area would also indicate excessive mucus and an increased tendency to chest and throat infections. When these marks are seen it is generally a very good idea to reduce the amount of fats in the diet, especially from dairy products such as cheese and milk. There is a theory that allergies to milk indicate unresolved issues with the mother; however, I certainly did not commonly notice this correlation in my practice. If it were the case, Bottlebrush would be the appropriate essence to correct this. Also humans are not biologically adapted to digest milk after the age of about twelve. It is a food best avoided after this age as the molecules of cow's milk are many times larger than the molecules found in human milk.

It is not uncommon to find lymphatic tophi all around the iris, not just in the lung and throat areas. When this occurs it is called a lymphatic rosary. If the lymphatic system becomes even more sluggish and chronic, the white tophi will change to yellow and, finally, a brown colour which indicates a very toxic system. Basically when this occurs the person is literally swimming in a cesspool of their own waste. Other symptoms of a sluggish lymphatic system would be fluid retention (especially around the feet), tiredness, lethargy and a tendency to skin conditions such as acne, eczema, etc. Apart from dietary deletions and more exercise, Bush Iris in particular should be thought of in treating the lymphatic system. It will invariably correct a sluggish or retrograde lymphatic system with marked benefit to the individual. If someone is continuing to eat dairy food, then the lymphatic system could be supported with a combination of Paw Paw, Crowea and Peach-flowered Tea-tree to help with the digestion of fats, together with Wedding Bush for commitment to go off them. Bottlebrush and Boronia could also be considered to help break an addiction to any dairy food. Many people crave dairy products such as cheese and icecream. Bottlebrush and Boronia will help break the physical addiction to these substances but please be observant of any underlying emotions that are then released. The addictive substance serves to suppress feelings or emotions that the person is usually uncomfortable experiencing. Five Corners could be given to clear any subconscious sabotage programs that force the person to continue taking substances that they know to be harmful to them. Flannel Flower would be an excellent essence to help people to be totally in their bodies and to enjoy expressing themselves physically, so that movement and exercise becomes pleasurable.

Nerve Rings

Nerve rings indicate stress and tension that is not being released from the body; rather this tension is stored in the area where the nerve ring occurs in the iris. Tightening or even cramping of the tissues will often occur in that area of the body. It is very common to see nerve rings in people with a busy and hectic pace of life living in urban areas. The nerve rings are found around the outside of the eye (please refer to the photograph of the nerve ring in the colour pages of this book), and are usually located in the zone of the iris corresponding to the neck and back, although it is not uncommon to find them in the chest, solar plexus and head areas. People with these markings often experience chest pain, poor digestion and headaches, respectively.

Stored emotional stress can also create nerve rings and these rings generally commence in the digestive organ area of the iris chart. A nerve ring commencing in the liver region would indicate unresolved anger and also the need for Dagger Hakea. The more rings and the deeper they are, the greater the degree of stress being stored in the body. Sometimes there can be up to five nerve rings in any one segment of the iris. To help treat the stored stress that these rings indicate, think of: Crowea, as it works on tight, tense and cramped muscles; Black-eyed Susan to slow down and help relax; Gymea Lily for tension around the spine and neck; and Emergency Essence for headaches (which also contains Crowea). Even the Meditation Essence would be useful for people with a lot of nerve rings to help them to slow down and allow them to go inwards.

Toxic Colon

As mentioned earlier, brown-eyed people are more likely to have problems with their colon than blue-eyed people. The large intestine, also known as the colon, is found close to the centre of the iris in a zone just above the stomach and small intestinal regions, which are found next to the pupil. One of the major reasons for health imbalances—from a purely physical point of view—is the reabsorption of metabolic wastes through the bowel wall into the bloodstream. This is a particularly common pattern that I have noticed in my practice. It leads to autotoxemia and is a forerunner to most degenerative health problems. In the iris, autotoxaemia will often show as a brown discolouration that often can be seen spreading out to different parts of the iris from the bowel region (please refer to the photograph of the toxic colon in the colour pages of this book). Whenever I see this pattern in the iris I always think of using Bottlebrush. After taking this essence a number of patients have actually said: 'It literally felt like a bottlebrush was put up inside me and cleaned me out!' Bottlebrush works on both physical holding on (constipation) as well as helping to let go emotionally, which is usually why someone is constipated in the first place. When there is prolonged diarrhoea, Kapok Bush should be thought of, although in many cases, diarrhoea can be a sign of irritation in the bowel as a result of constipation. If there is lack of tone in the colon then Crowea will help to restore good muscular tone and integrity to the colon.

Astrology, Health and the Australian Bush Flower —Essences—

by Louise Anderson, Dip. Med. Herb.

A quick look at the sites of the major ancient civilisations supports the theory is all the proof needed that our ancestors knew a lot about astronomy, and took the time and care to construct enormous structures to track the movement of the stars, structures still standing today and able to be used by those who know how. Stonehenge is perhaps the most famous. Dating back to 3000 BC, it is calculating solstices, equinoxes, eclipses and the risings and settings of the sun, moon and various stars as accurately today as it did the day it was built. So lost in time was its true reason for being that we didn't even know its purpose until the early 1960s, when the astronomer Gerald Hawkins fed its measurements into his primitive computer and confirmed his suspicions that it was in fact a giant star observatory.

All over the world it is a similar story. Stone medicine wheels, which serve the same purpose as Stonehenge, are dotted throughout North America. The Aztecs in South America built their pyramids for the same reason and the great pyramid of Cheops in Egypt was built in such a way as to allow the light from both Sirius and the Pole Star to shine down the two ventilating shafts into the royal burial chamber and on to the head of the king's sarcophagus. Further, Sirius does this at the start of the Egyptian Year, signalling the annual flooding of the Nile. This pyramid's measurements also reveal that its builders knew the circumference of the earth, the length of the polar axis, the mean distance between the sun and the earth, the specific gravity of the earth and the exact number of days in a year (accurate to four decimal places). The Babylonians had their ziggurats, the Chaldeans tracked the stars and so did the Chinese—and with a degree of accuracy our civilisation is only just beginning to appreciate and match. Archaeologists have unearthed 30,000-year-old bones with engravings marking the moon cycles, believed to be female fertility calendars. Detailed zodiacs from ancient Egypt, China, India, Mexico, Greece, Babylon, Assyria and Sumer have also been found. Fourteenth century Chinese zodiacs show the effect of planets and constellations on health. Confucius is quoted as saying: 'He who wants to understand man must first understand Heaven, for it is Heaven which gives man his nature and his law.' In ancient times, in every culture, the planets were named after and worshipped as gods and goddesses.

Why did they bother? Life was hard in ancient times. With no machinery or supermarkets there was soil to be tilled, crops to be grown and harvested. Why waste precious time gazing at stars and planets and building monuments to keep track of them? Let alone start philosophising about it all. Was it all superstition or pleasant hobby to pass the time, or something seen as so vital by every single major culture worldwide since time began that it couldn't be neglected? The answer is fairly simple in the end. Until the Industrial Revolution, human life was intricately woven with the cycles of nature. Through long observation the ancients worked out that the journey of the sun through the constellations coincided with the seasons and plant growth; the phases of the moon with the tides, and they lived in harmony with these cycles. If they didn't they starved. Herbs were an important part of medicine and the herbalists observed over long centuries that the medicinal qualities of plants were strongest, safest and could be stored longer if harvested at particular times. The sun and the moon marked these passages of time (and still do!). Any modern fisherman will tell you fish bite better and sometimes not at all on certain tides and moon phases. Many farmers still look to their 'Farmer's Almanac'—a moon ephemeris—before sowing or harvesting their crops. No self-respecting sailor will go to sea without first checking his Tide Chart. Then and now, people in close contact with nature have to work within its rules if they wish to survive and prosper.

Ancient cultures that included surgery in their medicine observed that operations on certain areas of the body invariably went wrong at predictable times in the lunar cycle. That women's fertility and menstrual cycles were linked to the moon phases. That people born at certain times of the year exhibited distinct character traits and were prone to illnesses in specific areas of the body. All this information evolved into the science and art of astrology—science because it is based on mathematical calculations of the movements of the stars and planets, art because there is definitely a knack to the interpretation. As far back as the first century AD, Ptolemy was writing of the correlations between a person's star sign and their physical health and there is evidence to suggest that he was simply the first to write down what had been known for some time. Since the Greeks used the astrologically advanced Egyptians as physicians until the sixth century BC and the Egyptians had in turn learnt from the Babylonians (5000 BC) with whom they traded, no one is quite sure how old this knowledge is. Certainly both these civilisations took care to hide their most advanced knowledge on the subject in the actual construction of their pyramids; very little was committed to either papyrus or clay tablet.

However, this system had progressed to such an extent by the height of the Greek civilisation that Hippocrates, 'the father of modern medicine' and founder of the largest and most respected medical school of the ancient world, had the following to say: 'Ignorant is the doctor who understands nothing of astrology. The role played by astrology in medicine is no small one; indeed it is very large.' 'A doctor without knowledge of astrology does not have the right to call himself a doctor.' 'He who practises medicine without the benefit of the movement of the stars and planets is a fool.' The Hippocratic oath, named after him and until recently taken by all medical doctors upon graduation, stated first and foremost that a doctor would not harm the health or wellbeing of his patients with his treatment. Hippocrates remains so highly regarded that his philosophies and teachings are the backbone of naturopathic principles to the present day.

In the seventeenth century, the English herbalist Thomas Culpepper assigned planets to each plant, which could then be used to heal problems associated with that particular planet. Like the sixteenth century physician, astrologer and philosopher Paracelsus, Culpepper believed that a plant's appearance and locale gave clues to its healing properties. Although for a time put aside as superstitious nonsense, this 'Doctrine of Signatures' is considered invaluable by many modern herbalists and makers of flower essences, including Ian White.

It is only since science took hold and scientists told us nothing was valid unless machines could measure it, that the marriage between spirituality, human nature, healing and astrology has dissolved. Our technology needed to advance sufficiently before we could fully appreciate Stonehenge. With new machines on the cutting edge of quantum physics just recently invented, hopefully we will soon be reading hard data on the energies of vibrational remedies and their effects on the human aura and body, and then these modalities can enter the healing mainstream with the blessings of both modern science and medicine.

Medical astrology can show us whether we are likely to enjoy good health or if we are prone to certain diseases. It shows us which parts of the body are ruled by each sign and planet. It can show us when we are more likely to suffer a health crisis and, traditionally, which herbal remedies will support our own unique constitution to help us avoid disease. Flower Essences can also be used to assist correction of these imbalances before (and even after) they manifest physically. Wholistic therapists believe that disease is the result of mental and emotional imbalances which, when left untreated, filter down to the physical body in order to be recognised. If neglected, the body will try another illness to bring the matter to our attention. The books *You Can Heal Your Life* by Louise Hay, and *The Body is the Barometer of the Soul* by Annette Noontil, cover this subject in detail.

The best way to know what your potential health problems may be is to have your complete birth chart cast using your exact time, place and date of birth and then interpreted by a competent medical astrologer. An accurate birth time is essential; if you don't know it there are various ways to obtain it, which a professional astrologer can help you do. Even without having your chart cast, however, you can still use this chapter to discover what general imbalances you are prone to according to your sun (star) sign.

Emotional imbalances

Each star or sun sign expresses distinct personality traits and people born under a particular sign will behave and react in fairly predictable ways. When an astrologer draws up your birth chart, they are actually making a map of the sky as it looked at the exact time of your birth in that exact place. All the planets (not just the sun) are placed in a birth chart. Many of these fall into different signs and as each planet represents a different part of our personality, we are all unique blends. This explains the differences between people of the same sun (star) sign, and also why we often feel as if some of the traits of other signs apply to us. The most important parts of our birth chart are our sun sign, moon sign and ascendant or rising sign. Sometimes this energy is not flowing freely and so begins to express in a negative way.

The good news is it doesn't have to stay like this. If your kitchen sink were clogged you wouldn't feel the need to put up with it indefinitely. You'd call the plumber and get it fixed. Your birth chart doesn't need to be any different. Flower Essences work on blockages and imbalances in the etheric body, so marry perfectly with astrology. You are not stuck with any of the imbalances within your birth chart. We are here on this earth to learn, heal and grow, to bring into balance the energies of our birth chart. The Australian Bush Flower Essences are an excellent tool for smoothing the path, making the process both easier and faster.

Each planet rules a sign and a specific area of our life (see the table below).

Planet	Sign	Areas in which it affects our attitudes and abilities
Sun	Leo	Identity, self-esteem, sense of self-confidence
Mercury	Gemini	Communication, self-expression, thought processes
	Virgo	Attention to detail, discernment, discrimination, service
Chiron	Virgo	Higher Self, healing self and others, service
Venus	Taurus	Sensuality, material possessions, perseverance, strength
	Libra	Relationships, intimacy, love, friendship, balance (creativity, art, music and beauty are ruled by both signs)
Moon	Cancer	Emotions, home, family, mother issues, nurturing, intuition, soul memories
Mars	Aries	Ability to initiate action, courage, sex drive, willpower
Jupiter	Sagittarius	Education, wisdom, fun, justice, long journeys, abundance
Saturn	Capricorn	Father/authority issues, responsibility, commitment, history
Uranus	Aquarius	Social/group/humanitarian issues, technology, change
Neptune	Pisces	Spirituality, compassion, reality, merging, dreams, addictions
Pluto	Scorpio	Power, passion, transformation, deep insecurities, death, grief

There are two ways to use this section. First, look up your sun sign in the following pages. Often imbalances will emerge as characteristics listed under the 'Excess' section of that sign; however if the sun energy is blocked by a 'difficult' angle to another planet, you may also experience some of the 'Deficiency' traits. It doesn't matter if you don't have your full birth chart: you'll probably recognise the traits within yourself anyway. The Flower Essences next to the trait can help you work through these issues.

Another way to use this section is to read through the list above. If you feel that a particular part of your life is not working as well as you would like, look to see which sign is influencing it. This may well be different to your sun sign, in which case it is quite likely that the planet ruling that sign is blocked. There is usually great opportunity for personal growth in this area, and overcoming any difficulties you have been experiencing is part of your life lesson. Turn to the sign that rules that area of life and see if any of the imbalances listed there apply to you (often these emerge as the traits listed in the 'Deficiency' section).

In both cases, look at the qualities that sign embodies when the energy is balanced; these are the character traits you are striving to make a part of yourself. The essences will help move you in this direction, and the process can be sped up by being aware of the nature of that energy when it is balanced and consciously trying to live it. Energy wants to be used. If you are not using your energy at all, nor using it positively, it has no choice but to emerge negatively. If you find yourself falling back into negative patterns, read through the section again to remind yourself what it is you are trying to learn and trying to be, and take the essences again to help you get there. For many of the imbalances there is more than one essence to correct it. See the book *Australian Bush Flower Essences* for ways to choose the best one for you.

Aries/Mars Blocks

Mars, the God of War, rules Aries. Well balanced Aries energy is fearless, pioneering, honest, ambitious, assertive, energetic, enthusiastic, independent, generous, confident, inspiring, optimistic, original, decisive, adaptable and idealistic. It creates natural leaders who are easily able to initiate action. Mars represents the physical body and the lower will; the ability to move through and operate in the world. Imbalances emerge in the following way:

Excess
Aggressive/angry ... Mountain Devil
Impatient/quick-tempered/frustrated ... Black-eyed Susan
Lacking diplomacy/blunt ... Kangaroo Paw
Restless ... Jacaranda
Difficulty completing projects ... Peach-flowered Tea-tree, Red Helmet Orchid, Wedding Bush
Bossy/dominating/arrogant ... Gymea Lily, Hibbertia
Easily bored ... Peach-flowered Tea-tree

Egocentric . . . Gymea Lily
Sexuality issues . . . Billy Goat Plum, Flannel Flower, Fringed Violet, Red Lily, Sturt Desert Rose, Wisteria
Insensitive . . . Flannel Flower, Kangaroo Paw
Bloody-minded . . . Isopogon, Kangaroo Paw
Intolerant . . . Yellow Cowslip Orchid
Overly competitive . . . Mountain Devil

Deficiency
Unable to initiate action . . . Kapok Bush, Red Grevillea, Red Lily, Silver Princess, Sundew
Stuck . . . Mint Bush, Pink Mulla Mulla, Red Grevillea
Lacking vitality . . . Banksia Robur, Old Man Banksia, Pink Mulla Mulla
Low self-esteem . . . Five Corners
Sexuality issues . . . Billy Goat Plum, Flannel Flower, Fringed Violet, Red Lily, Sturt Desert Rose, Wisteria
Aimless . . . Silver Princess
Lacking passion . . . Bush Gardenia, Mulla Mulla
Lacking courage . . . Sturt Desert Rose, Tall Mulla Mulla, Waratah
Fearful . . . Dog Rose, Dog Rose of the Wild Forces, Grey Spider Flower

Taurus/Venus Blocks

Taurus is currently ruled by Venus—Goddess of Love and Beauty—until its true ruler is discovered and assigned. This ruler is thought perhaps to be Vulcan, the smithy of the gods who had the dual Taurean traits of strength and artistic ability. Balanced Taurean energy is patient, strong, sensual, affectionate, practical, deliberate, dependable, tranquil, persevering, enduring, firm, grounded, loyal and artistic. Imbalances emerge in the following way:

Excess
Stubbornness . . . Isopogon
Depression/pessimism/despair . . . Sunshine Wattle, Tall Yellow Top, Waratah
Over-indulgence . . . Bush Iris
Fear of poverty . . . Philotheca, Sunshine Wattle
Feeling burdened/weighed down . . . Banksia Robur, Old Man Banksia, Paw Paw, Wild Potato Bush
Lethargy/sluggishness . . . Banksia Robur, Macrocarpa, Old Man Banksia, Pink Mulla Mulla
Stuck . . . Mint Bush, Pink Mulla Mulla, Red Grevillea
Resistance to change . . . Bauhinia

Overly cautious . . . Hibbertia, Little Flannel Flower, Sunshine Wattle, Yellow Cowslip Orchid
Controlling . . . Isopogon, Southern Cross
Possessive . . . Bluebell, Bottlebrush, Mountain Devil, Southern Cross, Sunshine Wattle
Intolerant . . . Freshwater Mangrove, Slender Rice Flower, Yellow Cowslip Orchid
Chauvinist . . . Wisteria
Prejudice without personal experiences . . . Freshwater Mangrove
Greed/materialism . . . Bluebell, Bush Iris, Rough Bluebell
Resentment . . . Dagger Hakea
Stale relationship . . . Bush Gardenia

Deficiency
Blocked sensuality . . . Billy Goat Plum, Flannel Flower, Wisteria
Blocked creativity . . . Turkey Bush
Unable to see beauty in others . . . Freshwater Mangrove, Slender Rice Flower
Unable to see the beauty in self . . . Billy Goat Plum, Five Corners
Lacking perseverance . . . Kapok, Macrocarpa, Wedding Bush
Insecurity . . . Dog Rose, Tall Mulla Mulla
Difficulty giving or receiving love . . . Bluebell, Philotheca

Gemini/Mercury Blocks

Mercury, the messenger of the gods, rules Gemini, and blocks here can cause problems with communication and difficulties with left-right brain co-ordination. When balanced, Gemini and Mercury energy is adaptable, witty, charming, quick, social, agile, dexterous, intelligent, curious, persuasive, irresistible, politically astute, industrious, multi-talented, communicative, playful and free-spirited. Mercury represents the left brain. Imbalances emerge in the following way:

Excess
Burnout . . . Black-eyed Susan, Macrocarpa
Scatteredness . . . Jacaranda
Feeling split/ungrounded . . . Red Lily, Sundew
Stress . . . Black-eyed Susan
Fickle/restless . . . Jacaranda
Rushing . . . Black-eyed Susan
Changeable/easily bored . . . Peach-flowered Tea-tree
Ungrounded . . . Red Lily, Sundew
Inability to tap into intuition . . . Angelsword, Green Spider Orchid, Hibbertia, Red Lily
Not trusting intuition . . . Bush Fuchsia

Distrust of inner wisdom . . . Angelsword, Green Spider Orchid, Hibbertia, Southern Cross, Sturt Desert Rose
Out of touch with Higher Self . . . Paw Paw, Red Lily
Listening to others, not inner self, resulting in giving power away . . . Southern Cross
Gossiping . . . Green Spider Orchid, Kangaroo Paw, Sturt Desert Rose
Uncommitted . . . Wedding Bush
Sarcastic . . . Rough Bluebell
Inconsiderate . . . Kangaroo Paw
Intolerant . . . Black-eyed Susan, Yellow Cowslip Orchid
Superficial . . . Jacaranda
Aimless . . . Silver Princess
Lying . . . Hibbertia, Rough Bluebell
In the head rather than the heart . . . Hibbertia + Yellow Cowslip Orchid
Mental superiority . . . Hibbertia

Deficiency
Communication problems, speech impediments, left-right brain co-ordination difficulties, or a blocked throat chakra . . . Bush Fuchsia
Poor memory . . . Isopogon
Learning difficulties/dyslexia . . . Bush Fuchsia
Poor concentration . . . Jacaranda, Sundew
Difficulty mixing with others . . . Dog Rose, Slender Rice Flower, Tall Mulla Mulla, Tall Yellow Top, Yellow Cowslip Orchid
Attention deficit disorder . . . Bush Fuchsia, Jacaranda, Paw Paw, Sundew
Clumsy . . . Bush Fuchsia
Lacking practical dexterity . . . Bush Fuchsia, Flannel Flower
Need assistance in improving handyman skills . . . Kapok Bush

Cancer/Moon Blocks

Cancer is ruled by the moon. In a birth chart, the moon represents our emotional nature, soul memories and intuitive connections. It also reveals how we perceive our own mother and our views towards mothering, nurturing, being nurtured and food. As our mother has such an enormous influence on us in our formative years, the moon and Cancer also influence our attitudes towards home and family. There are as many different ways for blocked moon/Cancer energy to emerge as there are emotions, but some of the more common ones are:

Excess
Emotional overwhelm . . . Crowea, Dog Rose of the Wild Forces, Mint Bush, Paw Paw, Red Suva Frangipani

Difficulty letting go of others emotionally ... Autumn Leaves + Bottle-
brush + Bush Iris + Lichen, Mint Bush, Sturt Desert Pea
Hypersensitive ... Dog Rose of the Wild Forces, Fringed Violet, Mint
Bush, Red Suva Frangipani, Yellow Cowslip Orchid
Worry ... Crowea
Insecure ... Dog Rose, Tall Mulla Mulla
Anxious ... Crowea, Dog Rose
Feeling abandoned ... Tall Yellow Top
Feeling rejected ... Illawarra Flame Tree
Living in the past ... Bottlebrush, Sundew
Difficulty breaking family emotional patterns ... Boab
Caregiver suffering emotional burnout ... Alpine Mint Bush
Resentment towards family members ... Dagger Hakea
Feeling used ... Southern Cross
Not feeling nurtured by others ... Bottlebrush, Red Helmet, Red Suva
Frangipani
Hoarding ... Bottlebrush
Prolonged grief ... Sturt Desert Pea
Pining ... Boronia
Psychic wound ... Pink Mulla Mulla
Psychic sponge ... Angelsword, Fringed Violet
Guilt ... Dog Rose of the Wild Forces, Sturt Desert Rose
Despair ... Waratah
Obsession ... Boronia

Deficiency
Cut off from feelings ... Bluebell
Unable to tap into intuition ... Angelsword + Bush Fuchsia + Bush Iris
+ Red Lily
Insensitive ... Kangaroo Paw, Rough Bluebell
Difficulty expressing feelings ... Flannel Flower
Constantly moving home ... Jacaranda
Mother issues ... Bottlebrush + Dog Rose
Unable to nurture self ... Philotheca

Leo/Sun Blocks

Leo is ruled by the sun and both are concerned with our identity, ego,
confidence and self-esteem. Positive Leo energy is courageous, strong,
confident, artistic, magnetic, entertaining, dramatic, enthusiastic, inspi-
rational, optimistic, vital, generous, ambitious, loyal, affectionate, cheerful, regal and fun. Leos are natural organisers and leaders and have hearts
of gold. Imbalances emerge in the following way:

Excess

Arrogant/domineering ... Gymea Lily

Vain ... Gymea Lily

Overly proud ... Gymea Lily, Slender Rice Flower

Intolerant ... Freshwater Mangrove, Slender Rice Flower, Yellow
  Cowslip Orchid

Quick-tempered ... Mountain Devil

Overly dramatic ... Illawarra Flame Tree

Narcissistic ... Gymea Lily, Kangaroo Paw

Overly focused on self in relationship ... Bush Gardenia, Kangaroo
  Paw

Difficulty sharing ... Bluebell

Superior ... Hibbertia, Slender Rice Flower

Feeling rejected if not centre of attention ... Illawarra Flame Tree

Jealous ... Mountain Devil

Deficiency

Low self-esteem ... Five Corners, Sturt Desert Rose

Lacking vitality/joie de vivre ... Banksia Robur, Crowea, Dog Rose,
  Macrocarpa, Old Man Banksia

Heart chakra blocked ... Bluebell, Waratah

Lacking joy ... Alpine Mint Bush, Five Corners, Little Flannel Flower,
  Sunshine Wattle

Depressed ... Tall Yellow Top, Waratah

Father issues ... Red Helmet

Blocked creativity ... Bluebell + Bush Fuchsia + Turkey Bush

Lacking passion ... Bush Gardenia, Mulla Mulla

Lacking courage ... Dog Rose, Dog Rose of the Wild Forces, Grey
  Spider Flower, Sturt Desert Rose, Tall Mulla Mulla, Waratah

Self-effacing ... Philotheca

Vulnerable ... Bluebell, Flannel Flower, Red Suva Frangipani

Pessimistic ... Sunshine Wattle

Exhausted ... Macrocarpa

Lacking generosity ... Bluebell

Avoiding close relationships ... Bush Gardenia

Virgo/Chiron Blocks

Traditional astrology holds that the planet Mercury currently rules both
Gemini and Virgo. Until the true ruler of Virgo is assigned, Virgos will
continue to suffer from some Mercury/Gemini imbalances. Debate con-
tinues in the astrological community, but in her pioneering book, *Chiron:
Rainbow Bridge Between the Inner and Outer Planets*, Barbara Hand Clow
puts forward a very good argument that Chiron is the true ruler of Virgo.
Her research shows that Chiron heals a chart under transit. In *Mythic
Astrology: Archetypal Powers in the Horoscope*, Ariel Guttman and Kenneth

Johnson also suggest Chiron is a co-ruler of Virgo, along with several asteroids. In mythology, Chiron was a healer who was wounded, so it seems logical that Chiron would rule both Virgo and the sixth house (the house of health and sickness). Chiron and Virgo do appear to figure prominently in the charts of many healers and as true healing comes through Spirit (the Higher Self), it seems fair to say that Chiron rules the crown chakra and that Virgo at its highest level is the sign of healers.

On a more day-to-day level, well balanced Virgo energy is analytical, technically minded, curious, reliable, highly moral and ethical, discriminating, organised, efficient, tidy, practical, industrious, considerate and reserved. It pays close attention to fine detail, is perfectionist in nature and is willing, able and gratified to provide a high level of service. Out of balance, this energy can manifest in the following way:

Excess
Nitpicking . . . Hibbertia, Yellow Cowslip Orchid
Critical of self . . . Five Corners, Hibbertia, Philotheca
Critical of others . . . Yellow Cowslip Orchid
Restless nervous energy . . . Black-eyed Susan, Dog Rose, Jacaranda
Overly mental/cut off from emotions . . . Hibbertia, Yellow Cowslip
  Orchid
Workaholic . . . Black-eyed Susan
Unable to relax . . . Black-eyed Susan
Hypochondria . . . Peach-flowered Tea-tree
Mental rigidity . . . Hibbertia
Fastidious . . . Billy Goat Plum, Boronia
Frugal . . . Yellow Cowslip Orchid
Irritable . . . Black-eyed Susan
Perfectionist . . . Hibbertia
Overly conventional . . . Bauhinia, Yellow Cowslip Orchid
Burnt out as a healer/care giver . . . Alpine Mint Bush
Focused on giving, not receiving . . . Philotheca
Unable to contact other realms . . . Green Spider Orchid

Deficiency
Lacking discernment . . . Angelsword
Lacking attention to detail . . . Sundew
Lacking spirit of service . . . Yellow Cowslip Orchid
Closed off to the Spirit . . . Bush Iris, Paw Paw
Out of touch with Higher Self . . . Paw Paw, Red Lily
Perception difficulties . . . Bush Fuchsia, Freshwater Mangrove

Libra/Venus Blocks

Like Taurus, Libra is ruled by Venus. Here Venus brings in not only her artistic ability, but also her love of beauty, harmony, balance, luxury and a sense of fairness. Venus also represents our attitudes towards relationships. Balanced Libran energy is polite, diplomatic, friendly, cheerful, harmonious, soothing, talkative, strategic, cultured, graceful, elegant, stylish, musical, unhurried, gracious, charming, gentle, kind, understanding, considerate, sharing and helpful. Librans like to weigh a question from all sides before making a decision. Imbalances can emerge in the following way:

Excess
Procrastinating/indecisive . . . Paw Paw, Red Lily, Sundew
Mood swings . . . Peach-flowered Tea-tree
Avoid confrontation . . . Dog Rose, Tall Mulla Mulla
Prone to excess/materialistic . . . Bluebell, Bush Iris
Need to have other people around . . . Illawarra Flame Tree
Need to be accepted and liked . . . Five Corners, Illawarra Flame Tree
Vain . . . Gymea Lily
Beauty issues . . . Billy Goat Plum
Co-dependent . . . Red Grevillea
Love addict . . . Flannel Flower
Confusion/perturbation . . . Mint Bush
Feeling out of balance . . . Crowea
Lazy . . . Kapok Bush, Sundew
Stuck . . . Mint Bush, Pink Mulla Mulla, Red Grevillea
Aimless . . . Silver Princess
Apathetic/unmotivated . . . Banksia Robur, Kapok Bush, Old Man
     Banksia
Lacking perseverance . . . Kapok Bush, Peach-flowered Tea-tree,
     Wedding Bush
Unsure of life purpose . . . Silver Princess
Fear of poverty . . . Sunshine Wattle
Dislike being told what to do . . . Gymea Lily, Isopogon, Red Helmet
Low self-esteem . . . Five Corners

Deficiency
Avoiding intimacy . . . Flannel Flower, Wedding Bush
Blocked creativity . . . Turkey Bush
Blocked sensuality . . . Flannel Flower, Wisteria
Difficulty receiving love . . . Philotheca
Insensitive . . . Kangaroo Paw
Argumentative . . . Isopogon, Slender Rice Flower, Yellow Cowslip
     Orchid
Unable to see the beauty in others . . . Slender Rice Flower, Yellow
     Cowslip Orchid
Prejudiced . . . Freshwater Mangrove, Slender Rice Flower
Need to develop impartiality . . . Yellow Cowslip Orchid
Feeling out of balance . . . Crowea

Stale relationship . . . Bush Gardenia
Monopolise conversations . . . Gymea Lily, Kangaroo Paw
Clumsy . . . Bush Fuchsia
Bloody-minded . . . Isopogon
Depressed . . . Little Flannel Flower, Sunshine Wattle
Shy . . . Dog Rose
Isolated . . . Tall Yellow Top
Lacking sense of fairness and personal integrity . . . Sturt Desert Rose

Scorpio/Pluto Blocks

Ruled by Pluto, Lord of the Underworld, Scorpios are involved with the so-called 'shadow' of the personality. Robert Johnson has written a wonderful book on this subject called *Owning Your Own Shadow*. Scorpio issues include power, sex, survival, psychology, research, reincarnation, transformation and the death, dying and grieving processes. Spiritually, a strong Scorpio chart is an excellent opportunity to burn off a lot of old karma, the challenge being to learn and practise forgiveness towards those who try to or actually do you harm. Scorpios willing to do this often find themselves in a state of transition, as they dig progressively deeper into their subconscious and unconscious fears, as well as their past life karmic issues, and release them. The highest manifestation of this energy is said to be as the eagle, soaring high above the earth, rather than the lower end where it can sting itself and others to death as animal Scorpions do. While moving from the scorpion to the eagle, I believe many Scorpios resemble snakes, periodically shedding their outgrown skins—or phoenixes, rising from the ashes, purified and renewed. Balanced Scorpio energy is quiet, discreet, composed, ambitious, assertive, intense, passionate, intuitive, hypnotic, magical, magnetic, intense, religious, sympathetic, protective, loyal, determined, persevering, probing, regenerative and transformative. Imbalances manifest in the following way:

Excess
Base chakra survival issues . . . Bush Iris, Waratah
Bitter/resentful . . . Dagger Hakea
Vengeful . . . Mountain Devil, Rough Bluebell
Difficulty with forgiving . . . Dagger Hakea, Mountain Devil, Slender
   Rice Flower
Suspicious/distrustful . . . Mountain Devil
Controlling . . . Black-eyed Susan, Gymea Lily, Southern Cross
Fearful of losing control . . . Dog Rose of the Wild Forces
Manipulative/ruthless/cruel/vindictive . . . Mountain Devil, Rough
   Bluebell
Self-destructive . . . Dog Rose of the Wild Forces, Five Corners,
   Waratah

Abusing of power … Gymea Lily, Rough Bluebell
Violent … Mountain Devil, Rough Bluebell
Fearful of psychic abilities … Bush Iris, Dog Rose of the Wild Forces
Fearful of psychic attack … Angelsword, Fringed Violet, Grey Spider Flower
Fearful of misusing psychic abilities … Dog Rose of the Wild Forces, Rough Bluebell
Secretive/scheming … Mountain Devil, Pink Mulla Mulla
Fearful of revealing self … Flannel Flower, Mountain Devil, Pink Mulla Mulla, Tall Mulla Mulla
Catharsis … Bottlebrush, Dog Rose of the Wild Forces, Fringed Violet, Mint Bush, Transition Essence
Burning off spiritual dross … Mint Bush
Clearing negative karmic connections … Boab
Difficulty with letting go of the past … Bottlebrush
Sexual guilt … Sturt Desert Rose
Sexual revulsion … Billy Goat Plum
Promiscuous … Bush Iris, Flannel Flower
Sex addict … Boronia, Wedding Bush
Grieving … Red Suva Frangipani, Sturt Desert Rose, Transition Essence
Melancholy … Bluebell, Little Flannel Flower, Southern Cross, Sunshine Wattle
Obsessive … Boronia, Bottlebrush
Emotionally intense … Crowea
Fanatical … Hibbertia
Intolerant … Freshwater Mangrove, Slender Rice Flower, Yellow Cowslip Orchid
Isolated/loner … Tall Mulla Mulla, Tall Yellow Top
Suicidal … Waratah
Lacking discernment … Angelsword
Jealous … Mountain Devil
Possessive … Bottlebrush

Deficiency
Avoid looking within … Bluebell
Fear of transformation … Bauhinia, Transition Essence
Give power away … Dog Rose, Five Corners, Southern Cross
Victim of violence … Fringed Violet, Southern Cross
Victim of sexual abuse … Billy Goat Plum, Flannel Flower, Fringed Violet, Wisteria
Fearful in general … Dog Rose
Terror … Grey Spider Flower, Green Spider Orchid
Blocked passion … Bush Gardenia, Mulla Mulla

Sagittarius/Jupiter Blocks

Ruled by Jupiter, God of Wisdom, Sagittarian interests include philosophy, religion, education, teaching, publishing, the legal system, justice, long journeys, other cultures, humour, rhythm and gambling. Positive Sagittarian energy is abundant, harmless, generous, fun, extroverted, confident, funny, dramatic, free-spirited, adventurous, optimistic, independent, intelligent, imaginative, creative, honest, idealistic, ethical, loyal, bold, fiery, playful, wise, fair, broad-minded, sentimental, protective, rescuing, well-intentioned, lucky and flirtatious. Jupiter/Sagittarius blocks include:

Excess
Clumsy ... Bush Fuchsia, Jacaranda, Kangaroo Paw
Tactless/blunt ... Kangaroo Paw
Uncommitted ... Wedding Bush
Spiritual seekers ... Angelsword, Bush Iris, Hibbertia, Red Lily
Mental superiority/fanaticism ... Hibbertia
Judging/prejudiced ... Freshwater Mangrove, Slender Rice Flower,
    Yellow Cowslip Orchid
Argumentative ... Mountain Devil, Red Helmet
Dominating ... Gymea Lily
Need to be right/know it all ... Hibbertia, Kangaroo Paw
Feeling trapped/tied down ... Banksia Robur, Red Grevillea
Rebellious ... Red Helmet Orchid
Irresponsible ... Illawarra Flame Tree, Jacaranda, Kangaroo Paw
Unrealistically optimistic ... Sundew
Maintain cheerful facade even in crisis ... Flannel Flower, Tall Mulla
    Mulla
Bored ... Peach-flowered Tea-tree
Take unnecessary risks/gambling ... Kangaroo Paw
Tendency to exaggerate ... Gymea Lily, Illawarra Flame Tree
Excessive/overindulgent ... Bush Iris, Flannel Flower
Extravagant/overly generous ... Philotheca
Difficulty keeping secrets ... Green Spider Orchid
Greedy ... Bluebell, Bush Iris
Arrogant ... Gymea Lily
Outspoken ... Red Helmet

Deficiency
Reading/writing difficulties ... Bush Fuchsia
Antisocial ... Pink Mulla Mulla, Tall Mulla Mulla
Serious ... Little Flannel Flower
Lacking abundance ... Southern Cross, Sunshine Wattle
Stuck ... Red Grevillea
Afraid to take risks ... Bauhinia, Dog Rose, Sunshine Wattle

Pessimistic . . . Sunshine Wattle
Closed mind . . . Bauhinia, Freshwater Mangrove
Blocked teaching ability . . . Bush Fuchsia, Green Spider Orchid

Capricorn/Saturn Blocks

Saturn, the Lord of Karma and Time, rules Capricorn. In a birth chart, Saturn represents our father, whose imprint determines our attitudes towards authority figures, society, work, structure and rules. Saturn is seen as restrictive in traditional astrology and as spiritual initiation in spiritual astrology. A good analogy would be the heat and pressure which changes carbon into diamond over a long period of time—not a pleasant process for the carbon, but a transformation that produces something of great value just the same. Capricorns embody the work ethic. The balanced energy is punctual, organised, realistic, disciplined, responsible, conservative, respectful, cautious, thrifty, traditional, quiet, tactful, reserved, ethical, committed, persevering, dependable, loyal, patient, practical, objective, rational, efficient, grounded, ambitious, successful and achievement oriented. Imbalances can emerge in the following ways:

Excess
Resistant to change . . . Bauhinia
Stuck . . . Bauhinia, Boab, Red Grevillea, Sunshine Wattle
Overly serious . . . Little Flannel Flower, Sunshine Wattle, Yellow
  Cowslip Orchid
Depressed/pessimistic/struggling financially . . . Southern Cross,
  Sunshine Wattle
Breaking karmic patterns . . . Boab
Spiritual initiation . . . Mint Bush
Breaking family emotional patterns . . . Boab
Rigid . . . Bluebell, Yellow Cowslip Orchid
Overly critical . . . Yellow Cowslip Orchid
Overly frugal . . . Bluebell, Yellow Cowslip Orchid
Workaholic . . . Black-eyed Susan
Perfectionist . . . Hibbertia, Yellow Cowslip Orchid
Overwhelmed or burdened by responsibilities . . . Banksia Robur, Old
  Man Banksia, Paw Paw
Feeling weighed down . . . Wild Potato Bush
Overly conservative . . . Yellow Cowslip Orchid
Resentful/bitter . . . Dagger Hakea
Remorseful/regretful/guilty . . . Sturt Desert Rose
Austerity/self-denial . . . Hibbertia
Intolerant . . . Yellow Cowslip Orchid
Sluggish . . . Old Man Banksia, Wild Potato Bush

Unimaginative . . . Little Flannel Flower, Turkey Bush
Frustrated with physical restriction . . . Wild Potato Bush
Fearful . . . Dog Rose
Fearful of mixing with others . . . Tall Mulla Mulla
Isolated . . . Tall Yellow Top
Cut off from emotions . . . Bluebell, Yellow Cowslip Orchid
Stubborn . . . Isopogon
Unable to let go . . . Bottlebrush

Deficiency
Ungrounded . . . Sundew
Difficulty with authority figures/father issues . . . Red Helmet Orchid
Can't persevere or commit/undisciplined . . . Kapok Bush, Macrocarpa,
    Peach-flowered Tea-tree, Wedding Bush
Unable to implement steps to achieve a goal . . . Kapok Bush
Avoiding responsibility . . . Bottlebrush, Pink Mulla Mulla, Southern
    Cross
Unreliable/lacking personal integrity and trustworthiness . . . Sturt
    Desert Rose
Irresponsible . . . Illawarra Flame Tree, Jacaranda, Kangaroo Paw
Lacking the strength to be successful . . . Gymea Lily
Impractical . . . Jacaranda, Kapok Bush
Immature . . . Kangaroo Paw
Not learning from mistakes . . . Isopogon
Lacking structure and ability to plan . . . Jacaranda
No goals . . . Kapok Bush, Sundew, Sunshine Wattle
Difficulty finding life purpose . . . Silver Princess
Unpunctual . . . Black-eyed Susan, Jacaranda, Sundew
Procrastinating . . . Sundew
Discouraged . . . Kapok Bush, Sunshine Wattle

Aquarius/Uranus Blocks

Uranus, the sky father and creator, rules Aquarius. This energy is
involved with science, astronomy, astrology, technology, aviation, space
travel, inventions, vibrations, electricity, the future and breaking down
existing forms. Balanced Aquarian energy is eccentric, bohemian, weird,
abstract, unique, curious, independent, freedom-loving, electrifying,
gentle, rebellious, unpredictable, innovative, pioneering, visionary, inspir-
ational, aloof, analytical, intelligent, intellectual, persuasive, politically
astute, group-minded, charitable, humanitarian, harmonious, friendly,
non-judgmental and sees 'the big picture'. Like the list, Aquarians are full
of contradictions. They walk to the beat of a different drum.
    As the earth has now moved into the new 'Age of Aquarius', we will

all now be asked to attune to this energy, regardless of our sun sign. This means we need to begin to embody the positive Aquarian traits listed above, rather than slip into or remain entrenched in the negative expressions, which include:

Excess
Emotionally detached ... Bluebell, Flannel Flower, Yellow Cowslip Orchid
Difficulty verbalising emotions ... Flannel Flower
Cut off from feelings ... Bluebell
Aloof/in head rather than heart ... Hibbertia, Yellow Cowslip Orchid
Rebellious ... Red Helmet Orchid
Absent-minded/on another planet ... Red Lily, Sundew
Difficulty accepting and expressing own uniqueness and individuality ... Five Corners, Gymea Lily, Illawarra Flame Tree
Non-conformist ... Bauhinia, Freshwater Mangrove, Red Helmet Orchid
Feeling restricted ... Red Grevillea, Wild Potato Bush
Rejection ... Illawarra Flame Tree
Alienation and isolation ... Pink Mulla Mulla, Tall Yellow Top
Destruction of old belief systems ... Mint Bush
Anarchist ... Illawarra Flame Tree
Erratic ... Jacaranda
Lacking focus ... Boronia, Sundew
Impatient ... Black-eyed Susan
Difficulty following through ... Illawarra Flame Tree, Kapok Bush, Macrocarpa, Wedding Bush

Deficiency
Uncomfortable around new technology and situations ... Bauhinia
Antisocial ... Tall Mulla Mulla, Red Helmet Orchid
Unable to see into the future ... Sunshine Wattle
Can't see 'the big picture' ... Yellow Cowslip Orchid
Lacking a sense of the community's needs versus individual needs ... Yellow Cowslip Orchid
Lacking a sense of charity ... Bluebell, Philotheca
Prejudiced ... Freshwater Mangrove, Slender Rice Flower
Lacking appreciation of others ... Gymea Lily, Philotheca, Slender Rice Flower, Yellow Cowslip Orchid
Difficulty articulating thoughts ... Bush Fuchsia
Blocked clairaudience/throat chakra ... Bush Fuchsia, Bush Iris, Green Spider Orchid, Old Man Banksia
Fearful of independence ... Dog Rose, Five Corners, Gymea Lily, Southern Cross
Stubborn ... Isopogon

Pisces/Neptune Blocks

Neptune, God of the Sea, rules Pisces. Pisces is the last sign of the zodiac, the energy where many of our earthly lessons have been learnt and we are reaching most for our spirituality. Pisceans are on a different wavelength to the other signs. As Paul Callinan said, in a lecture on medical astrology: 'Their ears are tuned to the celestial music.' Many of them find the earth plane too harsh to deal with and so look for ways to escape reality. Positive means of doing this are meditation, yoga, visualisation, dreams, creativity, dance, art, music and acting. Unfortunately, Pisceans sometimes find it easier to fall into drugs, alcohol and other assorted addictions. They also have a tendency to give away their power just to keep the peace. Balanced Piscean energy is compassionate, empathetic, prophetic, psychic, intuitive, serene, imaginative, graceful, gentle, sacrificing, humble, charitable, generous, sentimental, sensitive, romantic, inspired, mystical, adaptable and idealistic. On a beach, it's difficult to tell where the ocean stops and the shore starts and Pisceans often have the same problem with people. They tend to want to merge with others as well as with the divine and may not know what a personal boundary is, let alone how to enforce it. Their imbalances include:

Excess

Difficulty establishing and maintaining healthy boundaries ... Flannel Flower

Giving away power to keep the peace ... Tall Mulla Mulla

Unable to say no ... Bush Fuchsia, Flannel Flower, Illawarra Flame Tree, Old Man Banksia, Tall Mulla Mulla

Difficulty with asserting self ... Bush Fuchsia, Southern Cross

Ungrounded ... Red Lily, Sundew

Psychic sponge ... Angelsword + Fringed Violet

Overly empathetic ... Alpine Mint Bush, Fringed Violet, Old Man Banksia

Addictive personality ... Boronia + Bottlebrush, Five Corners

Drug use ... Angelsword + Fringed Violet

Overly empathetic ... Alpine Mint Bush, Fringed Violet, Old Man Banksia

Emotional burnout ... Alpine Mint Bush

Martyr/victim ... Southern Cross

Daydreaming ... Red Lily, Sundew

Escapism/unfocused ... Bluebell, Red Lily, Sundew

Spiritual confusion/feeling 'foggy' ... Angelsword, Red Lily

Crumbling belief systems ... Mint Bush

Lacking purpose ... Silver Princess

Lacking commitment ... Wedding Bush

Chameleon-like ... Jacaranda

Unrealistic/self-deceptive . . . Bluebell, Kangaroo Paw
Vague . . . Sundew
No attention to detail . . . Sundew
Impractical . . . Kapok Bush
Feeling trapped in the physical body . . . Wild Potato Bush
Victim to illness . . . Spinifex

Deficiency
Lacking faith . . . Red Lily, Waratah
Atheism . . . Bush Iris, Meditation Essence, Red Lily
Unforgiving . . . Dagger Hakea, Mountain Devil, Slender Rice Flower
Lacking compassion . . . Hibbertia, Kangaroo Paw, Yellow Cowslip
    Orchid
Difficulty accessing Higher Self . . . Angelsword, Bush Fuchsia, Bush
    Iris, Paw Paw
Difficulty contacting spirit guides . . . Angelsword, Bush Fuchsia, Green
    Spider Orchid, Little Flannel Flower
Blocked clairvoyance/brow chakra . . . Bush Iris
Creative block . . . Turkey Bush
Lack of dreams . . . Bush Fuchsia + Isopogon + Sundew
Difficulty attuning to other realities . . . Green Spider Orchid

Physical Imbalances

This section is not meant to replace professional medical or naturopathic advice. Whenever there are physical symptoms present it is advisable to seek outside evaluation from a qualified practitioner of your choice.

When we are sick, however, we also need to listen to our body: it's trying to tell us something is wrong. Wholistic practitioners believe that physical symptoms are the end result of us ignoring imbalances in our thoughts and emotions to such an extent that they eventually manifest physically. The Australian Bush Flower Essences can help correct the imbalances underlying the physical symptoms and are therefore a valuable tool in helping prevent and assist the recovery from illness.

Rulerships

Each astrological sign rules certain parts of the body. When our energy is low or we are under stress, these are the parts of our body that are most vulnerable. Supporting these areas at these times can help prevent and assist recovery from physical illness. These rulerships are shown in the table below.

Sign	Parts of the body
Aries	Head, face, brain, teeth, adrenal glands, spleen, arteries and oxygenation
Taurus	Neck, throat, thyroid, larynx, pharynx, carotid arteries, jugular veins
Gemini	Shoulders, arms, hands, fingers, nervous system, lungs
Cancer	Stomach, breasts and, to some extent, the uterus
Leo	Heart, back (especially thoracic spine), arteries, aorta
Virgo	Small intestine, ligaments and tendons, pancreas
Libra	Kidneys, endocrine system, homeostasis, hormone balance, veins
Scorpio	Reproductive organs, bladder, large intestine, rectum, anus
Sagittarius	Hips, pelvis, coccyx, buttocks, upper legs, sciatic nerve, liver
Capricorn	Skeleton, skin, knees, gall bladder
Aquarius	Lower legs, ankles, meridians, veins
Pisces	Feet, toes, immune system, lymphatics

This section is divided into the twelve sun signs. The accompanying paragraph in each sign is a guide to the appropriate Australian Bush Flower Essences to help support the most vulnerable body systems for that sign.

Unreliable body areas

Aries
Adrenals (Macrocarpa), Cheeks (Sturt Desert Rose), Chin (Tall Yellow Top, Five Corners), Eyebrow (Dagger Hakea, Mountain Devil), Eyes (Waratah, Sunshine Wattle, Bush Fuchsia), Face (Billy Goat Plum), Forehead (Paw Paw, Boronia, Crowea), Hypothalamus (Bush Fuchsia), Jaw (Dagger Hakea, Mountain Devil), Mouth (Bauhinia, Isopogon, Billy Goat Plum), Pineal Gland (Bush Iris).

Taurus
Adenoids (Red Helmet, Dagger Hakea), Cervical Vertebrae (Bluebell, Paw Paw), Ears (Kangaroo Paw, Bush Gardenia, Bush Fuchsia), Larynx (Red Helmet Orchid, Bush Fuchsia), Neck (Isopogon, Crowea, Kangaroo Paw), Nose (Illawarra Flame Tree, Bush Iris), Throat and Tonsils (Bush Fuchsia, Bush Iris, Flannel Flower), Thyroid (Old Man Banksia, Southern Cross).

Gemini
Arms (Paw Paw, Philotheca, Flannel Flower), Elbow (Bottlebrush, Bauhinia), Fingernails (Fringed Violet), Fingers (Sundew, Kapok Bush), Lungs (Sturt Desert Pea), Nerves and Central Nervous System (Flannel Flower), Ribs (Red Helmet Orchid + Fringed Violet), Shoulders (Waratah, Dog

Rose, Five Corners, Kapok Bush, Sunshine Wattle, Paw Paw), Thymus (Illawarra Flame Tree, Southern Cross).

Cancer
See also Scorpio for female reproductive problems
   Breasts (Philotheca, Banksia Robur, Bottlebrush, Alpine Mint Bush), Diaphragm (Crowea, Tall Mulla Mulla, Paw Paw, Black-eyed Susan), Sternum (Bluebell, Fringed Violet, Red Helmet Orchid), Stomach (Paw Paw, Crowea, Dog Rose).

Leo
Aorta (Bluebell + Waratah), Back (Gymea Lily, Crowea, Waratah, Paw Paw, Sunshine Wattle), Circulation (Bluebell, Flannel Flower, Tall Mulla Mulla), Coronary Arteries and Veins (Bluebell), Dura Mater (Tall Yellow Top), Heart (Bluebell, Waratah), Mitral Valve/Ventricles (Waratah), Spinal Cord (Gymea Lily, Sturt Desert Rose, Flannel Flower, Red Grevillea, Grey Spider Flower), Thoracic Spine (Crowea, Bottlebrush + Sturt Desert Pea).

Virgo
Colon (Bottlebrush, Spinifex, Kapok Bush, Peach-flowered Tea-tree), Duodenum (Crowea), Pancreas (Peach-flowered Tea-tree), Spleen (Dagger Hakea, Dog Rose).

Libra
Balance (Jacaranda, Bush Fuchsia, Crowea, Fringed Violet), Fluid Regulation (She Oak), Homeostasis (Crowea), Kidneys (Dog Rose, Red Grevillea, Grey Spider Flower), Lumbar Spine (Crowea, Southern Cross, Gymea Lily), Veins (Tall Mulla Mulla).

Scorpio
Anus (Bottlebrush, Sturt Desert Rose), Bladder (Dagger Hakea, Dog Rose), Blood (Bluebell, Dog Rose, Bottlebrush), Colon (Bottlebrush), Fallopian Tubes (She Oak, Spinifex), Ovaries (She Oak), Prostate (Flannel Flower, Sturt Desert Rose, Kapok Bush), Testicles (Flannel Flower, She Oak), Uterus (She Oak).

Sagittarius
Hips (Sundew, Sunshine Wattle, Dog Rose, Old Man Banksia), Liver (Mountain Devil, Dagger Hakea, Silver Princess, Slender Rice Flower), Ileum (Bottlebrush, Peach-flowered Tea-tree, Dog Rose, Crowea), Legs (Red Grevillea, Sundew, Bottlebrush, Wild Potato Bush), Sacrum (Boab, Crowea, Southern Cross), Sciatic Nerve (Flannel Flower, Red Grevillea, Spinifex, Crowea, Dog Rose).

Capricorn
Bone Marrow (Five Corners), Bones (Red Helmet Orchid, Fringed Violet, Sturt Desert Rose), Gall Bladder (Dagger Hakea, Mountain Devil, Southern Cross, Slender Rice Flower), Gums (Jacaranda, Peach-flowered Tea-tree), Joints (Hibbertia, Tall Mulla Mulla, Bottlebrush, Dagger Hakea), Knees (Isopogon, Macrocarpa, Wild Potato Bush), Skin (Five Corners, Billy Goat Plum, Bottlebrush, Fringed Violet, Jacaranda), Teeth (Paw Paw, Jacaranda, Sundew).

Aquarius
Ankles (Flannel Flower, Sturt Desert Rose, Isopogon), Circulation (Bluebell, Flannel Flower, Tall Mulla Mulla), Etheric Body (Angelsword + Fringed Violet; see also chapter on the subtle bodies), Lower Legs (Red Grevillea, Bottlebrush, Sundew), Meridians (Crowea, Five Corners), Nerves (Flannel Flower, Bush Fuchsia, Spinifex).

Pisces
Aura (Broken: Fringed Violet + Angelsword; Misaligned: Crowea; Weak: Fringed Violet + Angelsword), Feet (Sundew, Bottlebrush, Red Grevillea), Immune System (Bush Iris, Illawarra Flame Tree, Mint Bush, Macrocarpa), Lymphatic System (Bush Iris), Toenails (Fringed Violet).

The Australian Bush Flower Essences can also be used to help clear disease miasms—genetic disease imprinting—which doctors acknowledge is a major contributing factor towards hereditary disease. Boab frees us of our karmic ties to our ancestors both psychologically and physically. These and other potential health problems can often be seen in the birth chart using conventional medical astrology. Recurrent themes often appear in the charts of family members which, if left to their natural devices, can develop into the same mental, emotional and, ultimately, physical imbalances, suggesting that psychological and physical disorders are both genetic and environmental. Doctors are right when they say disease is inherited and natural healers are right when they say it's the result of how we think and what we feel. The Three in One branch of kinesiology joins the two by discovering negative emotional concepts and tracing their age of cause or age of best understanding, be it from conception onwards or generational (and so genetic). Astrology is another valuable tool for recognising our patterns and the Bush Essences provide a safe, gentle way of assisting their release.

Copyright © Louise Anderson
(For birth charts, taped readings or correspondence, write to PO Box 705 Newport Beach NSW 2106 Australia or at the following e-mail address: neptune@intercoast.com.au)

The Astrology of a
—Flower Essence—

by Kerrie Redgate

T here is certainly far more to creating Flower Essence tinctures than simply tossing picked flowers into a bowl under the sun. The professionals, such as Ian White, who have given us so many wonderful remedies, are people who have instinctively been training throughout their entire lives to do this. To begin with, this work requires a confident rapport with the spiritual devic realm—not an entirely common nor easy feat in itself. However, one of the major talents of the Flower Essence creator (or actually co-creator), which goes largely unsung, is the superb attunement that these people have to the energies of the Cosmos.

Planets and asteroids[1] emit particular tonal frequencies as they orbit the sun. The constellations, which are actually groups of distant solar systems and galaxies, also resonate with inaudible sounds. These frequencies, or perhaps I should say 'symphonies', directly affect the flow and manifestation of all life and matter throughout the Universe. There are twelve basic frequencies from the zodiac ring of constellations which seem to affect matter and which correlate (within many octaves) to the

---

[1] Huge rocks, orbiting in our solar system, which are believed to possibly be a potential planet that could not form due to Jupiter's enormous gravitational field.

twelve musical notes of the Western chromatic scale, also resonating with the twelve meridians of the human etheric body utilised in treatments such as acupuncture and shiatsu, etc. In fact, quantum physics has agreed with the ancient Eastern philosophic and religious belief that matter is empty of inherent existence: the inner core of matter is essentially made of charged waves of energy.

Water is always used as the base for vibrational remedies (whether they be homoeopathic medicines, gem elixirs or Flower Essences), as it is a wonderful conductor of energy, and is especially susceptible to the vibrational wave patterns from the Cosmos that occur at each moment in time. Of course, water and sunlight are essential to life.

Every event has its own signature of sound patterns (planets and asteroids), as well as being what the birth chart of a human baby represents: the actual instant when the energy of the Cosmos entered the body, independently of the mother, for the first time. This stamp is imprinted as a kind of electromagnetic etheric grid which affects our brain patterning throughout our lives. This is not an accidental event, but a moment of harmonic resonance which correlates to the evolutionary soul vibrations of the incoming child. Or, more simply put, to its karma. No two people, as no two moments, are ever the same. Every chart is superbly balanced. We need only avail ourselves, consciously, of all of the energies it contains to become balanced and whole.

An astrology chart can therefore be drawn up for the beginning or instant of any event or occasion to ascertain the cosmic influences affecting those concerned. An old Taoist phrase from the *I Ching* states that the beginning holds the seed of all that is to follow.

In regard to the birth of flower remedies, what has been remarkable is the accuracy of the timing of the decanting process of the essences. It is as if the Cosmos had been sounding a gigantic clock alarm that only the Flower Essence creator can hear. It is actually an attunement process. One needs to have a high degree of sensitivity to the vibrational patterns of the moment, to the devic kingdom, and to one's spirit guides who are always in attendance.

So, we can now see that timing is everything. Obviously, when an essence that may affect hundreds, if not thousands, of lives is about to be created, there is a tremendous amount of support from the spirit realm to aid the procedure. At this time there are many advanced souls in spirit, as well as extant on the physical plane, to help humanity evolve to the next plateau of awareness. Some of these beings in spirit may work through inspiration in the arts, or politics, or religious movements, etc. Others specialise in the healing of physical, emotional, mental or spiritual ailments. This last group has been guiding the preparation of Flower Essences in the Western world since the time of Edward Bach.

Our evolution is gaining momentum as our solar system moves into alignment with the energy of the constellation we know as Aquarius.

And it is becoming increasingly more challenging for us all to keep up with the pace. Aquarius is the fastest moving vibrational pattern that we experience from the zodiac belt affecting our planet. The current developments in Flower Essence therapy are a reflection of the energy of Aquarius. It is my belief that no other healing modality (apart from direct spiritual healing) can reach to the outer extent of the complex human aura as Flower Essences do. They are capable of resonating with the fastest of our vibrational bodies where past lifetime concepts and ancient traumas may be blocking our full potential on deeply unconscious levels. Naturally, there are also skills and talents from those lives that our Spirit needs to access for our work in this life. Flower Essences may also realign us to those talents.

Being both an astrologer and a Flower Essence therapist, it was a natural progression for me to be curious about the astrology chart of an actual essence. After much deliberation and experimentation, I made the decision to use the moment when the flowers are taken from the water as the birth time. This is the final point of astrological influence that the sun and planets may have on the water/flower combination. As this is the time when the water is decanted, it may be a powerful moment for the *intention* from the practitioner to also take effect. There is always a kind of 'mind-meld' that occurs between the essence and its creator. Both are in tune with the flow in the heavens above.

The precision of the timing, involving both the dates and the time to the minute, in the creation of these Mother Tinctures was proven to me when I looked at the birth charts of second generation Flower Essences that Ian White had prepared. The energies in the new chart were the same as those that had been proven to be the qualities of the original batch of the Flower Essence made years before!

A theory of mine in regard to the timing is that when the flowers wilt (which is often considered to be the 'readiness' of an essence), their actual Soul is released into the water. Some people take the compassionate view that cutting the flowers is really unnecessary. My own personal belief is that essences made from uncut flowers will have an impact on the subtle bodies in much the same way as homoeopathy: it is the sound frequencies from the flower's etheric web which will be captured in the water, and this is what directs the action of the essence, as a kind of attunement process, to a particular chakra, meridian or organ, etc. This may have a direct impact on the lower subtle bodies of the aura, being the physical-etheric template, the emotional and the mental bodies, but will not have a direct impact on the outermost spiritual body where our past life concepts are operating. The spiritual Light energy which, I believe, is responsible for the essences being drawn to the highest, or outermost field of Light in our aura, will be missing. Perhaps it is the Light, or Soul, of the plant which makes the essences so incredibly self-adjusting. I believe that neither system is right or wrong, but simply useful in their own ways.

This is a highly controversial and somewhat emotional topic, and is certainly open to future research!

So, with the Australian Bush Flower Essences, the flowers have undergone a transformational process, much like our own deaths will be, discarding their physical form. And instead of dissipating into the ethers as they wilt, the flowers' collective Soul *and* etheric imprint are captured in the water which then becomes the healing elixir. The flowers live on!

As a diagnostic tool, astrology can be utilised for any level of our being, from the physical constitution (especially when combined with a knowledge of the elements, as in the Eastern approaches to medicine and healing); or for psychological insights into the mental-emotional domain; and, more profoundly, at the level of the chakras and higher auric bodies. Many disease states originate from the field of energy at the outermost rim of the aura. This contains our unconscious concepts that have been created through past lifetime experiences.

There is one major difference between the birth chart of a Flower Essence and the chart of a human being. We have the capacity to evolve those vibrational dynamics, and to develop the entire chart's potential at our own pace, or not at all, if we wish. However, the chart of an essence remains what it is for its entire shelf life. To explain this point further, there are geometrical angles called aspects that form between the planets from earth's perspective (in a geocentric chart). On a spiritual and harmonic level, the most potent effect is caused by either the conjunction of two or more planetary bodies at the same degree of a sign of the zodiac, or the angles which are multiples of 30° that form between planets. That is, 30° (a semi-sextile), 60° (a sextile), 90° (a square), 120° (a trine), 150° (a quincunx) and 180° (an opposition). (Other angles are used by astrologers who are working on a different level of interpretation.) Each of these aspects has a specific meaning. Some of these will be discussed in the following interpretation of the Alpine Mint.

In a Flower Essence chart, the particular planetary angles which are of a more harmonious nature (trines and conjunctions mainly) would relate to the positive qualities that one would hope to develop through the ingestion of the essence. The more challenging aspects (such as the squares and quincunxes) represent the fears that one is trying to overcome through the use of the essence.

Planets actually have what is called an orb of influence around them, much like an aura, so that if two planets or asteroids are 124° apart, rather than exactly 120°, they are still considered to be trining each other. This means that the wider the orb, the less urgent the effect seems to be in terms of our phyche. We have a lifetime to pick up all the wider aspects as our complete potential. Human beings, with our karmic and ancestral baggage, are quite complex creatures. Not so with flowers. The aspects analysed in a Flower Essence chart must be kept quite 'tight'. Also, it is usual for the professionals in this field to make up several different flower remedies within days of each other, sometimes even hours. The exact timing as well as the latitude and longitude of the location are crucial in order to differentiate between the charts.

A brief and simplified description of the workings of an astrology chart is necessary at this point. First, I must stress that there are many different fields of astrology, with various methods of analysis within those fields. My way is only one.

Most people are familiar with the term rising sign, or ascendant. These are often used to refer to the same thing. However, the ascendant is the exact degree of the sign of the zodiac which is on the eastern horizon at the time of 'birth'. The rising sign is more the general sign on the ascendant, rather than the exact degree. The ascendant is a powerful part of the chart which indicates the *modus operandi* for this lifetime: the type of energy which has now become our present orientation to the world. We have been developing and mastering this energy for several incarnations. For a flower remedy, this may reveal an energy that the essence helps one to utilise and express through in the external world. The ascendant is the most powerful point of spiritual consciousness.

The ascendant point, in the system devised by Placidus, which I use, begins what are known as the houses. These are sectors of the sky which have been divided into equal portions of time to do with the *apparent* speed of the sun as it moves from the horizon to its highest point. The houses correspond exactly to the vibrational qualities of the signs of the zodiac. Most astrologers read them differently from the signs and see them as special domains of influence (for example, 'home', 'health', 'love affairs', 'marriage', etc.). I have found this ancient technique to be highly outmoded in this present century. Astrology is purely the effect of vibrational waves. And vibration is just vibration, and what we are motivated to do with it depends on how it interacts with our other frequencies. Therefore, the 1st house (just below the horizon) is purely an Aries vibration and it will be utilised by us according to the patterns of the other Aries-type themes in the chart. The next house below that one is Taurus, etc. And so on around the wheel (to where it finally makes the area above the horizon a Pisces vibration. So regardless of what constellation was in the sky at the time, if a planet is in the zone just above the horizon, it will be influenced by two energies blending together like ingredients in a cake—Pisces plus the constellational sign of the zodiac that is in that part of the sky).

The descendant is opposite the ascendant point (on the western horizon), and must be consciously integrated with the ascendant as one whole energy. The opposing signs are really the yin and yang extremes of each other. They are complementary forces.

The midheaven or MC (*medium coeli*, in Latin) is the degree of the zodiac which is above the birth location at the highest point reached by the 'sun's path' that day. This is our ultimate goal that we are reaching for. This energy must be developed and then utilised for the benefit of others. Traditionally, this point along with the area of the sky just to the east of it has been known as the 10th house of 'career'. To be more specific and practical, it is actually where we take on our ultimate responsibility in life. A key to self-mastery.

The IC (*immum coeli*) is directly opposite the midheaven (and under our feet, you might say). This is the foundation of the essence, and of our own lives. The polarity balance for the MC. We play a kind of 'snakes and ladders' game throughout life, trying to integrate these two energies. If we reach for the MC at the top before we have developed the energies of the IC, we will eventually slide back down to the beginning. It would be like setting up a law practice before actually going to university to study law. Foundations are extremely important in life. They prevent the impatience of the ego from steering us into blind corners and to dead-end cliff-tops.

The planets in our solar system work like 'chapter headings' for the chart. As planets may relate to many different things at different times, it is their special combination of energies, with the constellations as their backdrop, that creates the distinction. The asteroids fill in the real details within those chapters. According to Bode's Law, there should actually be another planet in orbit around our sun, between Mars and Jupiter. This is where we find what is termed the asteroid belt.

It is believed that these bodies were never able to form into one planet due to Jupiter's enormous gravitational field. These asteroids can vary in size from hundreds of kilometres in diameter to tiny pieces, with each 'rock' having a flavour of its own. Concentrated mineral deposits may make a difference energetically as does, of course, the individual orbital patterns which create a definite sound resonance from each asteroid.

Data for the movements and locations of approximately 7000 asteroids (at the time of writing) are available now on computer disks for astrologers. The numbers are increasing rapidly. For curiosity's sake, I might mention that it is usually the astronomers who name the asteroids once they have discovered them. This is a type of 'harmonic principle' at work. Only those asteroids vibrating to frequencies that resonate with the particular investigating astronomer will be sighted by that individual. It is therefore logical that the name the astronomer then chooses will be of the same vibrational frequency. All names, as words (sounds), have vibrational patterns; and these may echo the 'symphonic patterns' of the heavens at the moment of discovery. I would also be inclined to believe that more than a little intervention takes place from our friends in the realm of Spirit. (All astronomers, due to their natural affinity with the planet Uranus, are actually subtly clairaudient—they really are 'closet psychics', but don't try to tell them that!)

In our European-based languages, the planets have the names of mythological Roman gods (with the exception of Uranus, which is Greek) but the asteroids are now being named for historical characters, abstract qualities, countries, cities and mythological heroes and beings from every race, culture and era in the world. This now allows for a generous amount of accuracy in the interpretation of the themes within a chart. However, there is a trick to this. As there are so many asteroids in orbit (approximately nineteen for every degree of the zodiac!), it is imperative that we search for the 'common denominators' among them. In other words, we should seek out only the recurring themes that are produced by asteroids making tight angles to the planets, and to each other, reflecting the themes in the planetary relationships as well as the MC–IC and ascendant–descendant and other axes, etc. This is like playing only those keys on a piano that are part of the key signature scale for a particular piece of music. The other notes available to us are irrelevant and are not played. They will not even subtly resonate. I have marked the asteroids in the following text in italics, as they are often spelt slightly differently from their mythological or historical namesakes, especially if discovered by non-English speaking astronomers.

At the outskirts of our solar system, there are eight other planets that were discovered in the 1920s by a German man, Alfred Witte. They have never been sighted by telecope but were found through the study of the orbital changes in the then known outer planets, Uranus and Neptune. I have also done a great deal of research into the effects of these so-called 'hypothetical planets', often referred to as 'trans-Neptunian planets' or 'Uranian points'. They, too, have a strong influence in the charts of Flower Essences, but as this is new work, their dynamics are too complex to explore in any depth in this chapter. I will only be able to touch on some of them lightly. However, the important point is that they bring in a very high spiritual energy which directly affects our causal or outermost auric layer, and their position has always confirmed the planetary energies prevalent in the rest of the chart. A detailed analysis of their energies will be found in a forthcoming book of my own, *Astrology's Seventh Veil*.

I would never suggest that astrology *alone* should be relied on for data concerning the qualities of Flower Essences. I feel that the immediate intuition of the essence maker should be our first guide. He or she is the original interpreter for the plant deva. In the same manner, I do not believe in reading astrological charts for people who are not physically present for the reading. Dialogue is so important, as astrology can be interpreted and utilised on so many levels. This is also the case with Flower Essence charts. However, when astrology is added to the insights of the essence makers, it becomes a wonderful tool for confirmation, clarity and depth of information.

Through the science of astrology, we can now see that the spiritual properties of a flower, when captured as an essence remedy, are the manifestation of the dynamic energies of sky and Earth combined together in perfect timing, to be released through the bridge of the human heart, into the world.

Alpine Mint Bush

Made in the Jindabyne area, NSW, Australia
31 March 1993, 3:57:00 PM AEST

This essence, as far as I can ascertain, seems to be unique among flower remedies. It addresses specific issues that all healers, from surgeons to aura workers, must face in the course of their careers. I have found that the astrology chart for the creation of this essence not only perfectly echoes the intuitive and now clinical understanding of its properties, but also actually reveals more of the potential within this remedy for further applications.

The Alpine Mint Bush is known to bring enthusiasm and joy back into the hearts of healers and carers when it is all becoming 'just a bit too much'. Continually having to deal with other people's pain may lead to a shut down of the sensitivity that is required of a true healer. The signature of compassion is evident in this essence, from the chart. As Ian White has stated, this remedy works on the mental-emotional levels. However, there is another dimension to the Alpine Mint Bush that is apparent from its astrological make-up.

The main focal points of a chart are the ascendant–descendant axis as well as the midheaven–immum coeli. This gives us a basic background to work with. Leo (Ω), the sign on the ascendant, is always indicative of heart issues. This essence has the capacity to revive a heart that has been strained by the outside world. The opposite sign, on the descendant, is Aquarius ($\approx$). This is the sign of detachment. So here we have the axis which develops the open heart that gives without conditions or expectations.

The midheaven (MC) sign is Gemini (II), with a Sagittarian ($\nearrow$) IC. The midheaven as the goal that the essence helps us to achieve is, here, to do with the mind and open, concise communication. Sagittarius, on the IC, is the foundation of our own inner wisdom. We will return to this theme further on.

The asteroid *Arthur* (named for the legendary King of Camelot) had just risen when the Alpine Mint Bush was decanted. It sits right on the ascendant which amplifies the asteroid's qualities. Arthur was known not just for his democratic wisdom and responsible leadership, but also for his compassion, especially for his wife, Guinevere. When forced (through the weight of great responsibility) to execute her at the burning stake, he prayed that his best friend, her lover, Lancelot, would arrive in time to save her (which, of course, he did). As the legend states, Arthur forgave

Alpine Mint Bush Flower Essence

31 March 1993, 3.57 PM AEST
Jindabyne area, NSW, Australia
36°S30'30'' × 148°E16'00"

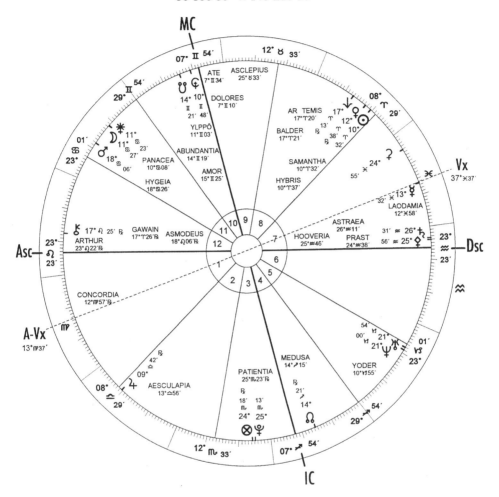

Geocentric – Tropical Zodiac – Placidus Houses – True Node

them both for their treachery and did not kill Lancelot when the opportunity was at hand. This clearly echoes the Leo/Aquarius theme of the
ascendent–descendant axis.

So we can first begin to synthesise the chart by following the theme
of compassion (which is the only true motivation for wanting to alleviate
the suffering of others). This leads us to the asteroid *Amor* which I have
found to always indicate compassionate, unconditional love. This asteroid is conjunct the south node (☋) where we always find the abilities
that have already been experienced. Also, an asteroid named *Abundantia*
sits at this point. This one simply brings in an abundance of whatever it

contacts which, in this case, is compassion. So, our first clue is that the person who needs to take this essence is someone who has already developed the quality of compassion.

Our next question, relating to that Leo ascendant and *Arthur* conjunction, might be: 'Is the theme of responsibility significant in this chart?' The development of the energies emitted by the planet Saturn (♄) lead us to develop self-mastery, and through self-mastery we are capable of accepting responsibilities. With *Amor* being in the 10th house of the sky (always a Saturn–Capricorn (♑) vibration), this compassion is to be maintained in the outer world in the area where one will take on responsibility.

We then look to Saturn, itself, which we find conjunct the asteroids *Pallas* (♀), *Hooveria* and *Astraea*. *Pallas* was named for Pallas Athena, the ancient Greek goddess. She was the protective deity of Athens, born with shield, spear and helmet already in place! And she was also the Goddess of Wisdom (picking up the theme of our Sagittarian IC). Her wisdom and inventiveness were always put into use in ways that benefited mankind. So she represents 'wisdom in action'. *Hooveria* was named for Herbert C. Hoover who organised the Belgian Relief Committee and later the American Relief Administration, which sent aid to Russia and other parts of Europe suffering famine following World War I. He was regarded by millions of people as a great hero who could feed the world. His reputation had spread even to the isolated yurtas of Mongolia. (This was before he became the thirty-first President of the United States.) One facet of the asteroid *Astraea* is to recognise the value of spiritual law over human law. So when we put this sentence together, it reads 'the opportunity to develop responsibility to help the suffering people, through accessing one's own spiritual wisdom by doing what we know to be right'. Saturn–*Pallas*, being in the sign of Aquarius, signify the ability to access this wisdom through detachment. This does not mean 'shut down', but emotional objectivity while keeping the heart open.

These asteroids are not far from another one named *Prast*, which is very near the descendant (another power spot in all charts). Martin Prast is a Vietnam veteran, a paraplegic, who founded 'Mobility Aids for Handicapped Persons'. He certainly sounds like a 'Pallas Athena' type to me!

As Ian White has suggested, Alpine Mint Bush Essence works on the mind as well as the emotions. At this Gemini MC point we have two asteroids. One is *Dolores*, a name which means 'sorrows'. This is obviously about dealing with depression. Next to her is *Ate*, the Greek Goddess of Evil. She is positioned at exactly the same degree as the midheaven itself. To put this into context, it may be beneficial at this point to first take a look at the planet Mercury (☿) which elaborates this MC theme for us. (Mercury is the lower octave tone to Gemini.)

The combination of Mercury being in Pisces (♓) (which can absorb the thought-forms of others, for good or ill) and in the 7th house (a

Libran (♎) vibration) usually produces a mind which is highly receptive to another person's communication and ideas. When we think about this in relation to *Ate* on the MC, it becomes clear that the goal of this essence is also to deal with other people's negativity. This is actually a prerequisite for being a healer. Therefore, I believe, the Alpine Mint Bush can be beneficial in protecting the healer's mind (and thus emotions) from absorbing too much negativity (*Ate*) from patients, through the ability to maintain detached objectivity.

People who have this particular Mercury placement have the potential to be wonderful listeners and counsellors, often focused on other people's issues rather than their own; and they have the natural ability to be compassionate in their thinking. It is very interesting to read Ian's initial description of this aspect of the Alpine Mint Bush in *Australian Bush Flower Essences*: 'This is a remedy for those in service, giving much of themselves emotionally, listening to people in pain and need …'

The Vertex (Vx) is a calculated point, rather than a planetary body, much like an ascendant. Suffice it to say, here, that my research has proven that its effect is always to highlight a past-life crisis that is bleeding through into this life, something that must be mastered before we can fulfil our purpose in this incarnation. Mercury is at this point and the asteroid *Laodamia* is conjunct the Mercury–Vertex in the Alpine Mint Bush chart. Laodamia appears in Greek mythology as a woman who committed suicide due to the intense grief she experienced after her husband had been killed in the Trojan War.

This is another facet that I have found within the Alpine Mint Bush: to allow healers to accept the inevitable death of some of their patients. The loss of a patient, of course, can trigger deep grief in any healer. Also, most healers have subconscious memories of 'failures' in past lives when they were practising some form of healing. They quite possibly were persecuted or even killed for not being able to save someone of prominence, let alone circumstances where they may have had to helplessly watch a loved one die, despite their own efforts. This is where the responsibility can weigh heavily. Grief versus compassion. Compassionate action can overcome grief.

Some healers may have been conditioned to view death, even from a subconscious stance, as a failure on their part, especially when under tragic circumstances, such as the untimely deaths of children and young people. There is a quality within this essence that can awaken in the healer a respect for death as a healing process in itself. Our Western approach to medicine has for too long been focused on 'keeping the body alive, no matter what'. In not respecting death's purpose, we have ignored the dignity within death that is so much a part of life. And no healer can work against karma. If a soul needs to leave, she will leave. There will be a time for each one of us.

This issue can reach a point of bringing up suicidal feelings in the healer at his/her perceived failure. The fear of responsibility may also result from this experience. I have successfully used this essence quite extensively, and in combination with other relevant essences, to help healers who have been blocked by the past-lifetime terrors which related to the responsibility of healing others. Sometimes this fear had developed through an experience of using innovative, alternative methods that had not been supported in those ancient incarnations.

Medusa is the terror which turns us to stone. Again from Greek mythology, Medusa had once been a beautiful woman who had been tragically turned into a hideous creature as a punishment for misusing a temple (that's another story!). Anyone who was to perceive her countenance would be immediately turned to stone. This asteroid appears next to the north node (☊) which is a vibrational point (always directly opposite the south node) relating to our soul's chosen path in this life. First, this node is in Sagittarius and in the 4th house. Apart from the gaining of wisdom, Sagittarius is the greatest 'rescuer' in the zodiac (a prominent signature in firefighters' charts, for example), and Cancer, being the energy generated in the 4th house sector of the sky, has the greatest protective instinct. This is an unusual place for *Medusa* to be residing, but I feel that she may represent, in this context, having to face our own past-life subconscious terrors, surfacing as phantoms in our psyche, while we are engaged in helping to heal the traumas of others, the source of their own disease. This essence could help a carer to access their wisdom and strength when counselling someone who is at a suicidal point in their lives. This is evident in *Medusa*'s 'square' to the Mercury–Vertex–*Laodamia* which is opposite an asteroid named *Concordia*. This makes what is known as a 'grand cross' formation. A crucial challenge in our growth.

Concordia (relating simply to 'concord, peace, harmony') sits on the anti-vertex (A-Vx), the balancing point for the vertex crisis. So this essence may be useful when having to counsel others, especially when required to give a prognosis relating to a condition, or news of the death of a patient to the family involved. This may be the inevitable shock that *Medusa* brings to others through one's words. The compassion from the *Amor* or the south node, which also squares the *Concordia*, completes this picture. One cannot deliver sad or tragic news sensitively without compassion.

This brings us to the planet Pluto (♇) (Scorpio's (♏) lower octave) which emphasises our 'survival' issues. Pluto was the Roman God of the Dead (as was his Greek counterpart, Hades), as well as the God of the Riches of the Earth. He sits here, in this chart, directly opposite *Asclepius* (the Greek counterpart of the Roman-named *Aesculapia*), and also squaring the Saturn–*Pallas*–*Astraea*. There is one other aspect of Medusa which may be relevant here. When she was killed by Perseus, the blood from her severed head ran in two streams, one a deadly poison, the other a miraculous healing agent. It was Asclepius who used the latter to heal others miraculously and to even raise the dead. However, Asclepius was killed by Zeus, for his arrogance at defying Hades's (Pluto's) domain.

Again we see a signature for those healers and carers having to make decisions and take responsibility in the deepest areas of others' life-and-death struggles. The square (from the Saturn–*Pallas*–*Astraea*) emphasises that the essence will give assistance in this difficult area. Pluto is also conjunct *Patienta* and the 'part of fortune' (⊗). Patience is undoubtedly a virtue. Our desire (Pluto is the planet which relates to all base chakra issues of attachment and desire) for results must be curbed. We cannot hurry the healing process in another. The part of fortune always leads us to develop our heart energies fully. It emphasises the Pluto, here, as the ability to transform negative energies (whether desires or fears) into positive ones, which is, of course, the role of the healer, but we need patience to fulfil this process. The wisdom of *Pallas* is the key.

This would be a marvellous essence for surgeons and paramedics who face the issues of death daily. They may feel the necessity to 'shut down' when overwhelmed with the pain they see around them. Complacency may then set in, especially when overworked.

Aesculapia is another asteroid corresponding to the issues of his Greek counterpart, *Asclepius*. Not surprisingly, this rock also figures strongly in this chart. Both these asteroids are, therefore, indicative of spiritual healing powers, and here *Aesculapia* makes a quincunx angle (a type of 'initiation trial') to the Mercury–Vertex. This is a challenge to access the power of the mind to heal. (We cannot achieve the power in our 'quincunxes' until we have worked through the emotions connected to our 'squares'.) To keep our minds centred on a perfect state of health for our patients is another task of today's healers. To project positivity is healing in itself. Thought forms are powerful energies.

One of the most important focal points of any astrology chart is the sun (☉). The sun's energies directly influence the condition of the heart chakra. This, much like the ascendant, is where our Spirit aspect emanates out into the world. We give to others via the heart. In fact, all of the energies in our chart are filtered through, and conditioned by, our heart chakra. The sun in this chart carries a further weight as the expression of the ascendant sign (Leo) itself.

There is an asteroid called *Samantha* exactly at the degree of the sun in the Alpine Mint Bush chart. This rock was named for a little girl in the USA who had a life-threatening disease. Samantha became famous for her dream of friendship between all people of the world. Her concern was not self-centred, but focused on others in the broadest way. It is fascinating to see the theme of the life-threatening disease emerging once again here, as well as selfless concern for others.

The sun is in Aries (♈) in the 8th house (which resonates with that Scorpio/Pluto vibration). A person with this combination can very easily burn out from overwork. Scorpio (♏) is determined and driven, and will do the work that no one else wants to do, while Aries (related to Mars (♂), the Roman God of War) believes he is indestructible! The lesson of Aries, for all of us, is to initiate *new* experience in this lifetime, rather than repeating the past which is a security pattern (no matter how painful) from the subconscious aspect of the mind. And Scorpio is the test of being immersed in the past. He must face his own inner demons. Aries is also the individual, the leader, who 'boldly goes where no one has gone before'. He is totally fearless.

Hybris is also conjunct the sun. This asteroid was named for the term 'hubris': 'insolence and excessive pride'. I have seen this asteroid, in clients' charts, relating to times of having to take the law into one's own hands. We are back to the Saturn–*Pallas* issue of trusting one's own judgment. This essence could be especially useful for doctors and herbalists who are fighting government departments. The recent euthanasia debate in Australia is a case in point. There is certainly a real strength in this essence. The combination of Aries and Scorpio influencing the heart is an unbeatable force.

The sun is opposite Jupiter (♃), the planet relating to our own inner wisdom (Sagittarius). Most of us have a tendency with oppositions to project them on to other people, which is not our evolutionary goal. This essence chart is again reiterating the value of our own judgment and wisdom when in a healing capacity. Perhaps the Alpine Mint Bush will prevent healers from blaming themselves when past decisions regarding treatments have 'failed'.

The trans-Neptunian planet Hades (♇) is an octave jump up from Pluto, by resonance. Through years of my own clinical research, I have found that Hades pinpoints a deeply unconscious area of our psyche that may hold us back from our full potential. (This is unconscious self-sabotage.) Yet, at the same time, it *is* our potential, our greatest gift. This is an extremely complex area and a full explanation of this energy body cannot be given here. However, the asteroid *Ylppö*, sits right next to Hades in this chart. *Ylppö* was named for a Finnish paediatric physician, Arva Ylppö. We can at least gather from this that the Alpine Mint Bush may be the essence remedy to help unblock people who continually sabotage careers in the healing professions.

We can also look to the planet Mars (♂) as resonating with the Aries influence on the sun. Mars is in Cancer (♋), the sign governing our inner emotional reactions as well as our capacity for sympathy; and it is in the 11th house, which is an Aquarian vibration: humanitarian detachment. Again, this is an interesting combination to nurture others while not getting drawn into their emotional experiences.

Sitting right next to Mars we have a very important asteroid named *Hygeia*. She is the Goddess of Healing (and *Asclepius*'s daughter), and represents a very powerful healing force, often of a spiritual nature. I have found that *Hygeia* in the charts of Flower Essences usually indicates the particular problem that the remedy will address. As Mars also activates the energy of a chart, and through being in combination with *Hygeia*, to heal others becomes an outward expression and drive. *Hygeia* may also be used inwardly to heal the physical energies of Mars when they are exhausted. It is the planet Mars which distributes our life force through the body via the spleen as well as the iron in the blood. As I understand it, one of the functions of the spleen *chi*, in Chinese medicine, is to move the *chi* (life force energy) up into the head (the head being traditionally ruled by Mars in classical astrology!). Excessive rumination, which we can associate with the Gemini–Sagittarius axis (the MC–IC here), can drain our spleen energy. As Ian's commentary continues:

> ...They are having to think of how to help or heal and be creative [certainly the Leo ascendant], as well as often feeling responsible for others. As a consequence, they can reach a point of tiredness, feeling that their life has lost its joy. There is a feeling of 'why bother'. This essence works on a mental and emotional level. It puts spring back into their life and into the work they do. This remedy helps to refresh and to revitalise when there is a feeling of mental and emotional exhaustion. Like other Mints, this is very aromatic, refreshing and cooling.

Chiron (⚷) is believed to be a comet which is caught in orbit in our solar system, mostly between the orbits of Saturn and Uranus. It seems to have the strongest effect on our crown chakra, and I believe that it represents the qualities that our Higher Self, or Spirit aspect, has been trying to develop and grow through on the earth plane. We are then to give this out as part of our gift to others. It is one of the major spiritual aspects of life purpose for any astrology chart. (Chiron was a master teacher of wisdom in Greek mythology.) Here we find Chiron in Leo (the sign most connected to the heart), just like the ascendant, and in the 12th house—our Piscean signature, which is also the influence on the Mercury/mind by sign.

The asteroid *Gawain* is exactly conjunct Chiron. Gawain was one of Arthur's knights of the Round Table at Camelot, and the protector of women, no matter what their station in life. A highly ethical and chivalrous character. He was devastated when he accidentally killed a Lady who was protecting her husband. Gawain then swore that he would become the most chivalrous and courteous of all the knights (important traits in any healer!). The asteroid *Asmodeus* is also conjunct Chiron. He represents the dark forces. So again we have a signature of having to deal with another person's negativity compassionately and with no reproach, as well as, through *Gawain*, having to confront responsibility issues in regard to another's death.

The Chiron is also trining Vulcan (↓), a (so far) 'invisible' and 'hypo-thetical' planet which is said to be closer to the sun than Mercury. (I have seen enough astrological evidence to vouch for its authenticity as a form of energy.) This little planet relates to our unique gift, from the pains of our deep past, that we are here to give in this lifetime. Like the sun, it brings in strength through being in Aries and the 8th house. It is conjunct the asteroid *Balder*, who is a character from Norse mythology. Balder was the God of Light and Truth, and he was also skilled in the use of herbs, so he was often called upon to heal others. Obviously, the theme of the healer is strong through this placement. But it is also con-junct the asteroid *Artemis*. She was the Moon goddess and protector of the young and helpless, also presiding over many other areas. However, by being in the 8th house (Scorpio influence), we must tie in that sig-nature which takes us to a particular episode in her story: she had acci-dentally killed Orion, the man she dearly loved, with one of her arrows. Again, the Alpine Mint Bush has the capacity to allow a healer to process inwardly the death of a patient.

Mars and *Hygeia* actually square the Vulcan–*Artemis–Balder*, suggesting that the essence may help to alleviate the tension created when we are faced with having to deal with difficulties in assisting the healing process of others. Their trine to Chiron tells us that this essence is for people who are usually strong individuals in charge of others but are just burnt out due to the emotional and psychic overload. The aspiration to heal may be there but subconscious fears may be getting in the way.

The overload may also be seen in the square of Venus (♀) (the Libran planet of relationship and receptivity) to the moon (emotions) which itself is in conjunction to *Panacea*! Venus can relate to our own needs in terms of what we subconsciously expect from others. Our work as a healer/carer often entails having to put others' needs before our own. This, too, can lead to burnout. The moon is also our self-identity as it relates to our past, our memories. With the *Panacea*, it strengthens our inner identity as a healer. But the balance (the proper use of Venus) in acknowledging our own needs, must be present.

However, this moon–*Panacea* also squares the sun. This is another aspect of the emotions directly affecting the heart. As squares are always fear challenges, it seems that the Alpine Mint Bush may restore one's faith in one's own abilities as the mentor and healer for others. I have added 'mentor' here as the sun is also square to a cute little asteroid called *Yoder*, familiar to most people as Luke Skywalker's mentor in the *Star Wars* trilogy. Yoder was the great guru for Luke. He was expected to have all the answers. The moon is also opposite *Yoder*, as though this quality has been pushed away. (How many times do we need to be told by the Alpine Mint Bush to trust our own judgment rather than project-ing it on to others?)

The asteroid *Juno* is very close to the moon. She brings in the principle of 'commitment under difficult circumstances'. (In Roman mythology, Juno was married to Jupiter who, even though the leader of the gods, was not exactly the perfect role model as a committed husband.) So this combination, with the 'mothering and protecting' instincts from the moon's energies, is the commitment to nurture others. Again the essence is saying it wants to revitalise people who have been emotionally influenced to a detrimental degree by other people who need healing. Again, for those times when we are expected to have all the answers. Mothers are often in this situation when their children are unwell; also professional carers, social workers and especially people involved in palliative care. Astrological counsellors can do with a good dose of this one as well!

This really is a strengthening essence which can help us to maintain our commitment to helping others by revitalising our original resolve. It can be all too easy for us to pick up and echo the negativity (which is suffering) in those who are in pain of a physical, mental or emotional nature. To remain detached without losing our compassion is a tricky task. Our own issues, no matter how deeply buried, are consistently mirrored to us through our clients and patients. This essence can obviously assist us in this important process as we cannot be true healers if we do not remember our own pain. It is the pain which motivates us to want to help others. And by *doing* this our pain mysteriously turns into joy.

—Case Histories—

Case 1

I have included two case histories: the first is by Louise Anderson and is written from the practitioner's perspective, while the other is of the patient's experience. They are both very typical of the results that can be achieved using these very powerful healing tools—the Australian Bush Flower Essences.

Case 1

Last October a friend was struck down with Gillian Barre syndrome, a fairly rare virus which attacks the myelin sheath around the nerves. This sheath is vital to the transmission of nerve impulses. Statistics of documented cases show 40% of people who contract this virus are permanently paralysed, 10% die and the remaining 50% experience a convalescence of one to two years as the nerve sheath slowly regenerates. A reasonable proportion of these do not recover to their previous level of health. The symptoms are similar to multiple sclerosis (MS) and vary according to the location of affected nerves. It has been noted that many sufferers have chickenpox before or after the virus.

This fit 35-year-old international airline pilot boarded a plane in Sydney in full health. Soon after he began to experience tingling and then complete numbness in his hands and feet, blurred vision, a migraine-type headache, dizziness and photophobia (unable to look at light). By the time the plane reached Bangkok nine hours later he was totally incapacitated and the examining doctor ordered him onto the first plane back to Sydney, where he was rushed to hospital and immediately transferred to intensive care. An exhaustive set of tests were run which eliminated a brain tumour, MS and a number of other things before the doctors finally diagnosed Gillian Barre and told him there was nothing they could do for him and sent him home. A week after the first onset of symptoms he had fully recovered the full use of his arms and legs but had significant blurring of vision in his right eye, was feeling extremely weak and was very concerned about his future in general and as a pilot in particular.

I prescribed Sunshine Wattle for optimism in the future. He is a fairly positive person by nature and I just put it in to support that, along with Flannel Flower for sensitivity because the initial symptom had been numbness and because I knew that he had difficulty expressing his feelings at times. I thought Flannel Flower would put him back in touch with feeling and sensuality on a physical level as well as work on the emotional cause behind the disease. This sparked more sharing of feelings in the next fortnight than in the previous two years, especially with the Bluebell which I also included. I had put Bluebell in because a lot of disease comes from having closed down the heart and it would help shift the disease state. A wonderfully open heart resulted which was beautiful to watch and be a part of.

Also in the mix I put some Macrocarpa as I believed the entire episode had been brought on by, or certainly not been helped by, back-to-back flying followed by a four week ocean sailing race, more flying, a poor diet, chronic jet lag and a few too many late nights. No wonder his body fell in a screaming heap. I'd been away when all this happened and so he'd been out of hospital for three weeks by the time I saw him. He'd been resting up, had eliminated meat and sugar from his diet and was eating lots of fresh vegetables, fruit, whole grains and juices but obviously wasn't feeling his usual self. A week after starting on the essences he declared he felt so much better he was going to sail in the Sydney to Hobart yacht race in four weeks' time and began dashing madly around town getting the boat ready (in between crew-training sessions out on the harbour).

Around this time I rang Ian White, who did some surrogate muscle testing and suggested a mix of Flame Tree, Spinifex, Gymea Lily and Crowea to be alternated with my mix. A bottle of each were tossed into a sail bag and Gary departed for Hobart, and I didn't hear much more for a couple of weeks while they and their owner sailed halfway to Hobart, drove back to Sydney in a bad mood, jumped on a plane to Hobart, had a Happy New Year on Constitution Dock and sailed back to Melbourne via the West Coast of Tasmania before flying back to Sydney full of beans. After telling me all about his adventures he said he though his eyesight was improving faster on the first mix than on nothing at all and demanded refills. In all he had three bottles of each and apart from a healthy diet, some Echinacea and the odd visit to his osteopath, he received no treatment for the virus other than the essences.

After two bottles of each mix he snuck off to an opthamologist who didn't know him and passed an eyesight test, but Gary still had a bit of blurring in his right eye so he decided to dust off his surfboard and, when he could ride that again without any trouble, to go back to work. A fortnight later he had a full medical with his company's doctors and was pronounced fit to fly. These doctors, going on case histories of other sufferers, had thought the very earliest they would be seeing him for assessment would be in another four months' time and were amazed at the speed and extent of his recovery.

Several months later he was sent to a workers' compensation doctor who was not given any medical history on him. This doctor just happened to be the world's leading expert on Gillian Barre Syndrome. After examining him, the doctor announced him to be in perfect health and after signing all the paperwork enquired whether the claim had been the result of an attack of Gillian Barre. On hearing how long ago the attack had been (eight months by then), the doctor just shook his head and said in all his years of working with people with the virus he had not seen a single case of a full recovery until this one. He also said that he had seen some people recover to about 95% but only after several years. Certainly no one had been fit enough to be back in the cockpit of a jumbo jet five months after such a severe attack.

One happy pilot now attributes his cure to the essences and is currently on Cognis while he is in flight school, learning how to fly a new sort of plane following his recent promotion. His heart is still open and he's still into communicating his feelings in between his Sagittarian jokes. His last medical revealed that his eyesight is now better than it was before he fell ill.

Case 2

(This case history is a testimonial from Mrs Dorothy M. Johnson from Christchurch, Dorset, in England.)

I had my fifth and last stroke in 1989, having a near death experience at the time. For seven years I went through every door which offered the slightest ray of hope of recovery, as I was certain that I hadn't been sent back to spend the rest of my life in a wheelchair. Then I was introduced to Australian Bush Flower Essences. In June 1996 I received my first essences—Tall Yellow Top and Crowea. After only three days I started to have strange feelings in my head as though something was being moved there. This continued for three nights. On the fourth morning I awoke to find the excruciating pain in my left hand and foot had gone. By the end of that month pain had gone from all my afflicted muscles.

The second month Black-eyed Susan was added, as I am a restless person whose sleep pattern was erratic. I became calmer and sound sleep followed this. The third month Bush Fuchsia was added. After a few days I had feelings in my head which were similar to when I had the stroke—but I felt there was no need to worry. On the fourth morning I was aware that my face no longer felt numb down the left side. That morning my husband found me in bed grinning like a Cheshire cat! Over the next couple of weeks my balance gradually improved.

Waratah was added in February 1997. The change was mental rather than physical—positive thought, optimism and more determination took over. In March Jacaranda was added. A muscle on the top of my foot which had contracted into a hard lump, and resisted treatment, began to shrink and grow softer. In April I went onto Bluebell. The contracted muscle continued to shrink and my foot moved into its proper alignment. At this time pain and stiffness in my neck, which had been there since my stroke, disappeared and I can now turn my head normally.

In May Sundew and Southern Cross were added but there was no specific change; but I continued taking essences until the end of 1997—and I became mentally stronger and positive. It is two years since I commenced taking Flower Essences and the symptoms have not returned—I feel I have been cured. I am so thrilled with these beneficial changes that I want to shout it from the house tops! Thank you for your wonderful Flower Essences and God bless you and your work.

Repertory
of Emotional,
Mental and Spiritual
—Conditions—

In this Repertory I have listed alphabetically major emotional and spiritual themes that people commonly experience and work through, and alongside I've provided a detailed description of every essence which is relevant to the specific theme being discussed. As well as bringing you valuable and helpful information in choosing remedies either for yourself, friends, family or clients, I hope that this Repertory will provide you with major distinctions between the remedies as well as new insights into the sphere of action of each and every one of the sixty-two Australian Bush Flower Essences.

abandoned, feeling
Illawarra Flame Tree ... where there is a sense of rejection
Tall Yellow Top ... feeling isolated, alienated, lonely

absent-minded (*see also* focus)
Isopogon ... for sharpening memory; senile dementia
Jacaranda ... where attention is scattered; for ditherers
Sundew, Red Lily ... procrastination; for focus and concentration

abundance, lacking

Abund Essence . . . aids in releasing negative beliefs, sabotage and fear of lack, thereby allowing you to receive on all levels

Bauhinia . . . where there is resistance to change, to new ideas

Bluebell . . . subconsciously thinking there is not enough for all

Boab . . . limiting beliefs inherited from family

Dog Rose, Bluebell . . . fear of lack

Five Corners . . . believing you're good enough to deserve abundance

Philotheca . . . being open to receiving

Sunshine Wattle . . . faith in Universal providence; that things can get better

abuse, victim of

Billy Goat Plum . . . disgust about your own body because of sexual abuse

Boab . . . for breaking family patterns of abuse

Emergency Essence . . . to deal with trauma of abuse

Five Corners . . . self-esteem

Fringed Violet + Flannel Flower . . . sexual abuse, males

Fringed Violet + Wisteria + Flannel Flower . . . sexual abuse, females

Little Flannel Flower . . . for children who are being abused

Mountain Devil . . . anger, attracting violence to themselves

Pink Mulla Mulla . . . for old, deep hurt and pain from traumatic abuse

Red Helmet Orchid . . . eases effects of male–child abuse; when brought on by rebellious behaviour

Southern Cross . . . blaming others; being in victim role

Waratah . . . dark depression after abuse; courage to move on

Wild Potato Bush . . . frustration from physical impairment arising from abuse

abusing others

Boab . . . where there is family history of abuse

Dagger Hakea . . . spiteful and revengeful behaviour

Flannel Flower . . . to increase sensitivity and gentleness towards yourself and others

Mountain Devil . . . for anger, hatred, jealousy

Pink Mulla Mulla . . . spiteful words

Rough Bluebell . . . maliciously manipulating and hurting others

Sturt Desert Rose . . . for guilt about past action

abusing self

Billy Goat Plum, Five Corners . . . loving and accepting your own self and body

Black-eyed Susan . . . for the person who is always on the go, not giving themselves enough rest or sleep; generally driving themselves beyond their own safe physical and emotional limits

Five Corners ... not nurturing yourself with good food and healthy life-style; not believing you are fully deserving of these things
Flannel Flower ... learning to be gentle with yourself and others
Hibbertia ... excessive self-denial, self-repression and self-driving
Kangaroo Paw ... for the immature person who takes unnecessary risks with no thought of the consequences
Philotheca ... always giving but not being able or willing to receive

acceptance
Bauhinia ... acceptance of optional change; of new ideas
Bottlebrush ... acceptance of inevitable change; ability to accept what has changed and move on
Hibbertia ... being content with own knowledge and how you are
Philotheca ... of praise from others
Southern Cross ... acceptance of life's experiences
Tall Yellow Top ... feelings of alienation and not belonging
Wild Potato Bush ... of physical restriction and limitation

acceptance, need of, by others
Five Corners ... confidence in self
Illawarra Flame Tree ... feeling, real or imagined, of rejection by others

acceptance of others
Bauhinia ... resistance to accepting anything or anybody different
Boab ... changing negative thought patterns taken on from family, ancestors
Freshwater Mangrove ... where there is pre-formed mental prejudice
Mountain Devil ... hatred and jealousy
Slender Rice Flower ... where there is prejudice learnt from experience
Yellow Cowslip Orchid ... critical and judgmental

acceptance of self
Five Corners, Confid Essence ... self-esteem and confidence
Illawarra Flame Tree ... will help those with sense of being rejected realise own potential
Southern Cross ... coming into own power
Tall Yellow Top ... where there are feelings of alienation, of not belonging

accident; disassociatedness after accidents
Sundew, Emergency Essence ... grounds; brings back to reality

accident-prone
Boronia ... stilling the racing mind
Bush Fuchsia ... improves co-ordination
Jacaranda ... helps focus energies and attention
Kangaroo Paw ... awkwardness and clumsiness in immature person; taking unnecessary risks

Mountain Devil . . . anger is the cause of many accidents
Sundew or Red Lily . . . lack of focus and concentration

accident trauma
Billy Goat Plum . . . embarrassment, as a consequence of accident
Black-eyed Susan . . . to calm down the tendency to rush that often results in accidents
Boronia . . . stills the active or obsessed mind
Emergency Essence . . . use frequently at time of accident
Fringed Violet . . . works directly on aura, repairing damage caused by trauma
Jacaranda . . . helps to gather scattered attention, energies
Mountain Devil . . . anger at person or situation which caused accident
Mulla Mulla . . . emotional trauma from burns or fire
Southern Cross . . . where there is a tendency to blame others for accident
Sundew or Red Lily . . . to help with focus, concentration; grounding after shock

accuracy
Bush Fuchsia . . . for brain function and integrating information
Sundew . . . increases focus and attention to detail

acknowledgment of self and others
Philotheca . . . being open to receiving; for receiving and accepting acknowledgment from others

adaptability
Bauhinia . . . opening up to new ideas and possibilities of living life to the full
Boab . . . where resistance to outside people and ideas is the family pattern; where abuse, mistreatment from other culture, nation, has gone on for generations
Bottlebrush . . . acceptance of, and coping with, change
Freshwater Mangrove . . . learning to bypass learnt family prejudice
Red Grevillea . . . when feeling stuck in a situation; strength to leave unpleasant situations
Slender Rice Flower . . . for those who have difficulty accepting those of another race or culture because of bad past experience
Waratah . . . courage to get through difficult situations

ADD (attention deficit disorder)
Black-eyed Susan . . . for intense, impatient behaviour
Bush Fuchsia . . . co-ordination; brain balance; speech and reading
Bush Fuchsia + Boab . . . clears cranial-sacral blockages caused by immunisation
Bush Fuchsia + Jacaranda . . . clearing vaccination toxins from body
Crowea . . . brings balance on all levels

Flannel Flower ... to encourage gentleness of touch, expression of feelings
Jacaranda ... poor concentration; scattered
Kangaroo Paw ... poor social skills; aggressive behaviour towards others
Paw Paw ... learning; integrating information
Sundew, Red Lily ... concentration and focus; bringing spirit into body

addictions
Billy Goat Plum ... sense of shame associated with addictive behaviour or substance use
Boab ... where an addiction is a family pattern
Boronia + Bottlebrush ... breaking the habit of the behaviour or the taking of the substance
Bottlebrush + Dog Rose + Dagger Hakea + Bush Iris + Wild Potato Bush ... for cleansing toxins from body
Five Corners ... builds up self-esteem; prevents sabotage of self or goals
Fringed Violet ... healing the aura after substance abuse
Hibbertia ... in relation to intellectual learning; 'workshop-aholics'
Mint Bush, Dog Rose of the Wild Forces ... for the intensity of emotions arising after stopping addictive behaviour or substance abuse which served to suppress those same emotions
Peach-flowered Tea-tree ... craving sugar; for chocoholics
Red Lily, Sundew ... grounding after drug use
Southern Cross ... blaming others; victim mentality
Sturt Desert Rose ... guilt associated with drug use
Waratah ... despair; 'dark night of the soul' during withdrawal period
Wedding Bush ... commitment to a regime to break addiction or to a healthy lifestyle

adolescence (see also anger; change; children; relationships; self-esteem)
Adol Essence ... for adolescence generally
Billy Goat Plum ... helps with acne; pimples; acceptance with body and sexual development; disgust of body
Boab ... breaks down negative family patterns; sets healthy boundaries
Bottlebrush ... for adapting to and coping with biological change; improves relationship with mother
Cognis Essence ... study; communication; public speaking
Confid Essence, Five Corners ... self-esteem; confidence
Five Corners ... self-esteem, self-love and acceptance
Flannel Flower ... for setting up healthy boundaries
Freshwater Mangrove ... when there is rejection of new people, foods, ideas, without experiencing or knowing them
Illawarra Flame Tree ... for rejection—real or imagined—by peers, teachers, parents
Isopogon ... for controlling behaviour; not learning from past mistakes

Kangaroo Paw . . . for immature behaviour; poor social skills; unawareness of others; unnecessary risk taking

Paw Paw . . . for overwhelm; assimilating information; helps with decision making

Red Helmet Orchid . . . deepens relationship with father; helps in dealing with authority figures; rebellious behaviour

Silver Princess . . . sense of life direction

Sturt Desert Rose . . . sexual guilt

Sunshine Wattle . . . helps to realise that although things seem grim, they can get better

Tall Yellow Top . . . where there are feelings of alienation, aloneness

adoption
Bottlebrush . . . helps bonding between mother and child

Illawarra Flame Tree . . . for feelings of rejection (real or imagined)

Red Helmet Orchid . . . helps bonding between father and child

Tall Yellow Top . . . where there is a feeling of alienation; of not belonging; of being abandoned

Wedding Bush . . . aids commitment to adoptive family, to adopted child

adventure, sense of
Boab . . . getting rid of negative family behaviour patterns of overconcern and conservatism

Freshwater Mangrove . . . opens to possibilities previously blocked by mental prejudice

Gymea Lily . . . daring to 'go out on a limb'

Kapok Bush . . . engendering a willingness to 'give it a go'

Little Flannel Flower . . . approaching life with joy and playfulness

Peach-flowered Tea-tree . . . for stimulation and challenge

Southern Cross . . . moving into own power

Sunshine Wattle . . . optimism; open to joy and excitement of future

Waratah . . . courage; sharpening of survival skills

adversity
Kapok Bush . . . resignation in face of

Sunshine Wattle . . . even though things are grim they can improve; trust in Universal providence

Waratah . . . courage to get through difficult situation; survival skills

aggressiveness
Bluebell . . . opening heart to love

Dagger Hakea . . . anger, resentment, bitterness to those close

Dog Rose of the Wild Forces . . . fear of losing control or temper; where there is danger of being carried along with aggressive behaviour of others in group

Mountain Devil . . . anger, jealousy and hatred generally

Rough Bluebell . . . deliberately hurting or manipulating others

aging (*see also* change; death and dying; grief)
Bauhinia . . . opens to whatever aging will bring on a physical, emotional, spiritual level
Billy Goat Plum . . . accepting and loving physical body at all times
Bottlebrush . . . change; accepting inevitable change
Crowea . . . for chronic worrying
Dog Rose . . . for general anxiety and fear
Dynamis Essence . . . tiredness; loss of enthusiasm and energy
Flannel Flower . . . joy in using and expressing the physical body
Hibbertia . . . rigid behaviour
Isopogon . . . poor memory; senility; controlling personality
Little Flannel Flower . . . flexibility of body and mind; joy, playfulness
Peach-flowered Tea-tree . . . overly concerned and worrying about aging
Red Lily . . . for vagueness; loss of concentration
Rough Bluebell . . . martyr, playing role of; manipulating others
Silver Princess . . . feeling that life purpose has never been realised nor attained
Southern Cross and Sunshine Wattle (alternating) . . . helps slow down aging process
Tall Yellow Top . . . where there is loss of identity after retirement
Wild Potato Bush . . . frustration with physical limitations, restrictions

agitation (*see also* anger; calmness; fear; peace; serenity)
Crowea . . . to help calm and centre
Dog Rose of the Wild Forces . . . where you are in danger of being swept up in the agitated emotions of others
Emergency Essence . . . eases panic and agitation
Jacaranda . . . nervous and scattered energies

agoraphobia
Emergency Essence . . . to help get through panic attacks
Flannel Flower, Boab . . . for setting up healthy boundaries
Grey Spider Flower . . . resolves extreme fear, terror

AIDS (*see also* death and dying; depression; *also* Physical Repertory: long illnesses; immune system)
Billy Goat Plum . . . for the feelings of self-disgust and self-loathing that can come up with this illness
Boab . . . helps to break patterns of behaviour taken on from family which are harmful to your present health situation
Bush Iris + Illawarra Flame Tree + Philotheca . . . to boost the immune system by working on the lymphatics
Dagger Hakea . . . when there is anger towards the person from whom you have contracted the disease

Detox Essence ... to clear the body of any toxins in order to enhance its ability to heal itself

Dog Rose ... for the continuing niggling fear about what is going to happen next in your life, and when

Dog Rose of the Wild Forces ... where there is a danger of emotions going completely out of control

Kapok Bush ... when there is a sense of giving up because it is all just too hard

Little Flannel Flower ... to bring joy back into your life at times when you seem to be completely taken over by the disease and its associated medical problems

Macrocarpa ... for physical exhaustion

Mountain Devil ... for anger at the world at large for the situation in which you are now

Paw Paw ... when there is a sense of overwhelm with advice coming from all sides; helps to tune into your Higher Self and make the necessary decisions

Peach-flowered Tea-tree ... where there is a tendency to become over-involved with your illness

Red Grevillea ... this will promote independence and boldness when you can see that things have to change in your life but you can't see how

Southern Cross ... helps you to come into your own power and not blame others or the Universe for your present circumstances

Spinifex ... where there is a sense of being a victim to the illness, this will help reveal the emotional cause that is creating the disease

Sturt Desert Pea ... for deep sense of loss or grief

Sturt Desert Rose ... for any guilt associated with the disease or any previous actions

Sunshine Wattle ... there will be many days when things look very grim. This essence will help you see that even though it has been hard in the past it *can* get better

Wild Potato Bush ... when there is frustration with the poor functioning of the physical body

Waratah ... for times when everything seems hopeless and there is no point keeping going

aimlessness

Jacaranda ... focusing scattered energies and ideas

Kapok Bush ... resignation; 'it's all too hard'

Paw Paw ... decision making; integrating information; listening to Higher Self

Silver Princess ... finding direction in life

Sundew ... for vagueness and procrastination

alcoholism *see* addictions

alertness (*see also* clarity of mind)
Cognis Essence ... for clarity and focus
Dynamis Essence ... for vitality and 'oomph'
Red Lily ... to stay grounded and in reality when involved in religious, spiritual, psychic practices
Sundew ... to help the dreamy person focus and ground

alienation, feelings of
Illawarra Flame Tree ... rejection (either real or imagined)
Tall Yellow Top ... feeling a 'stranger in a strange land'

aloneness *see* lonely

aloof, withdrawn
Bluebell ... opening heart to self and others; expressing feelings
Dog Rose ... shyness
Kangaroo Paw ... so focused on self that unaware of others
Pink Mulla Mulla ... putting out prickles to keep others away
Red Grevillea ... for those overly affected by the criticism of others
Tall Mulla Mulla ... prefers own company
Yellow Cowslip Orchid ... for the person who lives in the head, aloof from others

altruism, kindness (*see also* selfishness)
Alpine Mint Bush ... for people in caring jobs in danger of burning out
Bluebell ... generosity; opening heart and sharing
Philotheca ... helps natural givers to accept from others

amnesia *see* absent-minded

analytical
Bush Fuchsia ... integrating left and right hemispheres of the brain
Paw Paw ... for integrating new information
Sundew ... for focus and attention to detail
Yellow Cowslip Orchid ... for those who are 'nitpicking', overly intellectual

anarchy
Dog Rose of the Wild Forces ... when there is danger of losing emotional control in turbulent situations
Illawarra Flame Tree ... the fire element
Red Helmet Orchid ... for people who have problems with authority

anger (*see also* aggressiveness; fear (as anger is always associated with fear); love)
Black-eyed Susan ... impatience, irritability
Boab ... where anger, temper tantrums, raging is a family behaviour pattern
Dagger Hakea ... anger, resentment and bitterness towards those close to you; the 'forgiveness' remedy

Dog Rose of the Wild Forces ... fear of being carried away by anger of others in group situation; fear of losing temper and control

Dog Rose ... fear of anger

Kangaroo Paw ... immature and inappropriate displays of anger

Mountain Devil ... anger, hatred, aggression, envy, jealousy; opens to unconditional love

Red Helmet Orchid ... rebellious to, resentment of, authority

Rough Bluebell ... cruel, cynical; deliberately malicious; hostility

Slender Rice Flower, Dagger Hakea, Mountain Devil ... hostility

Yellow Cowslip Orchid ... critical; fault-finding; judgmental; intolerant; condescending

anguish *see* grief

annoyance at others (*see also* irritable)
Bauhinia ... accepting different, even unpleasant, behaviour of others

Black-eyed Susan ... impatience with others

Dagger Hakea ... resentment of or irritation at others who are, or have been, close to you

Freshwater Mangrove ... when closed to others because of prejudices that do not stem from personal experience

Slender Rice Flower ... prejudice towards others after bad previous experience with one or many of another race, culture or religion

anorexia nervosa *see* abusing self; confidence; depression; eating disorders

antisocial behaviour
Isopogon ... controlling behaviour

Kangaroo Paw ... immature or poor social skills

Mountain Devil ... for aggression and anger

Pink Mulla Mulla ... putting out prickles to keep others away because of a fear of being hurt. This fear is often the result of trauma in an early incarnation

Rough Bluebell ... deliberately manipulating or hurting others

Slender Rice Flower ... racial prejudice

Tall Mulla Mulla ... fear of social interaction

anxiety (*see also* fear; stress)
Crowea ... where there is chronic worrying

Dog Rose of the Wild Forces ... fear of losing control

Dog Rose ... for fear and shyness

Sturt Desert Rose ... for those with a sense of guilt

apathy
Kapok Bush ... 'it's all too hard'; giving up without trying; resignation

Old Man Banksia ... when physically weary; sluggish

apologetic, very *see* guilt

appetite disorders *see* eating disorders

appreciation of others
Bush Gardenia . . . to help reconnect and be aware of those around you; stop taking people for granted
Freshwater Mangrove . . . opens heart where there is learnt, but not experienced, prejudice
Gymea Lily . . . helps those who automatically take charge, riding roughshod over others, allowing them to be aware of and appreciate the needs of others to participate and contribute
Kangaroo Paw . . . being aware of the needs of others
Philotheca . . . praising and acknowledging others
Slender Rice Flower . . . overcomes racism, narrow-mindedness
Yellow Cowslip Orchid . . . to see the positive and not just the negative in people and their behaviour

apprehensive of others (*see also* fear)
Dog Rose . . . where there is fear and shyness around others
Five Corners . . . helps build up self-confidence
Gymea Lily . . . transforms the negative thoughts you have about your oppressor
Tall Mulla Mulla . . . feeling unsafe about confrontation and lack of harmony when with other people

arbitration
Slender Rice Flower . . . for group harmony
Yellow Cowslip Orchid . . . helps with impartiality

argumentative
Black-eyed Susan . . . irritation and impatience with others
Freshwater Mangrove . . . mentally prejudiced about others; being open to other ways of doing things
Hibbertia . . . rigid, inflexible attitudes
Isopogon . . . controlling-type personality
Kangaroo Paw . . . ignoring the needs of others
Mountain Devil . . . angry and aggressive
Rough Bluebell . . . demanding others give way; insisting on own way even if others are hurt
Slender Rice Flower . . . racist or narrow-minded because of bad experiences
Yellow Cowslip Orchid . . . focused in intellect; critical and intolerant of others

arrogance
Gymea Lily . . . for the enthusiastic person whose single-mindedness tends towards arrogance

Hibbertia . . . for the person addicted to learning who sees themselves as better than others

Rough Bluebell . . . dominating others and hurting them deliberately

Slender Rice Flower . . . for the person who judges others as being lesser beings because of their race, religion, sex or culture

assault, trauma after *see* abuse, victim of; accidents

astral travel
Crowea . . . aligns etheric and astral bodies if disturbed during astral travel
Red Lily . . . grounds and brings you back to reality

atheism *see* faith

attachment *see* bonding; co-dependence; detachment

attention, lack of *see* absent minded; ADD

attention-seeking
Gymea Lily . . . charismatic people used to being in limelight; glamour-seeking
Illawarra Flame Tree . . . needing to be noticed and appreciated

attention to detail
Sundew . . . helps focus on detail

attunement *see* spirituality

aura
Angelsword . . . clears negative energies and entities out of the aura
Crowea . . . for misalignment in the subtle bodies
Fringed Violet . . . for holes in; damaged or weak aura

austerity (*see also* abundance, lacking)
Hibbertia . . . excessive self-discipline and strictness
Red Lily . . . when the physical is ignored for total focus on the spiritual
Southern Cross . . . poverty consciousness; martyr, victim mentality
Yellow Cowslip Orchid . . . self-denial

authority
Gymea Lily . . . overuse of power; dominating and controlling people; oppression by those in power
Red Helmet Orchid . . . for those who can't deal with authority figures; rebelliousness against

autism (*see also* abundance, lacking)
Bluebell . . . for suppressed or cut off feelings
Boronia . . . repetitive and obsessive behaviour
Bush Fuchsia . . . awareness and orientation of self; brain function; speech and learning skills
Flannel Flower . . . helps express and communicate feelings

Green Spider Orchid . . . non-verbal communication
Red Lily, Sundew . . . focus and concentration; helps bring spirit into body

avoidance
Bluebell . . . avoiding, suppressing and denying feelings
Dog Rose . . . for the shy person who doesn't stand up for, or express, himself
Five Corners . . . avoids starting things because of fear of being seen as a failure
Illawarra Flame Tree . . . for fear and avoidance of responsibility
Jacaranda . . . always asking other people for their opinion, hoping to avoid making your own decision, and the consequences thereof
Kapok Bush . . . avoids things because they feel it is too hard
Red Lily, Sundew . . . use of drugs to avoid reality
Sturt Desert Rose . . . doing what you know you have to do, even when it is very difficult and you would rather avoid it, but you have to be true to yourself
Sundew . . . procrastination
Tall Mulla Mulla . . . for the 'people pleaser' who hates and avoids conflict and people, preferring to be alone

awareness (*see also* focus; spirituality)
Angelsword . . . works on whole energy field; cuts through confusion and misinformation; to hear the clear words of the angels and of your Higher Self
Bush Fuchsia . . . heightens awareness of, and trust in, intuition
Green Spider Orchid . . . increases awareness in communicating with other people, species and kingdoms
Meditation Essence . . . awakens spirituality and enhances intuition; allows you to deepen any religious, spiritual or psychic practice
Pink Mulla Mulla . . . clears past hurt from perhaps an early incarnation which has left you closed and defensive, and helps you re-learn that you really are a true spiritual being
Red Lily . . . opens the crown chakra; helps us to remember we are the loving children of a loving God
Sundew or Red Lily . . . for being vague and spaced out; being grounded and practical in your spiritual practice

awareness of others *see* appreciation of others; sensitivity to needs of others

babies *see* children; pregnancy and birth

baby, 'floppy'
Bush Fuchsia . . . improves brain function, co-ordination

Emergency Essence or Fringed Violet . . . for birth trauma no matter how long after birth

Sundew + Fringed Violet . . . brings spirit properly into body (apply to fontanelle at birth or later)

balance

Black-eyed Susan . . . brings emotions into balance; for stress

Bush Fuchsia . . . brain function left/right, front/back; masculine/feminine

Crowea . . . calms and centres; balances subtle bodies with physical body; balances major organs, glands and meridians

Peach-flowered Tea-tree . . . for balancing mood swings

Red Lily . . . balance between the spiritual and the physical

She Oak . . . balances hormones, ovaries and fluids in the body

Slender Rice Flower, Freshwater Mangrove . . . balances opinions, prejudices

Tall Yellow Top, Yellow Cowslip Orchid, Isopogon, Hibbertia . . . all create a balance between head (intellect) and heart

Yellow Cowslip Orchid . . . helps to see 'big picture' as well as the detail

being here, resistance to

Red Lily . . . connecting physical life with God; living in present

Sundew . . . helps to ground; brings spirit properly into body

Tall Yellow Top . . . for feelings of not belonging that keep you separate

belief in self (see also confidence; self-esteem)

Dog Rose . . . for the shy, fearful person

Five Corners . . . self-love

Illawarra Flame Tree . . . for the person who feels rejected

belonging

Five Corners . . . for believing you have the right, and deserve, to belong

Illawarra Flame Tree . . . for the feeling of real or imagined rejection

Tall Yellow Top . . . for building sense of connection with family, country

bereavement see death and dying; grief

birth trauma see pregnancy and birth

bitterness

Dagger Hakea . . . anger, resentment, jealousy towards someone close

Pink Mulla Mulla . . . hurt or abuse from the past

Southern Cross . . . blaming others; victim mentality

black night of soul see despair

blame

Hibbertia . . . being very hard on self; blaming self for not being better or for doing or knowing more

Mountain Devil . . . for anger which is often associated with blame

Southern Cross ... for the 'poor me' person; those with victim mentality who are not taking responsibility for what they create in their life and instead blame others for what happens to them

Sturt Desert Rose ... self-blame; regret; remorse

bluntness

Black-eyed Susan ... for the 'go-go-go' person who can be snappy when under pressure and stressed, upsetting people by saying things they later regret

Gymea Lily ... for the bossy, dominating person who controls others

Kangaroo Paw ... for unaware person who is insensitive to others

Mountain Devil ... helps diffuse anger that results in hurtful outbursts

Rough Bluebell ... for the person who prides himself on speaking his mind even though it may hurt others

body image

Billy Goat Plum ... where there is shame or disgust associated with an aspect of the body

Dog Rose ... holds the posture of a defeated or crushed person—drooped and round-shouldered

Five Corners ... helps build self-esteem about your overall appearance; drab or dishevelled appearance reflecting your lack of self-worth

Gymea Lily, Illawarra Flame Tree ... your dress and appearance are designed to be noticed

Hibbertia ... you are very strict with yourself and your disciplines to improve how you look

Old Man Banksia ... usually prefers clothing that doesn't accentuate the body or sexuality in public as they dislike intensely being the centre of attraction

Peach-flowered Tea-tree ... for hypochondriacs, always hypersensitive to any little change in their body

Red Helmet Orchid ... their dress and appearance is often calculated to shock or offend if in a rebellious stage

Red Lily ... for lack of attention to the physical as all emphasis is on spiritual

Wild Potato Bush ... for those who feel heavy or burdened with the physical body; for feelings of physical limitation

Wisteria ... allowing to enjoy and express sensuality

bonding

Bluebell ... opening heart to others; sibling bonding

Bottlebrush ... mother and child bonding

Bush Gardenia ... deepening interrelationships within families

Mountain Devil ... where there is sibling rivalry

Red Helmet Orchid ... father and child bonding

Wedding Bush ... for commitment to a relationship or family

boredom

Bottlebrush ... breaking old habits that keep you feeling in a rut; for letting go of the old and creating a space for new things to enter your life

Bush Gardenia ... for renewing passion and interest when boredom or staleness has crept into a relationship

Gymea Lily ... even though life may be comfortable there is still a sense of boredom if you are not fully and passionately pursuing your life's purpose and destiny

Hibbertia ... helps break up and loosen rigid and repetitive self-disciplines

Kapok Bush ... bored and resigned with life

Peach-flowered Tea-tree ... for the early enthusiast who quickly loses interest once there is no longer a challenge

boundaries, establishing healthy

Alpine Mint Bush ... for recognising and honouring their own emotional and physical limitations when working with others

Angelsword ... for using discernment with spiritual teachings and messages and other people; for disconnecting and clearing psychic cords of energy between yourself and others

Boab ... will support setting your own standards instead of following negative family patterns

Dog Rose of the Wild Forces ... where there is a danger of being carried beyond your own principles by being swept up by intense external emotions or activities

Flannel Flower ... helps define, operate and maintain healthy boundaries with others in physical and emotional intimacy

Fringed Violet ... for protection against being physically, emotionally, psychically drained by others

Kangaroo Paw ... being respectful of other people's needs and boundaries

Old Man Banksia ... for the generous, home-loving person who can't say 'no' to demands of family and friends

Red Helmet Orchid ... respect towards parents and older people

Sturt Desert Rose ... for personal integrity; allows a person to follow their own code of behaviour and to say 'no' without feeling guilty

brashness (see also arrogance)

Flannel Flower ... to enhance more articulate and sensitive verbal communication

Gymea Lily ... where they expect themselves, their needs and desires to be put first by everyone

Kangaroo Paw ... for the gauche, immature person who speaks without thinking

Pink Mulla Mulla . . . for those who can say spiteful or hurtful things to keep people from getting too close
Red Helmet Orchid . . . for over-cocky or deliberately confronting behaviour and language

broken-hearted *see* grief

bubbliness
Gymea Lily . . . stemming from the excitement and passion of going for your life 100%
Jacaranda . . . the positive aspect of this essence where there is a quickness and sparkle in thought and action
Little Flannel Flower . . . to release your playfulness, fun and joy

bulimia (*see also* eating disorders)
Billy Goat Plum . . . disgust with own body and behaviour
Five Corners . . . self-acceptance and self-love
Grey Spider Flower . . . fear, terror at consequences of overeating, bingeing and induced vomiting
Red Grevillea . . . knowing you need to stop this behaviour but not how to
Rough Bluebell . . . destructive behaviour to yourself
Wild Potato Bush . . . frustration with simply having a physical body

burdened, feeling (*see also* responsibility)
Banksia Robur . . . temporary physical tiredness and loss of enthusiasm
Old Man Banksia . . . where the physical body feels heavy, sluggish
Paw Paw . . . where there is a sense of overwhelm
Wild Potato Bush . . . feeling burdened in relation to the physical body

burnout
Alpine Mint Bush . . . for people in caring situations who are in danger of burning out
Angelsword, Red Lily, Mint Bush . . . for being drained spiritually
Black-eyed Susan . . . for the constant striving and rushing and busyness in your life which leads to burnout
Cognis Essence . . . for mental burnout
Emergency Essence . . . take frequently to get through any crisis situation
Macrocarpa, Dynamis Essence . . . for physical burnout
Red Suva Frangipani . . . for the emotional exhaustion while going through a rocky period in a relationship

busyness
Black-eyed Susan . . . always on the go, filling your life with activity, doing and achieving many things at once
Jacaranda . . . always busy but unfocused and rarely completing what you start; brings focus to scattered energies; for ditherers

calmness

Black-eyed Susan ... *the* stress remedy; helps a person relax, slow down and turn inwards

Boronia ... brings about calmness and stillness in a person when their mind is over-active, when they keep going over and over in their mind the same conversations or incidents

Bottlebrush ... adapting and coping with change

Crowea ... soothes emotional intensity; for worry; it balances, centres and brings about peace and calm

Dog Rose of the Wild Forces ... where emotions are in danger of going out of control in highly emotive situations

Grey Spider Flower ... for phobias, nightmares, extreme fear or terror; brings about courage, calmness, faith

Kangaroo Paw, Tall Mulla Mulla, Pink Mulla Mulla ... creates a sense of ease and calm; for those who are uncomfortable in social gatherings

Mint Bush ... brings calmness when there is turmoil, chaos and perturbation during times of releasing old spiritual beliefs and values or in spiritual initiation

Sundew or Red Lily ... for bringing back to earth and grounding those who are flying high mentally, emotionally or spiritually

carefree (*see also* fear; joy)

Alpine Mint Bush ... restores the juice that you allow to be dried out of yourself in giving everything to those you are looking after

Crowea ... helps the chronic worrier to stop worrying

Little Flannel Flower ... encourages joy and playfulness

Paw Paw ... eases feelings or sense of overwhelm; for resolution of problems or decisions

Red Lily ... for living in the moment

caring for others

Alpine Mint Bush ... helps sustain, emotionally and physically, professional or full-time home carers

Old Man Banksia ... for very empathetic people who always have a friendly ear for friends or family in trouble

Philotheca ... constitutional for many healers or carers who find it easier to give than to receive

Red Grevillea ... for those who feel they have no choice, that they are stuck in their situation of looking after an invalid or incapacitated family member

catharsis

Bottlebrush ... encourages acceptance of change and helps to let go of the old and the past

Dog Rose of the Wild Forces ... where you are in danger of taking on the agitated emotions of others and losing control or sense of self

Emergency Essence . . . to deal with any trauma associated with catharsis

Fringed Violet . . . releases shock after a cathartic experience; psychic protection when around or in cathartic situations

Mint Bush . . . for perturbation and confusion during tumultuous change

Sundew, Red Lily . . . for grounding after rebirth or a near death experience or any intense experience when a person has 'split'

Transition Essence . . . for letting go; allowing an aspect of self to 'die' in order to move forward

cautious (see also fear)

Freshwater Mangrove . . . for willingness to try things outside limited learnt prejudiced experience

Hibbertia . . . not putting learnt knowledge into practice in life

Kapok Bush . . . encourages willingness to 'have a go'

Little Flannel Flower . . . for those with a lack of joy in life; overly serious

Sunshine Wattle . . . holding back because of expectation of grim outcome

Yellow Cowslip Orchid . . . listening only to the intellect; ignoring the heart; 'nitpicking'

centre of attention

Five Corners . . . because of low self-esteem they can be very needy and act or behave to get attention even if it is negative strokes

Gymea Lily . . . for charismatic, dominating or arrogant people used to being the centre of attention and getting their own way

Illawarra Flame Tree . . . strong need and desire to be appreciated and noticed

Isopogon . . . for stubborn people who delight in getting others to give in to what they want

Old Man Banksia . . . for the water elements who feel very uncomfortable being the centre of attention, especially if it involves public speaking

Tall Mulla Mulla . . . people who dislike any fuss or bother which they often associate as coming when they are in the centre of attention. They much prefer to be alone

centred see balance

certainty see confidence; faith; self-assertion; trust

chakras

Bluebell, Rough Bluebell, Waratah, Illawarra Flame Tree . . . heart

Bush Iris, Green Spider Orchid, Boronia . . . third eye or brow

Old Man Banksia, Flannel Flower, Bush Fuchsia, Mint Bush . . . throat

Peach-flowered Tea-tree, Macrocarpa, Waratah, Five Corners, Crowea . . . solar plexus

Red Lily, Angelsword, Bush Iris, Waratah . . . crown

Red Lily, Kapok Bush, Green Spider Orchid . . . for higher chakras above
   crown
She Oak, Flannel Flower, Billy Goat Plum, Turkey Bush . . . second chakra
Waratah, Red Lily, Bush Iris . . . root or base

change
All flower essences bring about change!
Bauhinia . . . where there is resistance to change
Boab . . . by getting rid of your negative, inherited family patterns it can
   dramatically change your approach to life and to your family dynamics
Boronia . . . helps manifest change through visualisations
Bottlebrush . . . accepting inevitable, biological change; for those feeling
   overwhelmed by, or not coping with, change—whether it be situa-
   tional or biological
Freshwater Mangrove . . . opening to new paradigms of thought and
   being willing to accept that you can change the ways you have tra-
   ditionally thought about things
Mint Bush . . . for change in your spiritual guides; changing beliefs and
   values
Peach-flowered Tea-tree . . . sudden fluctuations and changes in mood
Red Grevillea . . . for those who know what the desired change or
   outcome is but who feel stuck, can't see a way of achieving it
Red Suva Frangipani . . . for when a relationship suddenly goes into crisis
Silver Princess . . . helps find new direction after the end of the failure of
   a previous scheme, job
Sunshine Wattle . . . a change from pessimistic to optimistic
Wild Potato Bush . . . a change resulting in becoming physically restricted,
   limited or encumbered, such as a stroke or broken leg

charity *see* altruism, kindness

chauvinism
Freshwater Mangrove . . . for those who dismiss others because of mental
   prejudice
Slender Rice Flower . . . for those with an exaggerated sense of superiority
   of their own race or group
Wisteria . . . helps males to realise that they have a feminine aspect to
   their personality and tones down excessive macho behaviour

children *(see also* ADD; adolescence; 'floppy' babies; inner child)
Billy Goat Plum + Dog Rose + Red Helmet Orchid . . . helps children
   with bed-wetting problems
Bluebell . . . helps children to share
Boab . . . helps prevent family enmeshment
Boronia . . . for children with compulsive behaviour patterns
Bottlebrush . . . helps with bonding to mother

Bush Fuchsia + Paw Paw + Isopogon + Sundew . . . for all learning problems

Bush Fuchsia + Sundew . . . where a child walks on tiptoe

Dagger Hakea + Dog Rose of the Wild Forces + Fringed Violet + Mountain Devil . . . eases temper tantrums and violent behaviour

Dog Rose + Five Corners + Pink Mulla Mulla + Tall Mulla Mulla . . . for the shy and fearful child or the child who is a loner

Emergency Essence, Red Suva Frangipani, Sturt Desert Pea, Sturt Desert Rose . . . for the child after the death of, or separation from, one or both parents

Flannel Flower, Fringed Violet, Sturt Desert Rose, Wisteria . . . for children experiencing acute sexual abuse

Freshwater Mangrove . . . for those who reject new food, etc., without even trying

Fringed Violet . . . for the child who is surrogating for their parents

Green Spider Orchid, Grey Spider Flower . . . for nightmares or night terrors

Illawarra Flame Tree . . . when children are excluded from 'in' crowd at school, sport; where there is feeling of rejection, real or imagined

Kapok Bush . . . for the child unwilling to try something new because it is too hard

Little Flannel Flower . . . for helping a child to reconnect with his or her Spirit guides; for the child who grows up too quickly, taking on the role of little man or little woman of the house

Mountain Devil . . . for jealousy and sibling rivalry

Red Helmet Orchid . . . improves bonding between father and child; can help where child is rebellious

Wild Potato Bush . . . for babies', toddlers' frustration with not being able to use or control their bodies as they would like

chronic disease (*see also* health threat)

Bauhinia . . . where there is resistance to implementing new healthy lifestyle or diet simply because it is different

Billy Goat Plum . . . for feeling shame or embarrassment that you are suffering from a particular condition

Boab . . . when it is a hereditary illness running through the family

Bottlebrush . . . helping to accept the changes that the illness brings

Dog Rose . . . fear of developing a specific illness; encouraging a love of life

Dog Rose of the Wild Forces . . . for when medicine can offer no explanation for why the person is suffering these symptoms or this illness: it could be past life-related

Flannel Flower . . . to stop the tendency towards becoming a couch potato as this remedy engenders a desire and love of physical activity and expression

Kapok Bush . . . where there is a sense of giving up because it is all too much

Little Flannel Flower . . . to engender fun, joy, flexibility

Peach-flowered Tea-tree . . . becoming too obsessed and preoccupied with your health problems

Southern Cross . . . for the sense of 'It isn't fair, why me?'

Spinifex . . . feeling a victim, and powerless against the disease; not able to recognise the lesson the illness is teaching

Sturt Desert Rose . . . for feelings of guilt that you are letting others down by not being able to do what you normally would; regret and remorse that your lifestyle has led to your present condition

Sunshine Wattle . . . realising that, even though things have been grim, they can improve

Wild Potato Bush . . . frustration of not physically being free to do everything you want

clairaudience

Angelsword . . . to hear the words of the 'angels' and your own Higher Self more clearly; cuts out negative entities and any of the messages they may be feeding to you

Black-eyed Susan . . . hearing on higher levels

Green Spider Orchid . . . aligning to higher learnings and insights; telepathy, attuning to other life forms and realms

Meditation Essence . . . to enhance psychic abilities and receptivity

clairsentience

Bush Fuchsia, Meditation Essence . . . sharpens intuition; opens you to, and increases your trust in, your own inner knowing; to be in touch with the rhythms of the Earth and nature

Bush Iris, Meditation Essence . . . opens you to higher perceptions

Fringed Violet . . . for those who are so empathetic with others that they know what they are feeling or thinking

Old Man Banksia . . . supports those with strong intuitive sense; a tree the Aborigines traditionally referred to as being for female spirituality

clairvoyance

Bush Iris, Meditation Essence . . . opening of the third eye

Green Spider Orchid . . . for the seeing and reliving of a past life in dreams, often occurring as a nightmare

Turkey Bush . . . for the prophetic creative 'flash'

clarity of mind *see* absent-minded; focus

clinginess *see* children

closed mind

Bauhinia . . . clears resistance to new ideas

Freshwater Mangrove . . . helps clear prejudices and expectations of how things or people should be

Slender Rice Flower . . . for those who are unable to see beyond the race, religion or culture of a person

Yellow Cowslip Orchid . . . helps a person to see the 'big picture' when they are caught up in bureaucratic details

clumsiness (*see also* focus)

Bush Fuchsia . . . improves co-ordination

Jacaranda . . . where accidents are a result of a person's attention being all over the place

Kangaroo Paw . . . for socially gauche, inept individuals

Red Lily . . . provides grounding, especially during or after any prolonged meditative or spiritual practice

Sundew . . . for focus and attention to detail and being aware of what you are doing

co-dependence (*see also* fear)

Angelsword . . . to disconnect any energy 'cords' between people

Billy Goat Plum . . . for releasing any shame about yourself and your behaviour in a relationship

Boab . . . breaking down any dysfunctional family behaviour or dynamics

Bottlebrush + Boronia . . . to help break addictive behaviour

Bottlebrush . . . projection of your mother and mother issues onto your partners

Dog Rose . . . giving you the strength to stand up for yourself

Five Corners . . . when you fully love yourself you are complete by yourself and don't need anyone else to make you whole

Flannel Flower . . . to be able to clearly articulate and communicate your feelings; for establishing healthy intimate physical and emotional boundaries

Gymea Lily . . . always needing love and adoration from others and to be the centre of attention

Illawarra Flame Tree . . . overly concerned about rejection and unhealthily go out of your way to please others and to get their appreciation

Isopogon . . . for not learning from past experiences and continuing to repeat the relationship scenarios over and over

Kangaroo Paw . . . for immature self-centred behaviour often attracting a 'parent' in relationship

Philotheca . . . always giving out and not asking for what you need or not being able to receive from others

Pink Mulla Mulla . . . stays distant and withdrawn in a relationship for fear of being hurt or used

Red Grevillea . . . feeling stuck in an unhealthy relationship that you don't know how to get out of; over-dependent on opinion, advice of others

Red Helmet Orchid ... for projection of your father and father issues onto your partner

Rough Bluebell ... for those who manipulate and hurt others

Southern Cross ... blaming others in a relationship, never taking responsibility for what is happening in your life; for those who are martyrs

Sturt Desert Rose ... always feeling guilty and blaming yourself for whatever happens to anyone else; being true to yourself, to your own beliefs and morality

Tall Mulla Mulla ... hiding your true essence and wanting to be a people pleaser in social situations

cold-hearted (*see also* love)

Bluebell ... opening heart to others; encourages generosity and sharing; helps get in touch with emotions

Freshwater Mangrove ... opening heart closed by mental prejudice

Hibbertia ... its final message in its Doctrine of Signatures, as its heart-shaped petals fall to the ground below, is to integrate head and heart in order to achieve wisdom

Pink Mulla Mulla ... they remain cold and aloof rather than showing their vulnerability to others for fear of being hurt again

Rough Bluebell ... hurting or creating pain for others without concern or regret

Tall Yellow Top ... for those living in their head, cut off from feelings, it links the head to the heart

commitment (*see also* goal setting)

Gymea Lily ... giving the strength and support to honour and fulfil your goals and life purpose even if they set you aside from mainstream society

Jacaranda ... for being able to finish the task at hand or the current goal before being distracted or lured to something else

Kapok Bush ... not giving up when things get too hard

Peach-flowered Tea-tree ... to complete things that you have started even when they have become somewhat boring or repetitive

Wedding Bush ... for making or deepening a commitment to someone or some thing such as a relationship, project, dietary program or sport training regime

common sense (*see also* balance; wisdom)

Hibbertia ... for those who are fanatical and rigid with their beliefs and behaviour and/or constantly devour information or philosophies in order to improve themselves, but don't truly integrate it

Isopogon ... to be able to learn from your past experience and not repeat mistakes

Kangaroo Paw ... being able to pick up clues and observe from others how to behave in new settings and situations

Kapok Bush ... when a machine or piece of technology is broken, it enables you to have an overview of how it normally works and then to work back step by step to locate the problem and then understand what is needed to solve it

Red Lily ... before enlightenment 'chopping wood, carrying water'; after enlightenment 'chopping wood, carrying water'; no matter on what spiritual level or path, this remedy helps a person to operate practically on a day-to-day level and to look after the physical

Sundew ... paying full attention to what you are doing

Yellow Cowslip Orchid ... you can't see the forest for the trees

communication (*see also* clairaudience)

Bauhinia ... where a person is resistant to anything or anybody new

Billy Goat Plum ... difficulty with communicating with someone to whom you are attracted because of feeling embarrassed or too self-conscious; a sense of shame about an aspect of yourself holds you back from interacting or communicating with others

Bush Fuchsia ... helps with speech by clearing stuttering, word salad (getting words back to front) and retarded speech development; increases fluency; improves your reading ability by integrating left and right hemispheres of the brain so that you are aware of the individual words you are reading, but also take in the context and meaning of the words, knowing when to add inflection and emphasis instead of reading in a monotone; eases the flow of words

Bush Gardenia ... for strengthening communication within a family situation

Dog Rose ... difficulty with communication because of shyness

Five Corners, Confid Essence ... for building confidence in yourself

Green Spider Orchid ... for telepathy even with a person in a coma or unconscious state; helps you to understand and then impart spiritual knowledge not only verbally but also telepathically; communication with other people, spirit beings, plants and animals

Kangaroo Paw ... for those who feel awkward or inept when talking or communicating, can't think what to say until the opportunity has passed; those who speak without sensitivity

Pink Mulla Mulla ... for those who put out prickles to keep others away

Slender Rice Flower ... for racist, narrow-minded people who restrict their social interactions to those of a similar ilk

Tall Mulla Mulla ... for those who aren't comfortable mixing in company, and often say things to appease and please other people in order to make their interaction more stress free

Yellow Cowslip Orchid ... for the nitpicking intellectual who tends to be aloof from others

community (*see* family and social interaction)

compassion *see* altruism, kindness

competitiveness
Black-eyed Susan . . . always striving and pushing themselves
Bluebell . . . when your underlying motivation is driven by a sense that there is not enough to go around
Dagger Hakea . . . resentful of anyone doing better than, or defeating you, rather than simply enjoying the competition
Five Corners . . . being driven to win because of low self-esteem
Gymea Lily . . . always has to be seen to be the best
Hibbertia . . . fanatical about being the best
Mountain Devil . . . where jealousy, sibling rivalry, aggressiveness promote competitive behaviour
Rough Bluebell . . . for those who display a ruthlessness and coldness in always wanting to win no matter at whose expense
Slender Rice Flower . . . where competition between individuals or groups is marred by feelings of superiority and excessive bipartisan fervour

complaining (*see also* criticism; victim)
Dagger Hakea . . . for people complaining about others behind their backs
Hibbertia . . . complaining that people are not following the example you believe you are setting
Kapok Bush . . . passive complaining through resignation
Mountain Devil . . . complaining your situation with aggressive or foul language
Paw Paw . . . feeling overwhelmed and burdened
Rough Bluebell . . . manipulating others by playing the martyr
Southern Cross . . . blaming others; 'poor me'; 'it's not fair'
Turkey Bush . . . for those who complain and argue that they are not creative

completion
Boab . . . for completing and terminating the continual passing down, from generation to generation, of the same emotional and behavioural patterns
Boronia + Bottlebrush . . . can be used after Dagger Hakea for releasing resentment, to physically and emotionally let go of an ended relationship and move on
Bottlebrush . . . helps in the moving on from one stage of life to another
Jacaranda . . . for being able to finish the task at hand or the current goal before being distracted or lured to something else
Kapok Bush . . . not giving up when things get too hard
Peach-flowered Tea-tree . . . to complete things that you have started even when they have become somewhat boring or repetitive
Philotheca . . . acknowledgment is a last step in the final completion of

a project that provides the emotional impetus and motivation to move on to the next goal

She Oak ... for the confirmation of pregnancy that finally completes the desire of the infertile woman to be able to have a child

composure *see* balance; calmness

compulsive behaviour *see* addictions

concentration *see* awareness; focus

confidence (*see also* inadequacy; shyness)

Confid Essence ... helps build self-confidence and a feeling of wellbeing

Dog Rose ... where lack of confidence is associated with fear, shyness

Five Corners ... *the* remedy to increase self-worth, self-love and self-esteem and self-confidence; for crushed-in personality; for those who sabotage their goals and dreams because they believe they are not good enough to deserve them

Flannel Flower ... confidence in being a man

Hibbertia ... helps you feel content with your own knowledge without always tending to get your knowledge through books or workshops

Illawarra Flame Tree ... indicated when a person is very sensitive about being rejected and their confidence is down when rejection does occur; for those who are overwhelmed by responsibility of achieving own goals

Isopogon ... for those who lack confidence because of poor memory

Jacaranda ... where you are always scattering your energies by jumping from one thing to another, always asking other people's opinion because you don't have the confidence to make a decision

Kangaroo Paw ... for the gauche, clumsy person; for those lacking social skills

Kapok Bush ... confidence in your ability to succeed in your plans and challenges

Mint Bush ... confidence when all your own references—beliefs and values—are falling away around you, you can have a sense of entering a void, while the 'dross is being burnt off', as you emerge to a new spiritual level

Paw Paw ... creates confidence by resolving indecision: by tapping into your own Higher Self where your wisdom is stored

Red Grevillea ... for those overly influenced by criticism

Silver Princess ... helps you discover your direction in life thereby giving a sense of purpose and confidence

Southern Cross ... empowers you person by helping you realise you can create your own reality

Sturt Desert Rose ... you feel bad about who you are because of something you have done in the past

Sundew, Bush Fuchsia ... where disorientation, poor communications

skills and lack of academic success rob a person of self-worth
Sunshine Wattle ... confidence that things will improve and get better
Waratah ... restores confidence and certainty that you are never given anything that you can't cope with in life
Wisteria ... confidence in being a woman

conflict (*see also* aggressiveness; family and social interaction)
Angelsword ... conflict in determining if a message is from your Higher Self or from mischievous or malicious entities wishing to confuse or influence you
Bauhinia ... avoiding conflict by being able to embrace differences in, and annoying aspects of, another individual
Paw Paw ... when there is a difficulty choosing between one or more options
Red Suva Frangipani ... difficulties and conflicts in intimate relationships
Slender Rice Flower ... whenever there is lack of co-operation and group harmony
Wild Potato Bush ... the conflict between what you want to do and what you are physically able to do
Yellow Cowslip Orchid ... conflict when others are seen to be breaking the rules and regulations

conforming
Bauhinia ... willing to consider and be open to new ideas or ways of doing things long before most others are
Boab ... stops you conforming and behaving with the same mental and emotional responses that have come through the family generation after generation
Freshwater Mangrove ... open to new paradigms
Gymea Lily ... gives courage to 'go out on a limb', to be different in your outlook, values and beliefs to that of the majority of those in society
Red Helmet Orchid ... for those who have problems conforming to rules, regulations and authority or authority figures
Yellow Cowslip Orchid ... for the conservative-minded person whose predisposition is to continue the time honoured way of doing things

confrontation (*see also* aggressiveness; avoidance)
Dog Rose ... overcoming fear and shyness so as to be able to stand up for yourself
Five Corners ... feeling strong enough in yourself that you can confront others if it is necessary to do so
Sturt Desert Rose ... being true to yourself and doing what you know you have to do, even when you may come into conflict or confrontation as a consequence

Tall Mulla Mulla ... for the 'people pleaser' who hates and avoids conflict, confrontation and people, preferring to be alone

Waratah ... gives great strength and courage to tackle anything extremely difficult

confusion (*see also* absent minded; focus)

Angelsword ... spiritual confusion; for the discernment to cut through misinformation and find your own truth

Cognis Essence ... for all learning difficulties

Mint Bush ... whenever there is chaos, perturbation and confusion as a result of spiritual growth or the crumbling of your old belief system

Paw Paw ... when unable to choose between a number of options

Travel Essence ... when your body systems are disturbed and disrupted through travel, especially long distance aeroplane flights

Waratah, Emergency Essence ... when unable to cope and not knowing where to turn

consideration, lack of *see* sensitivity to needs of others

controlling personality *see* dominating behaviour

conversation *see* communications; confidence; speech problems

courage

Dog Rose ... helps in situations where fear and shyness are preventing positive and courageous action

Grey Spider Flower ... maintains or restores courage when confronting frightening situations

Gymea Lily ... gives strength to those who are successful and achieving, helping them stay at the top and be unaffected by negative projections from others; gives courage to follow their own life passion

Pink Mulla Mulla ... courage to overcome the deep emotional blocks and old traumas that surface when following your spiritual path

Sturt Desert Rose ... gives people the strength and personal integrity to be true to themselves

Tall Mulla Mulla ... encourages personal interaction when there is fear of socialising

Waratah ... will give the courage to cope when you are going through a period of darkness and despair

creativity

Boronia ... enhances creative visualisation, which can be used to help manifest and create what you want

Bush Fuchsia ... excellent for tuning into own intuition, for hand/eye co-ordination and for expression of ideas

Crowea ... for calming and soothing the oversensitive and intense personalities that are typical of many creative people

Five Corners, Confid ... builds up self-confidence in your own artistic abilities

Flannel Flower ... for trusting that it is safe to let out and express your innermost feelings

Grey Spider Flower ... helps deal with terror of performing or displaying creative work in front of an audience

Red Grevillea + Fringed Violet ... will help artists in all mediums to deal with, and be less sensitive to, criticism by their peers, teachers or public

Silver Princess ... at the times when it is not clear what path to take in the creative world this essence will give direction

Southern Cross + Sunshine Wattle ... to release the commonly held beliefs among artists that all artists have to struggle and be poor

Sundew ... helps channel ideas and put them to practical use; it also helps artist stay grounded and in touch with reality, and deepens concentration and attention to detail

Turkey Bush ... renews artist's confidence in her ability by clearing creative blocks; supports inspired creativity and creative expression

crisis *see* shock; trauma

criticism *see* judgmental

crossroads, when at life *see* life direction

cruelty (*see also* family and social interaction)
Bluebell ... for the person who is mean and stingy and not sharing with others in need or with those under their care

Kangaroo Paw ... can help the immature, unaware person who can be quite cruel in their dealings with others without ever meaning to be, or even realising that they are

Mountain Devil ... transforms cruel behaviour, instigated by anger and jealousy, into unconditional love

Pink Mulla Mulla ... cruel in their words or actions, which they use as a defence, to push people away as they have a fear of being hurt if others get too close to them

Rough Bluebell ... helps bring through the love vibration for the person who deliberately hurts others in order to get their own way

cry, need to (*see also* grief; teariness)
Bluebell ... after heart surgery it is seen as a good sign for long-term recovery if the patients can cry a great deal, getting in touch with and releasing emotions that have been blocked for a long time—and a likely cause of the heart problem in the first place!

Sturt Desert Pea ... helps the person who keeps bottled up deep sadness and grief to release their hurt and pain

cynicism (*see also* negativity)
Bauhinia ... their inability to be open to new ideas or situations can

make them quite cynical towards these very same things

Bush Iris ... for those cynical of anyone pursuing a spiritual path or direction

Illawarra Flame Tree ... where an experience of rejection can lead to feelings of cynicism

Mountain Devil ... suspicious and cynical of people and society, rarely able to see or appreciate the basic goodness in people's behaviour and actions, believing that there always has to be an ulterior motive. For they come from the viewpoint that they are basically alone and that they can't trust people, and that everyone is out for themselves or to rip them off

Pink Mulla Mulla ... is cynical of people's attempts to get close to them, which conveniently lets them stay aloof and separate from others. They fear that if they do get close they will be hurt

Red Helmet Orchid ... cynical of the society in general, and its rules and regulations, as well as of people in authority

Rough Bluebell ... difficulty in being able to feel or express love makes them quite cynical

Slender Rice Flower ... for when a person has experienced a similar pattern in either the situation of the relationship or a quality of the partner, and they then tar with the same brush either all men or all women, believing them to be all the same

daydreaming *see* absent-minded; focus

death and dying (*see also* grief; suicide)

Bauhinia ... is about being open to the new and the unexpected; a willingness to face and accept whatever death will bring

Bottlebrush ... for a person who already feels comfortable with their understanding and awareness of the spiritual realm and that of the immortality of the soul, yet is going through a major transition; to let go of, but not forget, a loved one who has passed over

Bush Iris ... resolves the fear of death that can lead to a grim holding on to life; opens the third eye, allowing for more lucid perception of the spirit world and of the loved ones who have already passed over and are gathered around to help the person move peacefully from the earth to the spiritual plane at the time of death

Dagger Hakea ... anger and resentment towards the person who is perceived as having left you

Dog Rose of the Wild Forces ... for people who become hysterical around death or at funerals

Emergency Essence ... to bring calmness and peace and pain relief for anyone suffering an acute trauma, critical accident or severely painful symptoms just prior or leading up to their passing over; helps friends and family deal with any shock and upset due to a loved one dying

Lichen Essence ... helps the etheric body to separate from the physical;

helps a person to look for and go through the Light at the moment of death

Red Suva Frangipani ... for the initial intense upset and grief for the loved one passing over

Southern Cross ... for the feeling that fate or God has been totally unfair to take away someone you love

Sturt Desert Rose ... for remorse at anything left incomplete with a person who has died

Sundew ... helps to bring the soul back into the physical body if it is hovering and uncertain, whether or not it wants to

Tall Yellow Top ... coming from a child's reaction to the loss of one or both parents

Transition Essence ... helps a person to pass over with calmness, dignity and serenity

deception *see* honesty

decision making (*see also* goal setting)
Crowea ... decision making often creates worry and distress: this will help generate a climate of peace and calm in which a decision comes more easily

Jacaranda ... because of a fear of making the wrong decision, there is a lot of dithering and rushing about, achieving nothing

Paw Paw ... by improving access to our Higher Selves we are able to integrate information and come easily to decisions, without overwhelm

Silver Princess ... when our direction in life is made clear we are then able to make decisions easily

Sundew ... for grounding and focusing on the detail of the available information

deep hurt *see* grief

defeatist attitudes *see* optimism

defensiveness *see* confidence; fear

defiant *see* rebellious

delegating *see* trust

delinquency (*see also* adolescence; conforming; street kids)
Gymea Lily + Rough Bluebell + Mountain Devil + Dagger Hakea ... diffuses the angst in teenagers who are making life unbearable for their parents and teachers

Mountain Devil ... helps dispel the anger that often drives these teenagers and brings through their unconditional love instead

Red Helmet Orchid ... when rebelliousness results in trouble with school principals, police and other people in authority

Rough Bluebell ... for kids who behave violently to get what they want without caring whom they hurt in the process

Tall Yellow Top ... violent or antisocial behaviour stemming from a lack of any sense of belonging to a family group or community

denial

Billy Goat Plum, Five Corners ... denial of physical body

Bluebell ... when a person is in denial and totally cuts off their feelings

Yellow Cowslip Orchid ... can use intellect to rationalise away their feelings and emotions

Bottlebrush ... to recognise that material things or relationships have changed, are no longer needed or have moved on, and to let go of them and the past

Bush Fuchsia ... when ignoring or denying your intuition and gut feelings

Turkey Bush ... for denial of creativity

Bush Iris ... for atheism, and denial of the existence of anything spiritual

Flannel Flower ... those who deny their physicality, sensitivity, gentleness, sensuality and passion due to fear of physical or emotional intimacy

Hibbertia ... where over-emphasis on intellectual development, fanatical self-improvement or strict personal regime results in self-denial and self-repression

Little Flannel Flower ... a river in Africa

Pink Mulla Mulla ... denial of your spiritual path

Red Lily ... grounding; for those who tend to live in the ethers, ignoring their physicality

Sturt Desert Rose ... to honour yourself and your personal integrity

dependability *see* commitment; responsibility; trust

dependence, on others *see* co-dependence

depression (*see also* despair)

Alpine Mint Bush ... compassion burnout when joy and juice of life has been sucked dry

Dagger Hakea + Bluebell ... depression associated with unexpressed anger

Emergency Essence ... immobilising, severe depression and terror

Flannel Flower ... to generate the desire to move and use your body and be active and physically expressive (movement is one of the best antidotes to depression)

Illawarra Flame Tree ... rejection of self; feeling dejected

Kapok Bush ... despondency, gloom and resignation

Little Flannel Flower ... to be playful, fun and light and 'get out' of yourself

Mint Bush ... for when prolonged confusion and chaos can lead to depression

Old Man Banksia ... disheartened, feeling sluggish and weary

Peach-flowered Tea-tree ... for addressing the mood swings of a person suffering from manic depression or premenstrual syndrome

Peach-flowered Tea-tree + Fringed Violet + Waratah + She Oak ... for post natal depression

Red Grevillea ... when feeling stuck for a long time and unable to see your way out of it

Sturt Desert Rose ... associated with guilt

Sunshine Wattle ... where life is grim, full of struggle and difficulty without a sense of things getting better or being able to change

Tall Yellow Top ... depression; loneliness; alienation, sense of not belonging

Waratah ... despair, 'black night of the soul'

Waratah + Sunshine Wattle + Tall Yellow Top + Black-eyed Susan + Red Grevillea ... general formula

Wild Potato Bush ... as a result of physical restriction or limitation

despair (*see also* depression; suicide)

Mint Bush ... for the turmoil and void of spiritual initiation

Tall Yellow Top ... comes about from feeling like a 'stranger in a strange land', of never fitting in

Waratah ... for those going through 'dark night of soul'; for dark depression; gives the courage to keep going

detachment (*see also* spirituality)

Black-eyed Susan ... to be able to detach yourself from a busy outer world and find your own still inner sanctuary

Bluebell ... detached and cut off from feelings

Bottlebrush ... letting go of things you don't need; for parents, especially mothers, who need to let go of their children after they have grown

Bush Iris ... being able to let go of physical attachments and not making the physical your only priority

Fringed Violet ... to be with people but not take on their 'stuff'

Lichen Essence ... helps etheric body separate from the physical body, thereby assisting the soul to go through to the Light

Rough Bluebell ... detached from, and having difficulty in expressing, love

Yellow Cowslip Orchid ... staying detached from emotional intensity, and remaining clear and focused

detail, attention to *see* attention to detail

details, over-concern with *see* analytical; fanatical beliefs, behaviour

determination *see* apathy; commitment

developmentally delayed children *see* ADD

disgust *see* body image

direction *see* focus; life direction

disappointment
Banksia Robur ... a temporary loss of drive or enthusiasm due to a disappointment or setback
Bottlebrush ... being able to let go and move on from a disappointment
Freshwater Mangrove ... when a strong expectation about an outcome or a person is not met
Kapok Bush ... not giving up in the face of initial disappointment (Walt Disney went to hundreds of banks, one after the other, seeking a loan so he could create his vision of Disneyland, never letting the disappointment of each successive bank refusal hinder his quest)
Southern Cross ... to see the benefit and lessons to be learned from a disappointment, rather than merely seeing it as a negative experience

discernment (*see also* spirituality)
Angelsword ... allows you to find your own truth, by cutting through information, teachings or channelled messages to find the part, if any, that is right for you
Bush Fuchsia ... also listening to your intuition, to assess a person or situation
Kangaroo Paw ... to realise when and what is appropriate

discipline (*see also* commitment)
Hibbertia ... to be very strong and self-disciplined when the need or situation arises
Jacaranda ... moving from task to task without organisation or self-discipline to complete something
Peach-flowered Tea-tree ... to maintain interest and complete a project after the initial enthusiasm has waned
Red Helmet Orchid ... for individuals, especially adolescents, who rebel against and have trouble accepting authority, rules and regulations
Wedding Bush ... making a decision and sticking to it
Yellow Cowslip Orchid ... can often become disciplinarians because they believe in and love rules and regulations and hate them to be broken

disconnectedness *see* alienation, feelings of; denial; focus

discouragement *see* apathy; disillusionment; optimism

disgust *see* shame

disheartened (*see also* depression; faith; frustration; trust)
Alpine Mint Bush . . . when constant care giving and treating wears down the passion, enthusiasm and vitality of the care giver
Banksia Robur . . . temporary loss of enthusiasm
Kapok Bush . . . where discouragement results in apathy, in the feeling that it is all too much trouble or too hard
She Oak . . . for the disheartening realisation that comes at the beginning of each menstrual cycle to a woman who wants to conceive
Southern Cross . . . where incidents or setbacks occur and you feel 'it's just not fair' and lose interest
Spinifex . . . where no matter what physical treatment you try, the illness or condition, especially a so-called incurable one such as herpes, keeps reappearing and you don't know why, nor how to heal and cure it

dishonesty *see* honesty

disillusionment
Alpine Mint Bush . . . the idealism that carries a person into the work of caring for others can sometimes be snuffed out or replaced by the feeling or belief 'What's the point?', and they wonder if their work really does make any difference in the long run
Illawarra Flame Tree . . . feeling rejected
Isopogon . . . seeing every event in life as a lesson to be learnt
Southern Cross . . . there is always a higher reason behind everything that happens
Southern Cross, Old Man Banksia, Alpine Mint Bush . . . feeling used by others
Sunshine Wattle . . . helps to realise that there is light at the end of the tunnel

disorientation *see* confusion; focus

distancing from others *see* aloof, withdrawn

dithering
Jacaranda . . . for the person with scattered energies who lacks focus
Sundew . . . when procrastinating or vague and dreamy and in a world of your own

divorce *see* separation; grief; relationships

dogmatic *see* fanatical beliefs, behaviour

dominating behaviour
Black-eyed Susan . . . speedy, busy and often impatient people who, almost by osmosis, get other people caught up in their intensity
Boab . . . the conscious or unconscious family projections, especially from parents, onto a child's future and career
Gymea Lily . . . these charismatic, dominating, although sometimes

arrogant, people find it very easy to take control or charge of a situation or the people around them—whether they want to or not
Hibbertia . . . a hard taskmaster who expects others to follow the example they have set and be just like them
Illawarra Flame Tree . . . demanding attention because of fear of rejection
Isopogon . . . controlling, stubborn, sometimes bossy personality type
Rough Bluebell . . . can frequently play the role of martyr in order to control or manipulate others
Yellow Cowslip Orchid . . . they often attempt to impose their structure and models of behaviour, or rules and regulations, on to others

dreams
Bush Fuchsia . . . allows you to tune into and access the dream state
Green Spider Orchid . . . nightmares relating to past times
Grey Spider Flower . . . nightmares of unknown origin
Isopogon . . . dramatically improves dream recall the next morning
Red Lily . . . for grounding after being deep in the dream state
Sundew . . . alleviates excessive daydreaming
Sundew + Bush Fuchsia + Turkey Bush + Red Lily + Green Spider Orchid + Wedding Bush . . . as a special dream mix, these work together to create the clear intention of having, as well as manifesting, the specific theme, person or people you want to have in your dreams that night

drug abuse *see* abusing self; addictions

dutiful, too *see* guilt; responsibility

dyslexia *see* ADD; focus

easily influenced by others
Bush Fuchsia . . . allows person to trust their own intuition and way of doing things rather than doing how or what others tell them
Dog Rose . . . submitting to abuse from others; helps you take a stand when 'enough is enough'
Fringed Violet . . . those who are easily affected by the thoughts and projections of others
Gymea Lily . . . allowing oppression by powerful person or source, such as government or dictator
Illawarra Flame Tree . . . willing to please others to avoid rejection
Jacaranda . . . when insecure about making decisions and always seeking advice of others
Kapok Bush . . . when weak-willed and easily put off or discouraged by the opinions of others
Red Grevillea . . . overly affected by criticism of others
Sturt Desert Rose . . . gives courage to stand up for your own beliefs
Sundew . . . for the dreamy, vague person who is easily pushed or ordered around

eating disorders

Angelsword ... clears negative entities providing false information, such as in anorexia—telling the person not to eat, that they are too fat. It promotes clear communication with the Higher Self as well as discernment to objectively and clearly see, and be aware of, what is really happening (e.g. the person suffering from anorexia who looks in the mirror and falsely perceives herself to be disturbingly fat and alarmingly overweight)

Billy Goat Plum ... for healing any shame, self-disgust or loathing of self or body

Bush Fuchsia ... listening to own intuition about what it is right to eat and when

Crowea ... aids digestive process by regulating the amount of hydrochloric acid in the stomach as well as helping the chronic worrier to be calm, balanced and centred

Dagger Hakea, Mountain Devil, Rough Bluebell ... anger and destructive behaviour directed towards self as in the case of anorexia and bulimia

Dog Rose ... fear and anxiety around food and eating, such as the putting on of weight, or of eating and combining the wrong foods; improves digestion by helping the spleen to absorb the spiritual vapours or essence of the food that we eat, taking it to the pineal gland where it stimulates psychic awareness and perception

Five Corners ... by loving yourself more you engender a greater desire to nurture and honour yourself, to eat good food in sensible amounts and basically live a healthy lifestyle

Grey Spider Flower ... for coping with terror that is felt when realising what damage we are doing to the body by destructive eating habits, or in dealing with the terror of putting on weight or getting too fat

Illawarra Flame Tree ... for feelings of rejection by parents, doctors and friends which can be as a result of, or a cause of, the eating behaviour

Paw Paw ... getting maximum benefit out of food that is eaten

Peach-flowered Tea-tree ... over-preoccupation and worry about self and physical body; improves pancreatic function digestion

Pink Mulla Mulla ... clearing deep psychic scars and emotional blocks around food and eating that have been there a long time

Rough Bluebell ... helps those who are controlling others by abusing their own body, which may be a way of getting attention or of punishing or disturbing others

Sturt Desert Rose ... removes guilt from any binges or indulgences

Sunshine Wattle ... creates a sense of optimism and hope that things can get better

Waratah or Emergency Essence ... the despair, hopelessness and even suicidal feelings associated with anorexia

egocentric *see* dominating behaviour; selfishness

elemental body type
Illawarra Flame Tree ... fire; longish torso with short legs, face triangular
Macrocarpa ... earth; stocky build, square face
Old Man Banksia ... water; either very fine petite build and features or soft and larger build with a round face
Yellow Cowslip Orchid ... air; tall and thin, long oval face

embarrassment *see* shame

emotional blocks (*see also* communication; denial)
Bluebell ... where emotions are suppressed and cut off
Boab ... when you are enmeshed in the old dysfunctional family behaviour patterns where there is much emotional blockage
Flannel Flower ... trusting that it is safe to let out and share with another your darkest and scariest emotional blocks
Pink Mulla Mulla ... very old emotional blocks which have resisted previous clearing
Red Grevillea ... where there is a feeling of being stuck

emotional control
Dog Rose of the Wild Forces ... when in danger of losing control because of intense emotions or energies you are experiencing within or around you
Hibbertia ... to be very strong and self-disciplined when the need or situation arises
Mountain Devil ... for being in control of your temper and anger
Yellow Cowslip Orchid ... allows you to be in control of your emotions and stay very clear, mentally sharp and focused, during chaotic, dangerous or intense situations

emotional upheaval
Bottlebrush ... for coping with and going through major change
Crowea ... calming and centring
Dog Rose of the Wild Forces ... fear of losing emotional control
Emergency Essence ... use frequently in a crisis period
Fringed Violet ... so as not to pick up the energies of upset people around you
Grey Spider Flower ... addresses any terror felt during this time
Mint Bush ... for times of perturbation and confusion
Red Suva Frangipani ... emotional turmoil in relationship break-up or when newly disabled
Sundew ... to stay grounded during emotional upheaval

emotionally closed *see* withdrawal

empathy
Alpine Mint Bush ... carers becoming weary and burnt out from constantly being totally responsible for and worrying about those in their charge

Fringed Violet ... protects the sensitive person from being like a psychic sponge and taking on the problems, energies and feelings of others

Kangaroo Paw ... the positive aspect of this remedy is someone very much aware of the needs of others, especially the host who is able to put himself in the other's position and recognise and meet their needs and difficulties in advance

Old Man Banksia ... helps natural empathetic people to realise their limits and not get overburdened by the problems of others

empowerment (*see also* confidence)

Dog Rose ... gives the strength to stand up for yourself, especially when feeling shy, insecure or insignificant

Five Corners, Confid Essence ... engenders confidence in yourself and your own abilities

Gymea Lily ... gives you the strength to be successful and achieve your destiny despite the influences and reactions of others

Kapok Bush ... empowerment gained through being able to understand and repair machinery or equipment; also empowers by showing all the small steps necessary to achieve a large goal or desire that in itself looks too hard or daunting

Southern Cross ... by taking responsibility for and accepting that you create what happens in your life, it will empower you as you realise that you can also determine and create what you need and desire in your future

Spinifex ... empowers through emotional understanding of the causes of your physical symptoms and diseases

Turkey Bush ... empowerment from creating an amazing artistic piece out of nothing

endocrine system (*see also* hormonal imbalance)

For every endocrine gland there is an Australia Bush Flower Essence which balances it. The following is a list of the major endocrine glands and the corresponding Bush Essence:

pineal ... Bush Iris

hypothalamus ... Bush Fuchsia

pituitary ... Yellow Cowslip Orchid

thyroid ... Old Man Banksia

parathyroid ... Hibbertia

thymus ... Illawarra Flame Tree

adrenals ... Macrocarpa

pancreas ... Peach-flowered Tea-tree

ovaries ... She Oak

testes ... Flannel Flower

endurance

Banksia Robur ... energy levels are much lower than normal because of a setback or illness

Black-eyed Susan ... for the person who goes at top speed all the time and is in danger of emotional and physical burnout

Dog Rose of the Wild Forces ... stops a person from 'snapping' or losing control when being under prolonged stress

Macrocarpa ... for physical stamina and endurance

Mint Bush ... strength to cope with long periods of perturbation, chaos and confusion

Peach-flowered Tea-tree ... for the starter of projects who tends to give up after the initial enthusiam has waned

Sunshine Wattle ... for being able to endure very harsh and difficult circumstances

Waratah ... gives strength, faith and courage to go through a 'black night of the soul'

Wedding Bush ... the total commitment that allows you to go to the very end of your endurance and even past it

energy drain *see* protection

energy lack *see* exhaustion

enlightenment (*see also* spirituality)

Angelsword ... protects you from outside influences and entities so it is possible to receive clear information from your Higher Self without interference

Bush Iris ... helps to open people up to their own spirituality and to access the doorway to their higher perceptions

Red Lily ... for spirituality and connection with God in a grounded and centred way

enthusiasm (*see also* completion)

Banksia Robur ... temporary loss of energy and enthusiasm in the normally energetic person

Gymea Lily ... supports the person willing to follow their passion in life with dedication and enthusiasm

Little Flannel Flower ... helps adults and children to get very involved in all aspects of life with spontaneity and lightness

Peach-flowered Tea-tree ... encourages commitment and energetic follow-through with projects or relationships

environment (*see also* protection)

Black-eyed Susan ... very much an urban remedy for the very active, energetic person living in the fast lane

Boab + Lichen + Angelsword + Fringed Violet ... these essences can be

mixed together in a misting bottle and sprayed around a space or area
to cleanse and clear it of negative energies

Emergency Essence ... to help to strengthen and activate the earth's
energy gridlines, apply topically to the earth, at sacred sites or energy
vortexes, in the form of an encircled Celtic Cross over which you ask
to be used as an instrument for God or the Light, and direct healing
energy out through your hands

Fringed Violet ... to decrease your sensitivity to natural or man-made
pollution

Fringed Violet + Flannel Flower ... where overcrowding makes it difficult
to set healthy boundaries and to keep your own energies to yourself

Green Spider Orchid ... to help you become more aware of the devas,
nature spirits and angelic beings who maintain the balance and energies of the landscape

Mulla Mulla + Waratah + Fringed Violet + Paw Paw + Bush Fusscia +
Crowea ... the radiation combination—to negate or reduce earth radiation, electric radiation, solar radiation, nuclear radiation, X-rays and
radiation therapy used to treat cancer

Red Helmet Orchid ... helps people become aware of, and act respon-
sibly, to help preserve the environment of the whole planet

Tall Mulla Mulla ... helps the natural loner who may find the close
proximity of others when living in a crowded town or city stressful

Wild Potato Bush + Dog Rose + Bottlebrush + Dagger Hakea + Bush
Iris ... removes toxins and heavy metals from the body

envy *see* jealousy

erratic behaviour (*see also* focus; mood swings)
Crowea ... helps to centre, calm and balance
Jacaranda ... for those with scattered energies; dithering; all over the
place
Kangaroo Paw ... for immature, gauche, socially unaware, unpredictable,
unthinking people

escapism (*see also* addictions; denial; procrastination)
Bluebell ... when feelings, emotions are not being acknowledged
Sundew or Red Lily ... grounding; bringing thoughts into focus
Waratah ... gives the courage to face life

exhaustion
Alpine Mint Bush ... for the emotional and physical exhaustion that
comes with the long-term care of others or for the burnout of profes-
sional healthcare workers
Black-eyed Susan ... emotional exhaustion of the 'go-go-go' type of
person who doesn't know when to stop or slow down
Fringed Violet ... when psychically or emotionally drained by others
Macrocarpa ... physical exhaustion, burnout

Mint Bush ... exhaustion arising from being in a state of perturbation or confusion for long periods of time

Old Man Banksia ... exhausted from always being available to listen to or help friends and families when they are in need, or just from their continual ongoing day to day demands and routines

Paw Paw ... exhaustion of a more mental nature, stemming from feelings of overwhelm, whether at work or home

Peach-flowered Tea-tree ... fatigue, exhaustion stemming from low blood sugar levels

Red Suva Frangipani ... exhaustion as a consequence of the emotional upheaval, turmoil and rawness of a rocky relationship

Waratah ... totally drained and exhausted and at the end of your tether

expectation (see also manifestation)

Bauhinia ... you expect any new situation that you are avoiding to be painful on some level

Bush Iris ... when there is the expectation that all life and consciousness ends with physical death

Crowea ... you often expect the worst and worry about it

Freshwater Mangrove ... where expectation of how things are or should be or will be block out or prevent you perceiving other realms of reality

Grey Spider Flower ... expect to be traumatised and terrified whenever you come in contact with your phobia

Mountain Devil ... you expect everyone to be out to use or abuse you; that you can't trust people

Pink Mulla Mulla ... for the expectation that if you open up and get close to people you will get hurt

Spinifex ... where you expect your physical problem, especially any so-called incurable condition such as herpes, to continue

Sunshine Wattle ... helps those who expect life to be grim and an ongoing struggle because of bad past experience

Tall Mulla Mulla ... for those who carry the expectation that they can never have harmony or avoid confrontation when they are with people

experiences, failure to learn from life

Isopogon ... helps to both recall and learn from past experiences

Southern Cross ... for anyone who is unable to make the connection between how the words, thoughts and actions that they put out will come back to them in the creation of their reality. This essence enables a person to realise it is *they* who create their reality and that, if experiences keep recurring, it is not fate and that they can change it so that it doesn't happen again

Spinifex ... the continual reappearance of any illness or symptom picture is an indication that we have not learnt the lesson that it had to teach us

exploitation *see* abusing others

exploration *see* adventure, sense of

extravagance (*see also* abundance, lacking)
Bush Iris . . . where there is over-emphasis on material things
Illawarra Flame Tree . . . dresses and acts, often outrageously, to be noticed; loves creating extravaganzas
Kangaroo Paw . . . they often do things, which at the time can be quite spectacular, without any thought of the cost or consequences
Macrocarpa . . . this constitutional or elemental earth type loves to have things big, although is often more focused on the question of quantity than of quality
Peach-flowered Tea-tree . . . the manic depressive who, when on a high, can do anything
Philotheca . . . for people who are excessively generous

extrovert
Five Corners . . . when you really love yourself and have self-confidence you can fully express your essence. You appear to be extrovert only because you are in such sharp contrast to the majority who are not fully expressing or loving themselves
Gymea Lily . . . glamour seeking; over-enthusiastic about own ideas
Hibbertia . . . the individual who can be quite vocal and expressive in putting forward their ideas and, at the same time, their belief that everyone should be doing and following what they do
Illawarra Flame Tree . . . needing to be centre stage because of fear of rejection; demanding attention because of fear of rejection; dramatising situations
Little Flannel Flower . . . lightness, play and fun takes anyone out of their inhibited self
Macrocarpa . . . this earthy person is very yang in their expression: what you see is what you get; they usually have a strong presence and command their space
Peach-flowered Tea-tree . . . the manic depressive who, when on a high, can do anything

failure (*see also* confidence; discouragement; grief; resignation; success)
Dog Rose . . . where fear of failing manifests as failure itself; for fear of success which will lead to failure
Emergency Essence . . . to deal with the shock and trauma when failure is sudden and unexpected
Five Corners . . . rather than seeing failure as a learning experience, these people 'bash themselves up' and give themselves a really hard time and generally erode away their self-worth. When goals or projects into which a person has put a lot of effort don't succeed, this can often indicate that there is a subconscious sabotage occurring. The bottom

line behind most sabotages is that the person doesn't believe that they are good enough to deserve the goal or project

Isopogon + Southern Cross . . . helps us to learn from our mistakes and failures and move forward in our personal growth

Kapok Bush . . . where failure is a consequence of giving up because it all seemed too difficult, too much effort

Red Suva Frangipani . . . for the period of turmoil when a relationship fails

She Oak . . . failure to conceive

Silver Princess . . . works at helping to find a new direction in life during the period of let-down after something has failed

Sturt Desert Rose . . . to clear any feelings of guilt associated with failure

Sunshine Wattle . . . for when, after one or a series of failures, they feel as if nothing will succeed

Waratah, Tall Yellow Top . . . when depression or despair rises after a failure

fairness *see* justice

faith (*see also* spirituality; trust)

Bush Iris . . . fosters faith; opens up the door to spirituality; to believe in and perceive beyond that the five senses can reveal to you

Grey Spider Flower . . . restores faith and trust while bringing about courage and calm in the face of terror

Pink Mulla Mulla, Tall Yellow Top . . . for the awareness and knowledge that we are never, or never have been, abandoned by spirit

Red Lily . . . opens the crown chakra as well as your spirituality, connecting you to the deepest level of faith by allowing you to realise that you are a loving child of a loving God

Waratah . . . at times of the 'black night of the soul', this essence brings in and restores your spiritual faith and trust that you are never given more than you can cope with

family and social interaction (*see also* bonding; children; communication)

Alpine Mint Bush . . . for those in caring professions or looking after members of the group or family

Bauhinia . . . encourages opening to new ideas and ways of doing things

Bluebell . . . where feelings are not being expressed; opens heart to others

Boab . . . where there is repetition and enmeshment in family patterns and behaviour; for an individual to break the shackles of collective karma that befalls a religious, political or national group

Bush Gardenia . . . it helps to draw together a family who are moving away from one another, busy in their own world

Dagger Hakea . . . for anger and resentment towards partner, friends and family and others who are close to us; the 'forgiveness remedy'

Dog Rose of the Wild Forces ... where there is mass hysteria, frenzy or panic sweeping through a group or crowd

Emergency Essence ... for dealing with any crisis situation

Flannel Flower ... helps you trust and express, especially verbally, your inner feelings; healthy personal boundaries with others

Freshwater Mangrove ... opens heart to others where there has been mental prejudice which has no experiential back-up

Gymea Lily ... for the 'tall poppy' syndrome

Hibbertia ... helps make societal or family theoretical guidelines practical; for those who feel superior to others

Kangaroo Paw ... for immature or selfish behaviour

Slender Rice Flower ... helps people to see beauty in everything and everyone; group harmony and conflict resolution when individual egos get in the way; allows for greater co-operation between people for the common good

Tall Mulla Mulla ... prefer to be by themselves, dislike conflict

Wedding Bush ... deepens commitment to another or to the group

Yellow Cowslip Orchid ... when the society or group becomes too bureaucratic with too many rules and regulations

family feud (*see also* family and social interaction)

Bluebell ... when a feud arises over the issue of money or a will and there is a lack of generosity and sharing between the family members

Boab ... where there is an historical pattern of feuds occurring in the family

Bottlebrush ... when a feud arises between the mother and her children

Dagger Hakea ... anger and bitterness towards a family member or members to such an extent that communications and contact have been severed

Freshwater Mangrove ... where a dispute or feud in the family has continued for so long that younger family members, as a result of conditioning, have accepted one side's view without ever hearing or even meeting relatives from the other side

Mountain Devil ... when a feud that has its origins in early childhood jealousy arises between siblings

Red Helmet Orchid ... for family feuds involving the father and the children

fanatical beliefs, behaviour (*see also* rigidity)

Freshwater Mangrove ... where there is a closed or biased approach to people, places, concepts or things without any experience of them

Hibbertia ... for those fanatical acquirers of knowledge who are driven to improve themselves, which they believe will come about if they know a great deal. Sometimes they see themselves as being, or would like to be, mentally superior to others

Slender Rice Flower ... helps those belonging to one group who have racist or a superior attitude of themselves in regard to or towards other groups. This could, for example, be religious in nature: Protestants feeling they are better than Catholics; or racial: Scots better than the English; or even sexist: women better than men

fantasy *see* imagination

fastidious *see* perfectionist

fatherhood (*see also* adolescence; children; family and social interaction; love; motherhood)
Black-eyed Susan . . . for developing the patience to go at the child's pace rather than at the father's
Boab . . . letting go of all negative preceding family patterns of parenting
Bottlebrush . . . adapting to and coping with continual change
Bottlebrush, Bluebell . . . assisting the parent to lovingly release and let go of their children as they grow up and mature
Bush Fuchsia, Green Spider Orchid, Kangaroo Paw . . . helps build a father's awareness of his child's need
Bush Gardenia . . . for family bonding
Dog Rose . . . fear of not coping
Five Corners . . . helps build confidence in your own ability as a parent
Flannel Flower . . . to help a man express his gentleness and sensitivity and enjoy physical contact with his child
Illawarra Flame Tree . . . where there is a fear of responsibility of fatherhood
Isopogon . . . for very rigid, stubborn, controlling father
Paw Paw . . . to assist in making the best possible choices for the children
Red Helmet Orchid . . . bonding of father with child

fatigue *see* exhaustion

fear
Bauhinia . . . fear of new technology, new situations
Bush Iris, Transition Essence . . . fear of death and dying
Bluebell . . . for fear of lack
Dog Rose . . . for fear generally, niggling fears (e.g. fear of anger, fear of the dark; fear of being in a relationship), anxiety
Dog Rose, Bauhinia, Yellow Cowslip Orchid . . . fear of risk taking
Dog Rose of the Wild Forces . . . fear of losing control, whether that be of your temper, rational mind or experiencing nervous breakdown, being swept up in hysteria or panic
Flannel Flower . . . fear of physical or emotional intimacy
Green Spider Orchid . . . for nightmares from past lives; fear of blood
Grey Spider Flower . . . for extreme terror and immobilising panic (e.g. public speaking for water elements!); phobias; nightmares; or terror that comes on suddenly; fear of psychic attack

Grey Spider Flower + Flannel Flower ... for agoraphobia (fear of open spaces)

Illawarra Flame Tree ... fear of responsibility; fear of rejection

Jacaranda ... fear of making the wrong choice

Mulla Mulla ... fear of heat, fire

Peach-flowered Tea-tree, Dog Rose ... fear of aging; fear of specific illness

Pink Mulla Mulla ... for the person who puts out prickles to keep others away

Sunshine Wattle ... fear of poverty

Tall Mulla Mulla ... for those who fear social interaction; people pleasers

Wedding Bush ... fear of commitment

feeling flat after achieving *see* goal setting

female sexuality, sensuality *see* sexuality

fickle
Jacaranda ... changes mind frequently

fidelity *see* infidelity

flexibility *see* rigidity

focus (*see also* absent-minded)
Boronia ... accentuates the focus for creative visualisation, or whenever something needs to be kept squarely focused on in the mind

Gymea Lily ... the strength to stay focused on and passionately pursue your personal growth

Jacaranda ... where energies are scattered; these people dither and are easily distracted

Red Lily ... it is for spirituality and connection to God in a grounded and centred way. It can be used after any prolonged meditative or spiritual practice to ground and get you back to the day-to-day world

Silver Princess ... helps find direction and focus in life

Sundew ... it enhances attention to detail; for people who daydream, are vague or 'split off' easily, are indecisive and procrastinate

foreign or alien, cultures, problem with *see* adaptability; refugees

forgetfulness *see* memory

forgiveness (*see also* aggressiveness; hatred)
Bottlebrush ... letting go and moving on

Dagger Hakea ... for friends, family and those close to you; it is *the* forgiveness essence

Mountain Devil ... helps to develop unconditional love and acceptance, thereby opening the way to forgiveness of anyone against whom you

have a hatred, anger, suspicion or grudge; it is usually used for people not personally close to you
Sturt Desert Rose ... self-forgiveness

freaked out *see* fear; trauma, shock

freedom (*see also* fear)
Angelsword ... cuts off and frees you from michievous or negative entities
Boab ... free from negative thought and behavioural family patterns
Bottlebrush ... to be free from the shackles of the past and old habits or addictions
Wild Potato ... ability to freely move once again without physical restriction or impediment

frenetic (*see also* hyperactivity)
Black-eyed Susan ... being speedy and always on the go with lots of things happening all at once
Dog Rose of the Wild Forces ... to stay calm and not get caught up in panic or frantic and hysterical scenes
Jacaranda ... intense scattered energy, chaotically moving from one thing to another
Peach-flowered Tea-tree ... for addressing the manic phase in manic depression

frigidity *see* sexuality

frugal *see* abundance, lacking

frustration (*see also* boredom)
Banksia Robur ... for the frustration that these normally vibrant and energetic people feel when, as a result of disappointment, setbacks or poor health, they experience a temporary loss of drive, just not feeling their old selves
Black-eyed Susan ... speedy types who become impatient and irritated when projects, life or people don't go quickly enough for them
Jacaranda ... frustrated by their continued scatty dithering nature
Old Man Banksia ... more the phlegmatic or slower types than the Banksia Roburs and, when disheartened by setbacks and family demands, become weary and frustrated
Peach-flowered Tea-tree ... frustration with boring or mundane activities
Red Grevillea ... knowing change is needed and knowing what it is you want, but feeling stuck and not knowing how, or feeling unable, to do it
Sunshine Wattle ... frustration with life and not seeing it getting any better
Turkey Bush ... the frustration of creative block
Wild Potato Bush ... for people who feel burdened or let down by the

physical body, not being able to do what they want

fun *see* humour; joy

gambling *see* addictions

garrulousness (*see also* dominating behaviour; speech problem)
Bush Fuchsia . . . some children, after their speech difficulties were cleared using this remedy, would speak non-stop for days. Previously they had hardly ever spoken or were incapable of much speech. In a short time this too came into balance
Gymea Lily . . . for those who need to be the centre of attention and dominate conversations
Illawarra Flame Tree . . . these fire types are usually very good—and often dramatic—communicators, who love talking
Jacaranda . . . for the very excitable types, who when in this state speak non-stop, almost in a verbal frenzy. If there are more than a couple of people around they want to speak to everyone at once
Mountain Devil . . . able to rant and rave, curse and swear for very pro-longed periods of time!
Rough Bluebell . . . for the person who talks over others in order to manipulate them
Sturt Desert Rose . . . for those who go on and on apologising for this, apologising for that

gauche *see* immaturity

generosity *see* altruism, kindness

gentleness *see* sensitivity to needs of others

gives up easily *see* resignation

glamour-seeking *see* attention-seeking

gloom *see* depression; disheartened; joy

goal setting
Black-eyed Susan . . . for the 'go-go-go' type person, helping them to slow down and find their quiet inner space where they can become aware of, and know the best way to achieve, their goal
Boronia . . . greatly improves and deepens creative visualisation where you can see and focus on achievement rather than on failure
Bush Fuchsia . . . enhancing intuition so goals may arise from this intui-tive state
Five Corners . . . lacking confidence in own ability; to eliminate subcon-scious sabotage
Green Spider Orchid . . . to keep ideas within and share only when time is right and not dissipate the energy by talking about the goal or project before it is manifested or completed

Hibbertia ... for flexibility and adjustment

Illawarra Flame Tree ... know the goal but fear the responsibility of it

Isopogon ... to prevent repetition of past behaviour or experiences

Jacaranda ... to focus and be still and to complete

Kapok Bush ... giving up and not trying because it is too hard; breaking the goal into smaller parts or steps that can easily be achieved one by one, rather than just seeing one big overwhelming project

Paw Paw ... using own inner wisdom to make decisions; overwhelm from too many ideas

Peach-flowered Tea-tree ... to allay boredom in the middle of it all; for those who start off enthusiastically but later lose interest

Philotheca ... to accept and let in the acknowledgment for achieving the goal

Red Grevillea ... know what the goal is but don't how to achieve it

Silver Princess ... for clearing the let down, 'well, so what?' feeling that can commonly occur straight after the goal has been attained. It gives a sense of the next direction to move on to

Southern Cross ... to empower yourself to create what you want

Sundew ... focusing on what is needed to achieve goal and stopping any procrastination

Sunshine Wattle ... to realise that failure or struggle in past need not be repeated

Wedding Bush ... commitment to the goal

gossiping (*see also* garrulousness)

Green Spider Orchid ... speaking about information before the time is right

Kangaroo Paw ... inappropriate or immature talking about people or situations with a lack of awareness of the consequences

Rough Bluebell ... being indifferent about hurting others to achieve own ends

Sturt Desert Rose ... helps people follow their own inner convictions and morality

greatness *see* confidence; success

greed

Bluebell ... for those afraid to let go of possessions; opens heart to sharing

Bush Iris ... avarice; stuck in materialistic mode

Rough Bluebell ... for manipulative people who take from and use others to achieve their own wants

grief (*see also* death and dying)

Bluebell ... helping to express feelings; to cope with denial

Boronia + Bottlebrush ... pining for partner after relationship break-up

Bottlebrush ... when holding on to grief; helps accept inevitable changes

Dagger Hakea ... anger associated with loss of loved one, loss of job, failure of scheme, etc.

Dog Rose of the Wild Forces ... when emotions are in danger of going out of control

Flannel Flower ... for soothing hurt

Illawarra Flame Tree ... where there are feelings of rejection

Little Flannel Flower ... grief in child after separation from, or death of, parent

Pink Mulla Mulla ... where there was deep hurt that went back perhaps to first incarnation

Red Suva Frangipani ... raw emotions associated with relationship break-up or death of loved one

Sturt Desert Rose ... for guilt associated with loss

Sturt Desert Pea ... for ongoing hurt after loss of loved one; deep hurt going back a long time

Sturt Desert Pea, Red Suva Frangipani ... for sadness

Tall Yellow Top ... when grief is because of feelings of alienation, aloneness

grounding *see* focus

group harmony *see* family and social interaction

grudges, holding *see* resentment

guarding against hurt *see* protection

guidance, spiritual *see* spirituality

guilt
Boab ... the heavy 'duty' message often present in old family patterns

Five Corners ... for some people their self-esteem is so low that they apologise constantly for nearly anything or everything, even when they are not responsible at all

Hibbertia ... their fanatic-like drive to be better or perfect often stems from a sense that they have not done well enough up until now

Sturt Desert Rose ... sexual or religious guilt; guilt about anything you did or did not do in the past; guilt after death of child; young children are very egocentric and if they experience sexual abuse, their parents' divorce or one parent dying, then they often feel they are responsible for it, which produces a lot of guilt

gut feeling, ignoring (*see also* intuition)
Bush Fuchsia ... allows a person to trust and follow their gut feelings

hallucinogenic drugs *see* addictions

handyman skills, enhance *see* practicality

happiness *see* joy

harmony
Black-eyed Susan . . . letting go of impatience and irritation with self and others
Bluebell . . . opening up heart to others
Bush Gardenia . . . deepens relationship between partners and family members
Dagger Hakea . . . for forgiveness of those close to you
Gymea Lily . . . allowing others to contribute and share in group decisions without overriding them
Kangaroo Paw . . . to be aware of the impact of your behaviour on others and to be aware of the needs of others
Little Flannel Flower . . . to allow the qualities of play and spontaneity as well as a sense of humour to come out during interaction with others
Slender Rice Flower . . . helps create group harmony and co-operation
Yellow Cowslip Orchid . . . to be less critical of those around you

hatred (*see also* aggressiveness; love)
Dagger Hakea . . . intense resentment towards family and friends around them which is often bottled up
Dog Rose of the Wild Forces . . . when an individual gets totally swept up by anger or hatred and loses their self-control
Freshwater Mangrove . . . racial prejudice and hatred taken on from family vices and programming
Mountain Devil . . . anger, envy, jealousy and hatred generally; this essence helps to develop unconditional love and acceptance; absence of love
Slender Rice Flower . . . racial prejudice and hatred stemming from an individual's prior experience of that group

head, separated from heart
Hibbertia . . . they often wish to feel mentally superior, constantly devouring information and philosophies. The flower's final message in its Doctrine of Signature—where the petals fall from the dead flower creating a carpet of yellow hearts—is to show that wisdom comes from combining the intellect with the heart
Tall Yellow Top . . . where there is a sense of alienation, separation and you live purely in your head because there is so much pain getting in touch with your feelings
Yellow Cowslip Orchid . . . head cut off from heart as a result of living in your intellect and mind

healers
Alpine Mint Bush . . . those in full-time home caring or professional healing situations who are in danger of burning out from the constant demands and responsibility of looking after others

Angelsword . . . can be used to rub on to your hands when doing spiritual hands-on healing

Bush Fuchsia . . . to enhance your intuition when healing

Flannel Flower . . . to help establish healthy boundaries between them and their clients

Fringed Violet . . . to prevent healer taking on the negative energies of those with whom they work

Green Spider Orchid . . . helps a person to attune and be more receptive when healing or treating animals or plants

Paw Paw . . . to help them absorb and assimilate all the journals and research material they need to keep abreast of

Philotheca . . . for those who can readily give to others but find it difficult to receive

Sturt Desert Rose . . . for releasing any remorse or regret regarding any previous treatments

health threat (*see also* chronic disease)

Banksia Robur . . . brings about enjoyment and interest in life again after, or even during, a threat to your health

Bauhinia . . . to be able to accept and embrace any major physical or appearance changes which results from health changes, whether that be the wearing of glasses, crutches or a prosthesis, or being in a wheelchair

Bluebell . . . for when there is denial about an imminent or current health threat

Fringed Violet . . . to protect you from any negative projections or fears about your condition from people with whom you come in contact

Paw Paw . . . this essence eases any feeling of overwhelm when having to medically assess your current condition and all its implications. It is also beneficial when you need to make a major decision in regard to your health and any possible treatment

Peach-flowered Tea-tree . . . whenever there is over-concern about the physical condition or even hypochondria

Spinifex . . . to help understand the lesson behind the threat

Waratah . . . whenever there is a crisis in the body such as in rejection of a transplanted organ; threat of blindness or heart problems

Wild Potato Bush . . . whenever there is physical restriction or limitation

heart (*see also* love)

Bluebell . . . opens the heart to feelings and especially to love; helps people to share and let go of feelings and beliefs of lack and scarcity

Freshwater Mangrove . . . opens heart to others where there has been mental prejudice towards them

Heartsong Essence . . . opens the heart to love and creative expression

Mountain Devil and Dagger Hakea . . . opening the heart to forgive

Rough Bluebell . . . opening the heart to experience and express the love vibration within

heaviness, feeling of *see* depression

helpless (*see also* co-dependence; empowerment)
Five Corners . . . where there is such a strong sense of lack of self-worth and low self-esteem that an individual feels totally inadequate
Kapok Bush . . . for whenever there is a feeling of resignation or apathy, two emotions guaranteed to create a feeling of helplessness; helps a person to understand or repair objects, instruments or technological equipment—areas in which many people feel helpless
Paw Paw . . . to improve access to Higher Self—your own inner wisdom for whenever you have to make a decision for yourself
Red Grevillea . . . when feeling stuck and unable to achieve your desired outcome
Southern Cross . . . for those with a degree of victim mentality, allowing them to realise and come into their own power
Waratah . . . for courage to do what has to be done

Higher Self, attuning to *see* spirituality

hoarder of things (*see also* addictions; letting go emotionally)
Black-eyed Susan . . . for individuals who are unrealistic about time, believing that in the future they will have enough time to read or go through the things that they are hoarding
Bluebell . . . unable to share possessions, often because of their fear of lack which leads them to hoard things in case of future shortage
Bottlebrush . . . unable to let go of material things, even things of no intrinsic value, or for which they have no need
Sturt Desert Rose . . . for the perceived guilt you will either give to yourself or receive from others by throwing out objects or things that they have given you. This remedy removes any outmoded notions of duty you feel towards the person who gave you the object or towards their memory
Sundew . . . for procrastination which stops you from clearing things out

homesickness *see* lonely

honesty
Flannel Flower . . . for trusting that it is safe to openly and honestly express all that you are feeling
Rough Bluebell . . . for those who play the martyr role in order to deceive and manipulate others and get what they want; for individuals who lie or steal from others without remorse
Sturt Desert Rose . . . helps you be true to your own inner convictions; gives you the strength to publicly own any past actions

Tall Mulla Mulla ... for the people pleasers who say what they think people want to hear

hope (*see also* faith; struggle; trust)
Bush Iris ... fosters faith, hope and belief in life after death and in a spiritual realm
Dog Rose ... by overcoming fear, it restores faith
Kapok Bush ... it removes any feelings of hopelessness, allowing the bright rays of hope to shine
She Oak ... offers hope for conception and motherhood
Sunshine Wattle ... to counter expectation of grim future
Waratah ... for engendering hope in dark, 'black night of the soul' times

hopelessness *see* despair; hope; suicide

hormonal imbalance (*see also* endocrine system)
Bush Fuchsia ... very beneficial for those who have been on 'the contraceptive pill' or HRT for more than six months, as both of these treatments can affect and throw the hypothalamus out of balance: Bush Fuchsia corrects the imbalance
Crowea ... has a general balancing effect on the muscles, meridians, glands, organs and subtle bodies
Peach-flowered Tea-tree ... for mood swings associated with pancreas or ovary imbalance
She Oak ... hormonal imbalance in females resulting in, for example, infertility, PMS, menopausal symptoms

horror movies, after (*see also* protection)
Angelsword ... cuts out and releases any negative energies taken on by the person during the movie
Angelsword + Boab + Fringed Violet ... these three essences can be combined and used as a spray to clear a house or space of any negative energies that have been brought in as a result of the movie being screened or watched there
Boab ... clears negative thought patterns and entities emerging in a group or specific space
Dog Rose ... feeling nervous or fearful after horror movies
Fringed Violet ... for shock or trauma as a result of seeing horror movies
Grey Spider Flower ... for terror, fear that comes on suddenly
Sundew or Red Lily ... grounding for the spaced-out feeling after TV or movie, bringing back to reality

hostility *see* anger; aggressiveness

humility *see* arrogance

humour (*see also* seriousness)
Hibbertia ... very serious and often unable to laugh at themselves

Little Flannel Flower . . . to release the fun, spontaneity and lack of self-consciousness of the child within

Yellow Cowslip Orchid . . . very dry, sharp wit which can be cutting and sarcastic at times; can be laconic in their humour

hurt and pain *see* grief

hurt feelings, injured pride

Illawarra Flame Tree . . . feelings of rejection, real or imagined

Red Grevillea . . . for those overly influenced by the criticism of others

hurt, unable to resolve very old

Pink Mulla Mulla . . . for those who have suffered a deep spiritual wound long ago, which has led to a deep scar on the soul and psyche

hyperactivity (*see also* ADD)

Black-eyed Susan . . . helps to bring emotions into balance; helps to find still quiet place within

Bush Fuchsia . . . to balance brain activity; for learning problems

Jacaranda . . . for poor attention span and behaviour that is erratic, scattered and restless

Red Helmet Orchid . . . where there are problems dealing with authority figures, such as teachers in a classroom situation

Sundew . . . for focus and concentration

hypersensitivity (*see also* protection; sensitivity to needs of others)

Angelsword . . . to release any energies that have been taken on when the aura has been open

Dog Rose of the Wild Forces . . . taking on emotional turmoil from those around them

Fringed Violet . . . for period after birth, re-birth, catharsis or shock—when a person is very susceptible and sensitive

Illawarra Flame Tree . . . for those who are deeply hurt by rejection, real or imagined

Red Grevillea . . . over-sensitive to opinions and criticism of others

Red Suva Frangipani . . . for the red raw feelings associated with the end of, or turmoil in, a relationship

Yellow Cowslip Orchid . . . excessively critical and judgmental; 'nitpicking'

hypochondria

Peach-flowered Tea-tree . . . for preoccupation with own health

Spinifex . . . when over-concern for any health problem arises because of lack of understanding of the cause of the symptoms or condition

hypocrisy *see* honesty

identity (*see also* confidence, self esteem)

Angelsword . . . enables an individual to be aware if messages are coming from their own Higher Self or from entities outside of them

Billy Goat Plum ... for a positive physical sense of self and identity

Boab ... to be aware of what is you and what is the overlay of family and inherent emotional patterns

Bottlebrush ... to let go of old and outmoded self-images and identities

Bush Iris ... allows you to experience the spiritual and therefore see yourself as a spiritual being

Five Corners ... for a strong and positive sense of self

Philotheca ... allows you to both recognise and acknowledge your self for your positive attributes and achievements as well as allowing you to be open to receiving acknowledgment from others; consequently a strong self-image is created and/or reinforced

Tall Yellow Top ... for the person who has a sense of alienation from others; it engenders acceptance of themselves and where they fit in their society or family

imagination *see* creativity

immaturity (*see also* adolescence; fatherhood; motherhood)

Bottlebrush ... a first-time mother with the ongoing responsibility of a young baby will often, by necessity, mature quickly

Dog Rose ... many children, and even adults, who are shy and fearful developed these traits as a result of being intimidated and picked on by older siblings, or even one or both parents when they were small

Dog Rose of the Wild Forces ... the inability to keep your own balance and not get swept up in your own emotions or what is going on around you can sometimes be a consequence of immaturity

Kangaroo Paw ... for immature, gauche and naive behaviour

Red Grevillea ... in some instances the sense of 'stuckness' could be resolved with more life experience or a broader view of your situation

Red Helmet ... parenthood is a wonderful opportunity for a man to develop his maturity and sense of responsibility. This essence helps men having difficulty with both, which can manifest in a poor bond the man has with his children or in him being an absent father

Turkey Bush ... if a person starts painting or drawing as an adult for the first time since they were seven or eight, then their drawing will initially resemble an eight-year-old's. Turkey Bush will help them to accept their art and encourage them to continue with it

impartiality (*see also* awareness; justice; narrow-minded)

Alpine Mint Bush ... a good and effective care giver or healer needs to be able to keep separate their own issues from the person they are helping during a treatment or consultation

Freshwater Mangrove ... by suspending your preconceived ideas and prejudices you can then be open to new perceptions and experiences

Sturt Desert Rose ... helps you decide what is in your best interest to do, away from the bias, pressures and expectations of the people around you

Yellow Cowslip Orchid ... engenders the ability to stand aside from emotional issues and assess a situation objectively

impatience

Black-eyed Susan ... for quick thinkers and movers who become frustrated with others and themselves when things are all moving too slowly

Gymea Lily ... for natural leaders who are used to taking control of a situation, to assist them to step back and allow others to voice their opinions and have their input

Jacaranda ... allows them to be fully focused in what they are doing and not be distracted by, or become impatient to start, other projects—even if the current one is not finished

Peach-flowered Tea-tree ... they become impatient and bored when there is no longer a challenge in what they are doing

impulsiveness (see also extrovert; impatience)

Black-eyed Susan ... their impatience to complete things quickly can often lead them to making short-term decisions without necessarily taking the long-term consequences fully into account

Illawarra Flame Tree ... for those who are very impulsive talkers or communicators

Jacaranda ... where a person starts lots of different things but is scattered and lacks focus and direction

Kangaroo Paw ... for the person who jumps in 'boots and all' without any thought of the possible consequences

Peach-flowered Tea-tree ... where a person launches enthusiastically into a new scheme or relationship but loses interest once it becomes mundane

inadequacy see confidence

inappropriate behaviour see immaturity

incest (see also abuse, victim of; sexuality)

Billy Goat Plum ... for any feelings of shame or embarrassment as a consequence of incest

Bottlebrush ... helps balance the mother and child relationship when incest is involved

Fringed Violet + Wisteria + Flannel Flower ... for sexual abuse in females

Fringed Violet + Flannel Flower ... for sexual abuse in males

Little Flannel Flower ... for the child who is or has been sexually abused

Red Helmet Orchid ... helps balance the father and child relationship when incest is involved

Rough Bluebell ... putting your own needs first and not caring about the consequences to others

indecision *see* decision making

independence (*see also* co-dependence)
Boab ... where the traditional family pattern is to encourage dependence on the extended family unit, this essence will give the courage to break out and be yourself
Bottlebrush ... to help with letting go of the past and coping with the changes of life
Confid Essence ... will boost sense of self-worth and trust in your own abilities
Dog Rose ... where fear, shyness and apprehension of others prevents independence of action
Five Corners ... for anyone who, as a consequence of low self-esteem, lacks the courage to be up-front and be themselves
Gymea Lily ... strength to go out on a limb to follow your passion
Illawarra Flame Tree ... for self-reliance, self-approval and a willingness to accept responsibility
Red Grevillea ... helps reduce undue reliance on the opinion of others
Southern Cross ... for self-empowerment, no longer blaming others for life's vagaries
Waratah ... promotes courage when things are very black by calling on long forgotten survival skills

inferiority *see* confidence

infertility
Five Corners ... for some women their inability to have a child affects their whole self-worth as a woman
Flannel Flower ... when infertility is due to low sperm count or any other cause in the male
Flannel Flower + She Oak ... to clear any karmic blocks that may be hindering conception. She Oak should be taken by itself for six months before commencing this combination. If taken together straight away, as a short cut, it will not bring about the desired result
Flannel Flower + She Oak + Red Grevillea + Dagger Hakea + Slender Rice Flower ... whenever there are problems of incompatibility between the pH of the sperm and that of the vaginal secretions
She Oak ... inability to conceive, whether it be from a physical or an emotional cause. This essence rehydrates the uterus and regulates hormonal balance for women
Spinifex ... can help heal the scarring in the fallopian tubes caused by chlamydia. In Australia over 1000 women a year become infertile as a result of this problem
Sturt Desert Rose ... whenever there is any guilt, regret or remorse about

anything a woman did or did not do that might have affected her
ability to conceive (e.g. having a termination when she was younger).
This essence will also alleviate any feelings that she has let down her
partner or her parents who wish to be grandparents

Turkey Bush . . . works with creativity on all levels and having a child is
the most creative act of all

infidelity
Boab + Boronia + Bottlebrush + Bush Iris + Flannel Flower + Wedding
Bush . . . helping to heal sex addiction

Bush Gardenia . . . renewing passion and interest when boredom or staleness has crept into a relationship

Dagger Hakea . . . for those who seek to take out revenge on a partner

Wedding Bush . . . helps to deepen the commitment to a partner

Five Corners . . . to bolster self-esteem and prove to themselves that they
are still sexually attractive and capable

Flannel Flower . . . to increase honest, open sharing in communication in
a relationship; creates gentle and sensitive physical intimacy

Kangaroo Paw . . . where behaviour is immature, causing unrealised hurt

Rough Bluebell . . . deliberately attempts to manipulate and hurt others

Sturt Desert Rose . . . to help restore trust of your partner if you have
been unfaithful

inflexible *see* rigidity

inhibitions (*see also* boundaries, establishing healthy; extrovert;
introversions)

inner child (*see also* children; grief)
Bottlebrush + Red Helmet . . . addresses mother and father relationship
and related issues

Five Corners . . . the most important goal in our inner child work is self-
love and acceptance

Fringed Violet . . . will dissipate an old trauma that goes back a long way,
especially one associated with the birth process

Little Flannel Flower . . . helps people to get in touch with the child within
and to play and be playful—a great remedy for everyone

Red Lily . . . to realise you are a loving child of a loving God

Southern Cross . . . for whenever your inner child feels it's not fair, that
life is doing to you rather than you are creating life

Sturt Desert Pea . . . for old deep hurt and pain that is often carried but
not let out

Sundew . . . for when a young child has learnt to cope with trauma or
abuse by 'splitting' from their physical body

inner strength (*see also* commitment; confidence)

Dog Rose of the Wild Forces ... to find your own inner strength in order to stop you losing control in any situation
Sturt Desert Rose ... helps people follow their own inner convictions and morality
Waratah ... engenders strong faith and courage when things are at their darkest
Wedding Bush ... this essence helps you to draw on your inner strength in order to keep and uphold your commitments

inquisitive, open mind (*see also* closed mind; fanatical beliefs, behaviour; narrow-minded)
Bauhinia ... open and interested in anything new
Freshwater Mangrove ... opens an individual to perceptions outside the common reality
Kapok Bush ... helps to bring an appreciation of how things work
Little Flannel Flower ... helps to see things with the mind of a child—with openness, excitement and curiosity
Yellow Cowslip Orchid ... aids the ability to grasp concepts quickly and be aware of and interested in the detail

insanity (*see also* depression; mental illness; nervous breakdown)
Black-eyed Susan + Crowea + Peach-flowered Tea-tree ... for severe mood swings
Bush Fuchsia ... balancing brain function
Dog Rose of the Wild Forces ... fear of totally losing control
Emergency Essence ... for any crisis
Sundew ... disassociatedness; vagueness; sense of being split
Tall Yellow Top ... sense of abandonment, isolation and of just not belonging
Waratah ... going through 'black night of the soul'; despair; hopelessness; suicidal feelings
Yellow Cowslip Orchid, Isopogon ... loss of memory, weakening of the intellect

insecurity (*see also* confidence)
Dog Rose ... niggling fears; apprehensive with other people
Tall Mulla Mulla ... feeling unsafe when interacting with others

insensitivity *see* sensitivity to needs of others

insight *see* intuition

insomnia (*see also* sleep)
Black-eyed Susan ... for the 'go-go-go' type person who can't turn off; *the* stress remedy
Boronia ... to still the racing mind
Crowea ... for the worrier; brings calmness and helps to centre
Emergency Essence ... can help reduce stress and so induce sleep

Green Spider Orchid . . . where there are nightmares associated with past times
Grey Spider Flower . . . where there are nightmares or night terrors from this life or of unknown origin

instability (*see also* stability)
Sundew, Red Lily . . . to help ground and focus

integrity *see* guilt

intellect, living in (*see also* head, separated from heart)
Hibbertia . . . addicted to acquiring knowledge; inflexible, dogmatic
Isopogon . . . cut off from feelings; not learning from experience; may be powerful, demanding, intolerant
Tall Yellow Top . . . living purely in the head; cut off from feelings; isolated
Yellow Cowslip Orchid . . . focused in intellect; tends to be legalistic, judgmental

intensity
Black-eyed Susan . . . for the 'go-go-go' person who can't turn off
Dog Rose of the Wild Forces . . . where you are in danger of taking on intense emotions from others

intimacy *see* boundaries, establishing healthy sexuality

intolerance *see* closed mind

introversions
Dog Rose . . . for the shy person
Five Corners, Confid Essence . . . for confidence and feeling of wellbeing about self
Cognis Essence . . . for mental clarity and focus
Meditation Essence . . . to find quiet place within
Pink Mulla Mulla . . . for the person who puts out prickles to keep others at a distance
Tall Mulla Mulla . . . when not comfortable interacting with others

intuition (*see also* spirituality)
Angelsword . . . allows for clear communication with your Higher Self and angelic being and also removes negative or mischievous attached entities that are supplying false information to the individual
Boronia . . . helps find quiet place within by stilling repetitive thoughts
Bush Fuchsia . . . *the* remedy to enhance intuition: encourages sharpening of, and trust in, your own intuition
Bush Iris . . . opens the third eye, allows you to trust and be aware of the spiritual—what lies beyond the five senses
Green Spider Orchid . . . attunes you to be more receptive

Hibbertia ... helps apply learnt skills and inner knowledge and accept and utilise your own wisdom

Paw Paw ... accesses your Higher Self so you can better hear your own inner wisdom when there is a choice to be made between two or more things

Red Lily ... opens the crown chakra which in turn leads to greater awareness and intuition

irrational behaviour (*see also* mental illness; mood swings)
Angelsword ... where an individual's behaviour is influenced, even determined, by an entity or entities other than the self

Boab ... when the person's behaviour is masked or overshadowed by old family patterning and beliefs which can be out of character for that individual

Bottlebrush ... where addictive behaviour is out of character for an individual

Dog Rose ... when fear evokes unexpected and unusual behaviour from the individual

Dog Rose of the Wild Forces ... where something in the individual snaps and they lose control and do things they normally wouldn't

Jacaranda ... where your behaviour is very scattered and all over the place

Kangaroo Paw ... for the immature person who acts irresponsibly

Mountain Devil ... sudden and violent outbursts of rage

Peach-flowered Tea-tree ... for mood swings or fluctuations that can range from PMS to manic depression

irresponsible (*see also* responsibility)
Illawarra Flame Tree ... unwilling to take on responsibility (usually due to fear)

Jacaranda ... starting projects but rarely finishing them as you are easily distracted

Kangaroo Paw ... immature, erratic behaviour with no thought of the consequences

irritable (*see also* annoyance at others)
Bauhinia ... being irritated by a person or people who do things very differently to you

Black-eyed Susan ... annoyance or impatience with others who are less efficient or quick

Crowea ... where irritation comes from worry

Dagger Hakea ... irritation towards those immediately and intimately close to you

Dog Rose ... when fear or anxiety results in irritable behaviour

Paw Paw ... when irritability stems from being overwhelmed and stretched by events or situations

isolation *see* lonely

'it's not fair' *see* victim

jealousy (*see also* anger)
Mountain Devil ... jealousy, envy, suspicion or sibling rivalry
Slender Rice Flower ... envious of others on racial grounds; comparing
  with others

jet lag
Travel Essence ... take morning and night the day before and for a few
  days after a long flight, but hourly while awake on the plane. This
  combination enables you to arrive at your destination feeling balanced
  and ready to go. There are eleven essences in Travel Essence, including
  Bush Iris, which works specifically on the pineal gland (the pineal
  gland regulates the body clock)

joy
Alpine Mint Bush ... revitalisation of carers who have lost their joy
Banksia Robur ... enjoyment of life; energy and enthusiasm
Billy Goat Plum ... sexual pleasure and enjoyment of your body
Bluebell ... opening heart and joyful sharing
Five Corners ... love, acceptance and celebration of the self, leading to
  joyousness
Little Flannel Flower ... releasing child within; carefree and playful
Red Lily ... the joy that stems from the awareness and knowing that
  you are the loving child of a loving God
Silver Princess ... the tremendous joy of knowing that you are on track
  in your life, knowing that you are doing what you came here to do
Sunshine Wattle ... optimism; acceptance of beauty and joy in the
  present

judgmental
Five Corners ... for the person who is overly critical of themselves
Freshwater Mangrove ... for those who judge others because of learnt
  mental prejudice
Slender Rice Flower ... for the narrow-minded person, the racist; helps
  with seeing beauty in others
Sturt Desert Rose ... being true to yourself in your own choices, not
  being swayed or influenced away from that by anyone or anything
Yellow Cowslip Orchid ... *the* remedy for judgmental people. They can
  be highly critical and bureaucratic. They have a lot of *inner* as well as
  outer rules and regulations, and become very upset and critical of those
  transgressing them. Often the criticised people aren't aware of these
  rules they have broken. This essence brings about awareness of the
  bigger spiritual picture, that everyone is doing the best they can and

attempting to express themselves in a more positive way—even the most 'evil' person on the planet

justice (*see also* balance)

Gymea Lily . . . helps powerful people treat those in their power fairly

Southern Cross . . . to realise that nothing happens by chance or coincidence. We reap what we sow and we pull in the experiences that we need in order to grow

Yellow Cowslip Orchid . . . allows an individual to be emotionally impartial, see both sides of the situation and take all this into consideration with existing laws to reach a fair judgment

karma

Bluebell, Red Lily, Waratah . . . for opening the crown and heart chakras to the greatest magnitude of love which in turn can transmute much karma

Boab . . . will clear lines of karma between people so that they do not need to interact with each other and pay-back old scores this lifetime

Flannel Flower . . . can be added to She Oak if, after taking the latter for six months, no conception has occurred. It will then help to clear any karmic blocks that may be preventing conception

kindness *see* altruism, kindness

laughter *see* humour; joy

laziness (*see also* apathy)

Kapok Bush . . . giving up; unwilling to try because it seems too difficult

Rough Bluebell . . . manipulating others to do things for you

Sundew . . . dreamy, vague, ungrounded

leadership

Black-eyed Susan . . . slowing down and finding that still centre within, where abides your inner guidance of what needs to be done, then expressing that out in the world with decisive action

Bush Fuchsia . . . to clearly express and project yourself to others; being open to your own intuition and inner guidance when making your decisions and actions

Dog Rose of the Wild Forces . . . the ability to stay calm, centred and in control in times of inner or outer turmoil is a quality of great leaders

Five Corners . . . the inner strength expressed by one who is self-loving and confident will always inspire those people around them

Gymea Lily . . . enhances an individual to make decisions and take control, at the same time allowing strong, natural leader types to allow others to contribute without being overridden

Illawarra Flame Tree . . . to inspire and enthuse others with a vision or quest or higher purpose

Macrocarpa . . . these earth elements have a strong sense of presence and command; they can be easily used to galvanised those in their command

Sturt Desert Rose ... being true to yourself, making a decision and not being swayed away from it by others

Yellow Cowslip Orchid ... they make effective leaders by being able to see both the big picture and the detail, consequently their choices are usually wise and beneficial

Waratah ... their strength and courage in a crisis can inspire others

learning (*see also* ADD; children; focus)

Bush Fuchsia ... clears dyslexia by integrating left and right, front and back hemispheres of the brain; improves co-ordination, speech, reading and all learning skills

Cognis Essence ... for strengthening all areas of learning

Isopogon ... where there is inability to learn from past experiences; aids memory and helps to improve it

Kapok Bush ... helps you to learn and understand how technical machinery operates by bringing an awareness of its overall function, and then of each individual step or component that is incorporated to achieve this

Paw-Paw ... will improve the absorption and integration of new ideas and information

Southern Cross ... realising that every obstacle in life is a lesson to be learnt

Sundew ... helps particularly with children who have not united well with Spirit; where there is a feeling of being split; especially when they are vague or dreamy, helps with focus and concentration

Yellow Cowslip Orchid ... where aloofness and withdrawal result in weakened intellect

let down after the end of a project (*see also* goal setting)

Black-eyed Susan ... for the 'go-go-go' person who can't stop even though the job is complete

Boronia ... for someone who can't stop thinking about what they have just completed

Silver Princess ... helps to formulate new direction and goals, thereby resolving any flatness or let-down that commonly occurs when one goal has been achieved—especially if the focus has been on the outcome of the goal, not so much the journey within it

lethargy (*see also* apathy; tiredness)

Banksia Robur ... for temporary loss of energy and enthusiasm in people who are usually dynamic and full of vitality. A great one for chronic fatigue or ME

Kapok Bush ... lack of motivation and enthusiasm

Macrocarpa ... physical burnout; increases stamina and endurance

Old Man Banksia ... for phlegmatic or ayuvedic kapha constitutional types who are low in energy and weary

letting go emotionally (*see also* emotional blocks)
Boronia ... helping those who are infatuated with or obsessed by someone else
Bottlebrush ... coping with life changes and the ability to let go what was; breaking old habits and letting go of things that are no longer needed
Bottlebrush, Red Helmet Orchid ... work to release any old unresolved mother and father issues an individual may have
Fringed Violet ... releases the shock and trauma of any previous incident which can keep the person, on some level, back at that time
Mint Bush ... helps cope with the burning off of the dross—an essential process which almost invariably precedes you moving to new higher spiritual level
Sturt Desert Pea ... dealing with and releasing old, deep hurt
Sundew ... releasing any preoccupation with the past or future to be fully present in the now
Transition Essence ... as well as being used to assist an individual pass over gently, calmly and with dignity, it can also help an old part of yourself to 'die' so as to clear the way to move forward

life direction (*see also* goal setting)
Bauhinia ... where there is an unwillingness to venture into new areas of life
Boab ... to clear the family patterns and beliefs around career, money, etc. that can swamp the essence of a person and their knowing of what they are here to do
Boronia ... when your options about a life decision keep going round and round in your head
Bottlebrush ... when, in following your life purpose, you are led into a brand new area or phase of life. This essence assists the transition and any associated difficulties with it
Five Corners ... for people who believe they are not good enough or don't deserve to be what they want to be
Gymea Lily ... giving support to go 'out on a limb', to aim high
Kapok Bush ... for the child or adult who won't try to achieve and fulfil their dreams and visions because it all seems too hard and difficult
Paw Paw ... helping with the overwhelm in making decisions about a new direction in your life
Silver Princess ... for finding your life direction when you are at a cross-road and not sure where to go, or when you are still seeking what it is you are here to do
Sturt Desert Rose ... to galvanise your inner strength to follow your

own career and dreams and not be talked out of it, especially by parents projecting their own expectations on to you

listening
Alpine Mint Bush ... for individuals worn out and burdened by constantly listening to the problems of those in their charge

living in present (*see also* absent-minded; focus)
Bush Fuchsia ... to listen to and trust your intuition
Bush Gardenia ... improves interest in communication and awareness of what your partner or family are saying and doing
Green Spider Orchid ... helps you to attune and listen to other people, species, life forms and kingdoms
Kangaroo Paw ... improves sensitivity to really hear and be aware of the needs of others
Philotheca ... enables you to hear and accept praise, acknowledgment from others
Spinifex ... to listen to what messages your Higher Self and body are conveying to you through physical symptoms

lonely
Flannel Flower ... where any sort of closeness or intimacy is uncomfortable and difficult
Gymea Lily ... feeling very alone when striving to totally fulfil your highest life purpose and reach great heights, or when breaking away from concensus reality and realising there aren't too many like-minded people there with you
Illawarra Flame Tree ... for any feelings of rejection or being unappreciated
Pink Mulla Mulla ... for those who won't let others get close through fear of being hurt again
Tall Mulla Mulla ... feeling unsafe about mixing with other people
Tall Yellow Top ... feeling isolated, alienated or abandoned

long-term illnesses *see* chronic disease

love (*see also* caring for others)
Bluebell ... opening the heart to love and sharing, especially useful for those who feel there is a limit to the amount of love they have available to give out and therefore withhold themselves, and their love, from others
Dagger Hakea ... creates love and forgiveness by releasing any stored resentment to those people to whom you are close
Dog Rose ... to quote: 'Love is letting go of fear'
Five Corners ... everyone can do with a little bit more self-love and self-worth. This is the essence just for that
Flannel Flower ... allows you to trust that it is safe to express yourself

and your feelings to others. The more you are able to reveal yourself, the more you are able to be loved by those to whom you have revealed yourself

Freshwater Mangrove ... allows the love vibration to destroy previously held prejudice towards other people or groups

Mountain Devil ... transmuting anger and resentment to unconditional love

Philotheca ... encourages an individual to be open to receive and accept love and acknowledgment from others and Spirit

Pink Mulla Mulla ... when a person chooses to move away from love and contact with others from a fear of being hurt again

Red Lily ... to help you realise that you are a loving child of a loving God

Red Helmet Orchid and Bottlebrush ... establishing and re-opening loving bonds and connections between children and fathers and mothers, respectively

Red Suva Frangipani ... for the immediate intense pain and turmoil you feel when there is the threat or the reality of a loved one leaving through separation or even death

Rough Bluebell ... for the release of your inherent love vibration from within

Slender Rice Flower ... for the realisation that we are all one and for engendering unconditional love

Tall Yellow Top ... these people have a chasm in their hearts from abandonment or alienation which has cut them off from love and other people

lying *see* honesty

male sexuality *see* sexuality

maliciousness *see* aggressiveness

manifestation
Boronia ... enhancing the ability to hold fully present in front of you a strong clear image in creative visualisation; the more you can see and focus on what you want and the more you see yourself in that situation, having or doing it, the quicker and easier it is to manifest it in your life

Dog Rose ... whatever you focus on and especially fear, you will attract, so if you are manifesting snakes in your life it is usually because you are focusing on or fearing them

Silver Princess ... having a sense of your direction in the next stage of your life, even in your life purpose, makes it much easier to manifest and move along your path

Sundew ... allows for great attention to detail: the more specific and clear you can be in writing down what it is you want, the easier it is to manifest your goals; if you tell the Universe you want a car, it is happy to give you one, but it is not its fault if it gives you an old rusty bomb when you really wanted a new Jaguar sports convertible—just because you forgot to be specific!

Turkey Bush ... empowerment from creating an amazing artistic piece out of nothing

manipulative behaviour *see* abusing others; dominating behaviour

marriage *see* family and social interaction; relationships

martyr *see* dominating behaviour; victim

materialism (*see also* greed)
Bluebell ... unable to share possessions because of fear of lack
Bush Iris ... for the person stuck in a purely materialistic way of life—the 'sex and drugs and rock'n roll' remedy

maths, problems with *see* **learning**

maturity *see* immaturity

meditation (*see also* spirituality)
Boronia ... enhances the ability to maintain intense focus during creative visualisation or in guided meditation. It also clears the mind of thoughts, especially any obsessive repetitive ones
Bush Fuchsia ... to access and trust your intuition
Bush Iris ... allows you to go deeper in any religious, spiritual or meditative practice
Green Spider Orchid ... to attune and to be more receptive to other people, plants or animals while in a meditative state
Meditation Essence ... to meditate more deeply and in a totally protected space
Paw Paw ... to be open to your Higher Self and so your own inner wisdom

melancholy *see* depression; grief

memory (*see also* absent-minded; learning)
Isopogon ... to boost memory; opens subconscious to retrieve previously learnt information and forgotten skills
Red Lily, Sundew ... helps with focus and concentration
Waratah ... helps retrieve forgotten survival skills in times of crisis

menopause (*see also* Repertory of Physical Symptoms)
Bottlebrush ... for accepting and adapting to such a major change within your body and psyche
Illawarra Flame Tree ... where there is a fear of rejection from your partner

Macrocarpa ... to boost the action of the adrenal glands which produce small amounts of oestrogen

Mulla Mulla ... for hot flushes

Peach-flowered Tea-tree ... for mood swings

She Oak ... balances the ovaries and female hormones, maintaining sufficient levels of oestrogen to offer a viable alternative to hormone replacement therapy without the risk of increased breast or cervical cancer. (It is used in this way in hospitals in South America and Europe.)

mental clarity *see* focus

mental illness (*see also* depression; insanity; nervous breakdown; obsessiveness; phobias; psychosis; schizophrenia)

Sturt Desert Pea ... where there is stored such deep grief, hurt and pain that the person becomes disassociated and splits and their emotional self becomes suppressed and cognitive function fuzzy

Sundew ... for grounding, steadying, bringing back to reality

Tall Yellow Top ... where there is a sense of isolation, alienation and depression. It gives you a sense of belonging and spiritual nurturing

Waratah ... for black despair

mental retardation

Billy Goat Plum ... for any feelings of shame or embarrassment at being different from others

Boab ... where there is an inherited or genetic factor

Bush Fuchsia ... integrates the hemispheres of the brain

Fringed Violet ... whenever there has been birth trauma, such as the umbilical cord being wrapped around the throat and blocking oxygen supply to the brain of the newborn

Green Spider Orchid ... to help with communication where retardation affects hearing or speech

Sundew ... whenever there is a sense of disconnectedness

Yellow Cowslip Orchid ... it brings the pituitary gland into balance which can help in some cases

Wild Potato Bush ... for dealing with the frustrations of not being able to express yourself or communicate as easily as others

mind, overactive

Black-eyed Susan ... for the very active person who cannot slow down; always thinking of things to do or to be done

Boronia ... helps stop the same thought from going over and over in your mind

Crowea ... where worries keep turning over in your mind

Hibbertia ... for the over-disciplined person who concentrates too much on intellectual pursuits

Jacaranda ... where the mind is all over the place; no focus of attention

Yellow Cowslip Orchid . . . for the intellectual who ignores the heart and works solely from the head

money *see* abundance, lacking

mood swings
Black-eyed Susan . . . carried away by own enthusiasm and so becoming impatient, irritable
Jacaranda . . . scattered energies where interest and attention can quickly fluctuate
Peach-flowered Tea-tree . . . for any mood swings, ranging from premenstrual tensions to manic depression; where early enthusiasm dissipates because there is no longer any challenge
Sundew, Red Lily . . . for grounding and concentration

morality (*see also* commitment; guilt)
Bottlebrush + Red Helmet Orchid . . . exercising the full morality of parenthood by teaching the children through embodying and displaying your ethics, virtues and philosophies in your actions
Bush Iris . . . having a spiritual overview and awareness in which to frame your philosophies and morality, and be guided beyond mere physical pleasures and gratification
Crowea . . . for concern and consideration of others
Gymea Lily . . . helping to remain within your own morality when in a position of power; the commitment to fulfil yourself to the highest level
Hibbertia . . . striving to develop your ethics and virtues to their highest level
Mint Bush . . . when in the process of redefining your values and beliefs as you grow so that the previous ones become redundant and obsolete
Red Lily . . . allows the purity of spirit and humanity to evolve to their highest level
Rough Bluebell . . . of being aware and conscious of not hurting anyone by your actions, thoughts or words
Sturt Desert Rose . . . the strength to follow your own convictions and morality, to do what you know you must do
Wedding Bush . . . to add strength and commitment to maintaining your values and morality when faced with temptation
Yellow Cowslip Orchid . . . reinforces your commitment to doing the right thing and being very honourable; of putting values that benefit society before your own wants and needs

motherhood (*see also* adolescence; children; family and social interaction; fatherhood; love; pregnancy and birth; relationships)
Alpine Mint Bush . . . for any mental or emotional weariness or exhaustion arising from being in a constant caring role

Bluebell + Bottlebrush ... assisting the parent to lovingly release and let go of their children as they grow up and mature

Boab ... letting go of preceding negative family patterns of parenting

Bottlebrush ... bonding of mother with child; adapting to continual inevitable change

Bush Fuchsia ... to trust and follow their intuition and instinctive wisdom while mothering

Bush Fuchsia, Green Spider Orchid, Kangaroo Paw ... help build parents' awareness of the needs of the child

Bush Gardenia ... for family bonding

Dog Rose ... fear of not coping

Five Corners ... helps build confidence in own ability as parent

Flannel Flower ... to establish healthy boundaries with the child; to engender an easy, comfortable and loving, touching and physical relationship with the child

Illawarra Flame Tree ... where there is a fear of the responsibility of parenthood

Isopogon ... for overly rigid, stubborn, controlling parents

Paw Paw ... to assist in making the best possible choices for the children

Philotheca ... to be aware of and acknowledge their own needs, not just giving to others

Red Grevillea ... addresses the sense of frustration and restriction of being stuck at home with a young family

She Oak ... to help realign a woman's hormones and physical body after birth

motivation *see* focus; goal setting

music
Bush Fuchsia ... helps with rhythm, clear projection and timbre of the voice; also heightens good musical ear and hearing capacities; improves co-ordination for learning and playing musical instruments

Heartsong Essence ... a combination essence which helps with voice and creativity in music

Little Flannel Flower ... letting go of inhibitions and really feeling the music

Turkey Bush ... for boosting confidence in own inherent creativity

nail biting
Boronia + Bottlebrush ... for breaking addictive habits

Crowea ... for the worrier

Dog Rose ... when nail biting arises from fear or anxiety

naive behaviour *see* immaturity

narcissistic *see* selfishness

narrow-minded (*see also* fanatical beliefs, behaviour; racism)
Bauhinia ... closed to new ideas, new ways of doing things
Freshwater Mangrove ... whenever there is a preconceived concept about how things are or should be
Slender Rice Flower ... racial prejudice resulting from an individual's direct experience with that group

nature awareness, attunement (*see also* environment)
Billy Goat Plum .... to be aware of and appreciate the exquisite, inherent beauty in nature
Black-eyed Susan ... take before bushwalking to be aware of the subtleties of the area and nature
Bush Fuchsia ... deepens your connection to your own natural rhythms and the rhythms of the earth and nature
Bush Iris ... opens the psychic clairsentient and clairvoyant perceptions so as to be more aware of the spiritual kingdoms interacting through and in nature
Green Spider Orchid ... enhances communication with the plant and animal kingdoms as well as the devas, nature spirits and landscape angels

near death experience
Bluebell ... helps to keep the heart open as much as possible to match the intensity of the love they experienced while in the Light
Bush Iris ... clearing any residual fear of death as a consequence of this experience
Flannel Flower ... trusting that it is OK to share such an incredibly powerful experience with the appropriate people
Fringed Violet ... for the shock and trauma of the experience
Green Spider Orchid ... it helps stop dissipating such a special experience by talking about it too quickly before the experience has been integrated, or by discussing it too frequently afterwards
Mint Bush ... it assists the person going through such a tremendous change in priorities as well as in beliefs and values after such a life-altering experience
Red Lily ... after such a profound experience this essence grounds, and connects them back to physical reality in a gentle and effective way
Waratah ... for the despair and 'black night of the soul' some experience in being separated once more from Spirit and pure love
Wild Potato Bush ... helps to accept the limitations of the physical body once more, especially if the physical body has been hurt or badly damaged in the events leading up to the experience

negativity (*see also* love; optimism; protection; stuck)
Kapok Bush ... couldn't be bothered trying because everything is too hard; giving up easily

Mountain Devil ... cynical and suspicious attitude to life and other people

Red Grevillea ... feeling stuck and not seeing any way out from your current situation which is leading you to be progressively more negative

Red Helmet Orchid ... for rebellious 'chip on the shoulder' behaviour and attitude

Southern Cross ... blaming others for your own misfortunes or situation; exhibiting the attitude 'it's not fair'

Sunshine Wattle ... expecting the worst of life because of past experience

nervous breakdown

Angelsword ... where there are false and dangerous messages and energies being conveyed by attached entities that are severely disturbing the wellbeing of the individual

Banksia Robur ... for normally energetic people who are extremely flat, lacking enthusiasm and energy

Black-eyed Susan ... for burnout arising from excessive striving and over-activity. Also for patiently accepting that they must slow down and allow time and rest to be important aspects of the healing program

Dog Rose of the Wild Forces ... whenever there is a sense of something 'snapping' and losing control

Emergency Essence ... for use in any crisis period; for panic attacks

Fringed Violet ... repairs damage to the aura from past unresolved trauma which can lead to a complete drain of energy, both emotional and physical

Jacaranda ... where energies are scattered; sense of panic when making decisions

Kapok Bush ... where every task seems just too hard and tiring to accomplish

Macrocarpa ... for physical stress and burnout; helpful where endurance needed

Old Man Banksia ... for strongly family-oriented people who over-give of themselves and go beyond their physical and emotional limits

Paw Paw ... where there is overwhelming information or work that needs to be done, or decisions that must be made

Peach-flowered Tea-tree ... to stop any excessive morbidity or self pre-occupation, pity and hypochondria

Southern Cross ... after a traumatic or turning point experience such as this you would reevaluate how you lead your life and implement changes; if not and there is only a 'why me?' attitude, then think of this remedy

Spinifex ... to help understand and learn the lessons that led to this condition

Tall Yellow Top ... feeling very isolated and separate from everyone else

Wild Potato Bush ... frustration of not being able to fully express themselves on a physical plane in this point in time

Waratah ... for the despair and hopelessness, and even suicidal feelings, that can arise from this condition

nervousness (*see also* fear; stress)

Black-eyed Susan ... nervous intensity, restlessness and agitation, all of which can be caused or exacerbated by stress or by pushing yourself too far; or it can just be the constitutional make-up of this individual

Crowea ... for excessive worry

Dog Rose ... when caused by shyness, anxiety, fear or phobias

Jacaranda ... triggered by the worry and responsibility around decisions

nightmares (*see also* fear; sleep)

Dog Rose ... for bad nightmares or fear of their recurrence

Green Spider Orchid ... for nightmares associated with a past life experience

Grey Spider Flower ... for nightmares, usually of an unknown origin

'no', learning to say (*see also* boundaries, establishing healthy; confidence)

Alpine Mint Bush ... for the health professional who is in danger of burning out because he can't say 'no' to requests for his services, even when it is in his best interests to do so

Bush Fuchsia ... saying 'no' because you intuitively know

Confid Essence ... helps a person to come into their own power and to stop pleasing others

Dog Rose ... for the shy person who doesn't dare refuse the requests of others

Five Corners ... building up confidence so as to feel strong enough in own self to say 'no' to others

Flannel Flower ... for setting up healthy boundaries in relationships

Illawarra Flame Tree ... helping to overcome fear of rejection which influences your own behaviour towards others

Old Man Banksia ... for the heavy, slow, family loving person who continually gives of self

Sturt Desert Rose ... gives strength to honour self and have your own integrity even if it means saying 'no' in testing situations where you are expected to say 'yes'

Tall Mulla Mulla ... for the person who dares not contradict nor question what others suggest because of a fear of disturbing the peace or creating a scene

nurturing

Bluebell ... by opening your heart and sharing your love, you too are bathed in love which nourishes the psyche

Bottlebrush ... improves bonding, and so nurturing, between mother and child

Five Corners ... when you really love yourself you will also nurture yourself

Philotheca ... for the person who gives to others but can't let in others or easily receive from others or give to self

Red Helmet Orchid ... improves bonding, and so nurturing, between father and child

Red Suva Frangipani ... provides nurturing support when relationship is breaking up or going through a difficult period

Sturt Desert Rose ... by being true to and honouring yourself you will nurture your soul immensely

obsessiveness (*see also* addictions; mental illness)
Boronia ... breaks the pattern of obsessive infatuation and repetitive thoughts

Boronia + Bottlebrush ... helps where there are addictive behavioural patterns

Hibbertia ... for the workshop-aholic who keeps acquiring, but not necessarily applying, knowledge

Yellow Cowslip Orchid ... for anyone overly obsessive about rules and regulations or bureaucratic procedures

optimism (*see also* negativity)
Bush Iris ... the faith that there is a spiritual life beyond this plane

Mint Bush ... reinforces the belief that at some point the perturbation will cease and clarity will emerge

Southern Cross ... once you accept your thoughts and beliefs create your reality, it enables you to optimistically and cheerfully create the future you want

Sunshine Wattle ... for joyful expectation in spite of grim past events

Waratah ... for spiritual trust and faith that we are never given anything with which we can't deal

organisation (*see also* goal setting)
Jacaranda ... helps the scattered, dithering person to focus their energies

Kapok Bush ... allows for an awareness and overview of how a machine or structure is sequentially composed and how it functions

Paw Paw ... for effective decision making

Sundew ... for grounding and being focused

Yellow Cowslip Orchid ... for implementing systematic structure and organisation and attention to detail

out of sorts, feeling (*see also* balance)
Crowea ... when a person does not quite feel right, as this remedy brings the physical body and subtle bodies into balance and alignment

outspoken *see* dominating behaviour; garrulousness

over-achiever (*see also* frenetic)
Black-eyed Susan . . . for the 'go-go-go' type of person who doesn't know when or how to have a break or to slow down
Boab . . . where parents are pushing their children into achieving in areas where they are not comfortable, happy or even wanting to go. Usually it is because the parent is attempting to fulfil their own unachieved desires and ambitions
Hibbertia . . . for the person who is addicted to acquiring knowledge

overindulgence *see* addictions; greed; extravagance

overweight (*see also* addictions; commitment)
Billy Goat Plum . . . to accept and enjoy the physical body
Boab . . . to remove inappropriate old family beliefs and attitudes about food and physical appearance
Bottlebrush . . . breaking old dietary habits
Five Corners . . . to allow a person to love themselves without having to find that same love through food; to help a person feel good about their own physical body, to accept it and to care for it, and to clear any subconscious sabotage they have which may be stopping them losing their excess weight
Fringed Violet + Sturt Desert Pea . . . where overweight is associated with held-in emotional pain or trauma
Mulla Mulla . . . where fear, associated with heat and fire, manifests as a protective layer of fat
Old Man Banksia . . . for the heavy, sluggish person who lacks energy
Sexuality Essence . . . where the excess weight is a way of making themselves unattractive to a sexual partner because they feel uncomfortable about physical intimacy due to past sexual trauma or abuse
Wedding Bush . . . for commitment to a diet or exercise regime
Wild Potato Bush . . . where this is frustration with the physical state, and functioning, of the body

overwhelm, emotional
Bottlebrush . . . overwhelmed by major life changes
Crowea . . . for bringing the subtle and spiritual bodies into balance when worry results from emotional upheaval
Dog Rose of the Wild Forces . . . when in a situation of high emotional intensity in which one is in danger of taking on the energy of the other people involved
Mint Bush . . . where overwhelm and perturbation occur in times of powerful spiritual change
Paw-Paw . . . for overwhelm, particularly of information or work schedule and in making choices between two options
Peach-flowered Tea-tree . . . overwhelmed by responsibility

Red Suva Frangipani . . . for the often overwhelming red, raw emotions that erupt during a relationship break-up
Sturt Desert Pea . . . for overwhelming grief
Waratah . . . for times of overwhelming despair and hopelessness
Yellow Cowslip Orchid . . . helps a person step back from emotions and make impartial assessments or decisions

pain *see* grief

panic (*see also* fear)
Dog Rose of the Wild Forces . . . where there is danger of being taken over by your own panic or that of others
Emergency Essence . . . take frequently till panic subsides
Grey Spider Flower . . . for immobilising fear or extreme terror
Yellow Cowslip Orchid . . . can help a person stand back and detach from a situation which they know would usually lead them to panic

paranoia *see* schizophrenia
Angelsword . . . where their psychic possession leads them into this state
Dog Rose . . . fear of what others could do to you
Mountain Devil . . . for a paranoid and suspicious personality; where there is the feeling that others are criticising you and talking about you, even conspiring to take your possessions and rip you off

parenthood *see* fatherhood; motherhood

passion
Banksia Robur . . . to reconnect you with your vitality, drive and energy
Bush Gardenia . . . for renewing passion and interest in relationships
Flannel Flower . . . to fully enjoy expressing yourself physically
Gymea Lily . . . helps a person to achieve, with great passion, the most important thing in their life
Kapok Bush . . . not involved in life; they give up too easily and won't try because it seems too hard. This essence gets them back in touch with life and drive and motivation
Little Flannel Flower . . . this will release the inner child, opening you up to play, aliveness, fun and spontaneity
Pink Mulla Mulla . . . to open yourself to love and other people without any fear of being hurt or abused
Sexuality Essence . . . allows an individual to fully and passionately express their sexuality by clearing the effects of previous sexual abuse or trauma
Silver Princess . . . finding and following what makes your heart sing
Sturt Desert Pea . . . to passionately embrace without any concern of hurt and pain that might eventuate
Turkey Bush . . . to tap into and enjoy your creative expression
Wisteria . . . generates feelings of sensuality and passion

past lives

Angelsword + Isopogon . . . to help remember and recall instances and aspects of previous lifetimes

Boab . . . will help clear negative lines of karma between people which emanated in previous incarnations

Fringed Violet . . . for resolving any disorientation, shock or trauma arising from past life regression therapy or re-birthing sessions

Green Spider Orchid . . . fear, terror, nightmares which emanate from experiences in past lives

Meditation Essence . . . to heighten awareness and recall of events from a past life—where it is appropriate and beneficial to do so

Mulla Mulla . . . trauma associated with fire that arose in a past life such as, for example, being burnt at the stake. Nine million women and one million men were burnt as witches over a three hundred year period in Europe. Nine generations of children saw their mothers being burnt at the stake. This brutal and barbaric practice was an attempt by the Church to take healing out of the hands of women who were the traditional healers and herbalists of that day. Many healers today have been in that profession many times previously, quite likely during the 'burning of the witches' period, and still carry the scars and fear today of being publicly recognised as a healer in the community because of having been burnt in the past for such activity

Sturt Desert Pea, Tall Tellow Top . . . two essences that commonly address emotional states, grief and alienation, respectively, that have been carried into this life from a previous incarnation

peace *see* calmness

peer pressure

Confid essence . . . peer pressure does not have as much impact on you if you are confident and content with who you are. It has most impact on those who are insecure and looking for approval and acceptance from outside themselves, from the group

Gymea Lily . . . wanting to dominate and bully others into what you or your group want to do; being prepared to be different and separate from the majority of society in pursuing your life and goals to your own standard, not necessarily the values of the mainstream

Illawarra Flame Tree . . . being able to say 'no' without fear of rejection by your peers

Sturt Desert Rose . . . adhering to own standards of behaviour and personal integrity, doing what you know you have to do

perception *see* discernment

perfectionist *(see also* fanatical beliefs, behaviour)

Billy Goat Plum + Boronia + Yellow Cowslip Orchid . . . for the person who is overly fussy about their body, possessions and environment

Boronia ... for someone obsessively following perfection. Being a perfectionist is one of the most frustrating and senseless dispositions to have as perfection can never be achieved and will always lead to suffering and frustration

Hibbertia ... for fanatical self-improvement and excessive self-discipline

Yellow Cowslip Orchid ... for the 'nitpicking', intellectual, excessively critical person who is so focused on the details that they can often fail to see the bigger picture

perseverance *see* commitment

perturbation *see* confusion

pessimism *see* depression; optimism

phobias (*see also* fear)
Dog Rose ... mild phobias
Green Spider Orchid ... phobias relating to a past life
Grey Spider Flower ... the specific remedy for phobias and terror

physical disability
Bauhinia ... to be open and to embrace all the new situations, adaptations and outlooks that are needed as a result of the disability

Billy Goat Plum ... addresses any shame or embarrassment they feel about themselves

Bottlebrush ... helps one to accept the often unexpected incidents or events that have led to their disability and consequent life changes

Emergency Essence ... to help release and clear any residual shock or trauma from the incidents or events that originally led to the disability

Five Corners ... to realise that one's self-love and self-acceptance are not a product purely of their physical body

Kapok Bush ... when there is a sense of giving up in the face of their challenge

Mountain Devil ... where there is jealousy and envy of people who are not so disadvantaged

Southern Cross ... for excessive self-pity or victim-like response to their situation

Wild Potato Bush ... helps to accept the limitations of the physical body

pining, for recent lost love (*see also* grief; relationships)
Boronia ... for coping with repetitive or obsessive thoughts and longings about your previous lover or relationship

Red Suva Frangipani ... where emotions are tender and raw after a relationship break-up

planning *see* goal setting; organisation

positivity *see* optimism

possessiveness
Bluebell ... not willing to share because of fear of lack
Bottlebrush ... unwilling to let go
Bush Iris ... an over-emphasis on the material side of life; holding onto possessions because they believe the physical is all that there is
Mountain Devil ... jealousy and tight control and holding on to people for fear of them being taken from them

poverty consciousness
Bluebell ... hanging on to possessions because of lack of faith in future abundance, or fearing that there is not enough for everyone
Boab ... releasing negative and limiting family belief systems around money, prosperity and abundance
Five Corners ... clears any sabotage they have to being prosperous and abundant by enhancing self-love and allowing the individual to profoundly realise, that they deserve to have prosperity
Philotheca ... helps people to be open to receiving the gifts of the Universe
Southern Cross ... enables the individual to realise that they can create their own reality, full of abundance and prosperity. And all that is needed is for them to change their beliefs and thoughts
Sunshine Wattle ... for those with a strong belief that life is grim and will stay that way

power (*see also* co-dependence; empowerment)
Dog Rose ... allowing fear to prevent you from asking for your rights and desires; simply sticking up for yourself
Five Corners ... lacking the confidence to stand up for yourself
Gymea Lily ... helping those in positions of power to be aware of, and sensitive to, those under their control
Rough Bluebell ... controlling, hurting and manipulating others to achieve own ends
Southern Cross ... denying personal responsibility for life's lessons
Tall Mulla Mulla ... being a 'people pleaser' and so not being true to self

practicality
Bush Fuchsia ... improves co-ordination in physical activities
Jacaranda ... helps people with scattered energies to focus and achieve
Kapok Bush ... engenders an awareness and overview of how a machine or structure is sequentially composed and functions so they can repair it
Sundew ... staying grounded and in the present and paying attention to detail
Turkey Bush ... helps to adopt a creative approach to the job in hand

praise *see* acknowledgment of self and others

pre-exam nerves *see* learning; stress; worry

pregnancy and birth

Bauhinia + Bottlebrush + Crowea ... helps a woman having difficulty moving from the first to second stage of labour

Billy Goat Plum ... to accept changing body shape

Boab ... ideally it should be given to the child as soon as it is born, as the Aborigines do in the Kimberley region of north-west Australia in order to counteract as much as possible the negative emotional patterns of previous generations being passed on

Bottlebrush ... for adapting to changes in body and lifestyle; also for the bond between the mother and the new baby

Bottlebrush, Bush Iris, Swamp Banksia, Philotheca ... for the breasts

Bush Fuchsia ... to trust and follow one's intuition and instinctive wisdom in mothering

Bush Fuchsia, She Oak, Yellow Cowslip Orchid ... work on hormones which influence mammary glands and uterine contractions

Confid Essence ... to inspire confidence in ability to cope

Crowea + Dagger Hakea + Dog Rose + Paw Paw ... for morning sickness

Dog Rose ... for niggling fears, sense of insecurity about being pregnant; fear about something going wrong; fear of labour which is a common cause of morning sickness

Emergency Essence ... use frequently during labour, after a difficult labour or where there has been a big loss of blood

Flannel Flower ... to increase sensitivity and gentle touch in the new parent, especially the father

Fringed Violet ... in last trimester, to protect against negative influence of people sharing with them traumatic or negative birh experiences; shock of unwanted or unplanned pregnancy; apply to baby's fontanelle soon after birth for birth trauma and psychic protection

Grey Spider Flower ... for terror about coming birth process, often from past life experience; encourages calmness, courage, faith

Illawarra Flame Tree ... where there is fear, overwhelm about responsibilities of parenthood

Kapok Bush ... in the middle stages of labour when there is a feeling of giving up

Macrocarpa ... for stamina, endurance and to remedy physical exhaustion during labour

Red Helmet Orchid ... to help the father bond to the baby during pregnancy

She Oak ... helps conception; also for balancing hormones early in the pregnancy and afterwards

Slender Rice Flower ... helps heal any tearing, or stitches from an episiotomy or caesarian section

Sundew ... to bring spirit of the newborn properly into its body
Waratah ... helps where a child is stillborn
Wild Potato Bush ... use near end of pregnancy for any frustration the
    woman may be feeling due to physical restriction and limitation, such
    as feeling big and cumbersome, not being able to sleep comfortably.
    For the unborn child it will also greatly help with their physical restric-
    tions within womb before birth, and with the frustration due to the
    lack of control of their own body after the birth. It also addresses the
    frustration of having gone from being a spiritual being in the cosmos
    to suddenly being crammed into a non-responsive body in a third-
    dimensional reality

prejudice *see* narrow-minded; racism

premenstrual tension
Crowea ... to bring body into balance and ease period pain
Peach-flowered Tea-tree ... for mood swings
She Oak ... to balance hormones

prickly people (*see also* family and social interaction)
Dagger Hakea ... for those who are prickly with others and whose words
    can be sharp due to held in resentments
Mountain Devil ... overt anger and hostility
Pink Mulla Mulla ... for those who put out prickles to keep others at a
    distance for fear of getting too close to people and being hurt

pride (*see also* arrogance)
Five Corners ... the rising pride and joy you can feel for your family
    and their achievements
Gymea Lily ... engenders pride in the best sense of the word, without
    arrogance
Philotheca ... being able to acknowledge and enjoy achievements
Slender Rice Flower ... unleashes humility as part of deeper understanding
    that we are all equal even though we may be evolving at different rates

procrastination (*see also* avoidance)
Paw Paw ... to assist when there is a major decision to be made between
    two or more options
Red Grevillea ... for the person who knows a change is needed but
    doesn't know how to bring it about
Sundew ... for dreamers out of touch with reality and for those who
    keep procrastinating instead of just doing it

protection
Angelsword ... releases negatively held psychic energies
Boab ... helps release and clear earth-bound spirits from space and envi-
    ronment when used topically as a spray. Especially effective when
    combined in this manner with Angelsword, Fringed Violet and Lichen

Dog Rose ... by releasing the fear you have of something you will then stop attracting it into your life

Fringed Violet ... provides psychic protection

Grey Spider Flower ... fear of supernatural and psychic attack

psychic abilities *see* meditation; spirituality

psychosis

Boronia ... breaks pattern of obsessive, compulsive thoughts and behaviour

Mountain Devil ... for paranoia

Peach-flowered Tea-tree ... for manic depression

Rough Bluebell ... for violent and destructive behaviour as described in the Diagnostical and Statistical Manual used by psychiatrists and psychotherapists

Sundew ... addresses catatonic states

public speaking

Bush Fuchsia ... for clarity in speech and projection of the voice

Grey Spider Flower ... for the paralysing fear that can come when standing in front of an audience

Red Grevillea ... corrects imbalances in the temporomandibular joint of the jaw, thereby allowing you to open your mouth when speaking and project your voice to an audience

punctuality *(see also* focus; rushing)

Black-eyed Susan ... for an individual who is usually filling their life up with so much activity that they always, even at the best of times, have trouble completing all that they have scheduled. Plus they often underestimate the amount of time something will take so that they find themselves behind time and rushing

Jacaranda ... for those whose attention is scattered so that they are not focused on things like time and punctuality

Sundew ... helps with focus; for daydreamers and ditherers who are often unaware of what the time is and when it is time to leave in order to be punctual

punishing self *(see also* abusing self)

Billy Goat Plum ... where there is disgust at own body or a part of the body as in anorexia, where the individual response to the aversion is quite negative

Dagger Hakea ... where holding grudges is resulting in bitterness which is held in the body as toxicity

Sturt Desert Rose ... where guilt or regret from past actions is preventing you from having a positive self-image and sense of self

quietness *(see also* calmness)

Black-eyed Susan ... enables a person to slow down, to reach that still centre within and find calmness, inner peace and guidance

Boronia . . . to still and quieten the racing, chattering mind. It allows one to have total pinpoint concentration to fully hear or see whatever you are focusing on or listening for, regardless of what is going on around you

Dog Rose of the Wild Forces . . . to find the inner peace and calmness within you when all around there is turmoil and intensity

Green Spider Orchid . . . to value the energy of silence and its appropriate position in life

Meditation Essence . . . for creating a quiet and protected space in which to go deeply into meditation

racism

Bauhinia . . . where anybody different or new is not easily understood, accepted or included into the society

Boab . . . where there has been a long ongoing karmic pattern of persecution or prejudice, involving either a race or a religious group, such as the Black Africans or Jewish people

Freshwater Mangrove . . . for the person who has been taught by family to hate persons of a particular race or religion but who has had no personal experience to bring about this view or to feel this way

Slender Rice Flower . . . helps a narrow-minded person belonging to a group that has a racist or superior attitude towards other groups with whom they have had a negative experience. This could, for example, be religious in nature: Protestants feeling they are better than Catholics; racial: Scots better than the English; or even sexist: women better than men

radiation therapy

Mulla Mulla . . . reduces not only the amount of burning and scarring and the healing time, but also the emotional trauma and fear—even terror—that many patients experience when they get close to, or can smell, the treatment room on subsequent treatment days

rape (see also abuse, victim of; sexuality)

Billy Goat Plum . . . addresses the sense of feeling unclean and dirty after rape. It can be used to resolve any feelings of shame, revulsion or disgust a person may have about their own body after being raped

Emergency Essence . . . to be administered as soon as possible after the rape to ease the life-shattering trauma of the event

Fringed Violet + Flannel Flower . . . this combination is used for men who have experienced rape. Fringed Violet removes the shock and trauma of the incident while Flannel Flower helps establish ease, pleasure, and feeling safe and trusting with physical touch and intimacy once more

Fringed Violet + Flannel Flower + Wisteria . . . for women we have included Wisteria along with the combination we have used for men experiencing rape. Wisteria adds the elements of feeling, enjoying and sensuality, and trust to surrender to themselves and to their partner in their sexuality

Fringed Violet + Wisteria + Dog Rose + Grey Spider Flower ... when there is a fear of being raped again

Mountain Devil ... to help a person move from hate and plotting violent revenge against the perpetrator to a point where he or she can forgive him

Red Helmet Orchid ... increased awareness, concern for rape that is occurring on the planet; lack of respect, appreciation and working in harmony with nature

Slender Rice Flower ... hatred against all men that a victim of rape may feel after the experience

reading (*see also* ADD; focus; learning)

Boab ... where reading problems arise from cranial-sacral blockage after immunisation

Bush Fuchsia ... helps the brain integrate information coming in through the eyes when the eyes are focusing on a different direction—i.e. left–right, up–down. For some people the information reaching the brain when the eyes are focused in a particular direction can get scrambled at the point of the optic chiasma, and the brain is literally switched off to that information. This is why some people get quite sleepy when they read at night after just a few pages or have trouble remembering what they have just read. It will also improve speaking ability and voice projection when reading aloud. It is especially beneficial for people who read in a flat monotone voice. Basically they are dyslexic with a lack of integration between the left and right hemispheres of the brain. Once Bush Fuchsia integrates the hemispheres then the left can see all the individual words while the right can then see the bigger picture and have a sense of the meaning of the sentence. For now, it is no longer merely a group of unconnected individual words, so while reading they will know when to put inflection, tone and timbre into their voice; they will also remember what they have just read

Bush Fuchsia ... will help with not only reading difficulties but also with all writing and speech problems

Bush Fuchsia + Fringed Violet + Sundew ... can help where birth or other trauma has resulted in learning difficulties

reality (*see also* dreams; focus; horror movies, after)

Bush Fuchsia + Sundew ... for people feeling 'spaced out' after watching TV, videos and computer games for long periods

Bush Iris ... allows us to be aware of the spiritual world and what lies beyond the perceptions of the five senses

Freshwater Mangrove . . . opens new filters and opens us to new paradigms which allow us to perceive reality totally differently

Green Spider Orchid . . . for tuning into, merging with and experiencing directly the reality of a different life form, whether it be human, plant or animal

Mint Bush . . . when our major beliefs fall away, as if pulled out from beneath us like a rug, and we are left with a brand new way of viewing our life and the world

Red Lily . . . for keeping in touch with reality and practical day-to-day life while pursuing one's spiritual practice

Sundew . . . for grounding and living in the present; brings one's consciousness fully back to the present after drugs, general anaesthetic or after being unconscious

Yellow Cowslip Orchid . . . allows a judge to see the actions of a person who has broken the law through that individual's reality and so helps him or her to impartially assess their ruling on the case

rebellious (*see also* family and social interaction; fatherhood)
Gymea Lily . . . daring to be different
Mountain Devil . . . for anger at the world at large
Red Helmet Orchid . . . for those with problems with authority figures; improves father–child relationship

re-birthing (*see also* protection)
Emergency Essence . . . a good calming and settling remedy after a session where any catharsis has occurred
Fringed Violet . . . helps close the aura off if a person has been taken back a long way during a session
Tall Mulla Mulla . . . the specific essence for breathing and breath work

recognition
Gymea Lily . . . for those who crave attention, recognition and glamour
Illawarra Flame Tree . . . continually needing to be centre stage and have an audience with which to communicate because of the fear that you will be rejected or life will be boring if you are not noticed
Kangaroo Paw . . . the positive aspects of this essence encourage generosity within individuals and give recognition to those immature or inexperienced people around them, that they can feel important and at ease
Philotheca . . . the ability to give recognition and acknowledgment to self and others
Yellow Cowslip Orchid . . . your work is of the utmost importance to you and you will feel upset if it doesn't receive its due recognition

reconciliation (*see also* forgiveness)
Bluebell . . . opens the heart so it can have the capacity to love others
Boab . . . can help bring about reconciliation between groups where there

has been abuse, persecution or suppression for many generations. Often the players are incarnating over and over again into that same situation

Boab + Bottlebrush + Red Helmet ... a great combination for parents to take so they can withhold or remove their projections on to their children about what they should be or do. The parents can then embrace, accept and come to terms with the lives the children have chosen

Dagger Hakea ... helps the forgiveness process with those who are, or at some point have been, close to you

Freshwater Mangrove ... where there has been prejudice, not based on personal experience, that has precluded your interaction and reconciliation with others

Slender Rice Flower ... will resolve the situation where a direct experience with an individual or group has led to your prejudice against them

refugees (*see also* abuse, victim of; adaptability; confidence; depression; self-esteem)

Bauhinia ... to be able to embrace and accept such a new environment and new way of living, and all the other changes now occurring in your life

Billy Goat Plum ... helps resolve a sense of shame

Bluebell ... helps unexpressed emotions to be released; opens up the heart

Boab ... to clear long-held negative family thought patterns; for those who have experienced abuse or prejudice for generations

Boronia ... for obsessive thoughts

Bottlebrush ... to help let go of the past and all the things you have lost from your life

Five Corners ... to find your own self-worth without relating it to your possessions or former career

Grey Spider Flower ... for the terror of being a mere individual caught up in war or catastrophic change

Kapok Bush ... the strength to persevere and not give up in the face of such adversity

Little Flannel Flower ... to help keep your sense of humour or lightness, even in such heavy and dark moments

Mountain Devil ... clears anger, hatred directed against the situation or against people who have led to a change in circumstance

Paw Paw ... the overwhelm of having to start anew with all the things that are needed to rebuild your life

Pink Mulla Mulla ... for those who put out prickles to keep people away; where injustice is carried like a scar on the soul

Slender Rice Flower ... helps overcome racism or prejudice resulting from your own experiences

Southern Cross . . . for those with victim mentality; helps people see that each obstacle in life is a lesson to be learnt

Sturt Desert Pea . . . for deep hurt and sadness even when they have been stored a long time

Sturt Desert Rose . . . relieves remorse or guilt resulting from past actions; religious guilt

Sunshine Wattle . . . for constant struggle and difficulty in imagining things ever improving

Tall Yellow Top . . . for the sense of alienation; feeling a 'stranger in a strange land'

Waratah . . . for the utter despair, hopelessness of having lost every-thing—your home, possessions—and for all the other suffering

rejection

Illawarra Flame Tree . . . for feeling of rejection, real or imagined

relationships (*see also* family and social interaction; sexuality)

Bluebell . . . opens heart to love of, and sharing with, others

Boab . . . looking for and attracting, usually subconsciously, partners who mirror strong features and behaviour of your parents, in which case there will be many projections you will make on to the partner

Boronia . . . for mental obsession about another—either as infatuation or pining for a lost love

Bush Gardenia . . . helps deepen emotional attachment in relationship by renewing passion and interest in it. Great if the relationship is becom-ing a little stale

Dagger Hakea . . . transmutes into love and forgiveness any anger, resent-ment, bitterness towards an ex or current lover

Five Corners . . . when you are at the point of loving and accepting your-self and having a healthy sense of self-worth, then you will attract an equally balanced and emotionally healthy person to have as a mate and with whom you can create a loving relationship. For then you are not coming from a needy place of having to get your confidence and self-love topped up from or by your partner

Flannel Flower . . . transcending fear of emotional or physical intimacy and difficulty in communicating your feelings to your partner

Gymea Lily . . . inhibits the tendency of a dominant and more powerful person in a relationship to override and weaken the essence of their partner, who will then often become similar to their mate rather than that unique and different individual they were in the beginning of the relationship. Once this occurs, boredom and dissatisfaction will quickly arise in their partnership. For a healthy relationship each partner must be allowed the freedom to express their own unique gifts and interests

Kangaroo Paw . . . helps the gauche, selfish person develop maturity in themselves and their relationships, where they recognise and meet the needs of their partner, not just their own

Red Suva Frangipani ... for the great emotional intensity, grief, sadness and upset people can go through when a relationship is ending, close to ending or going through a very rocky period

Relationship Essence ... just about covers it all!

Wedding Bush ... deepens commitment in a relationship

relaxation (*see also* nurturing; stress)

Black-eyed Susan ... *the* stress remedy; for the super active person who isn't able, and doesn't know how, to slow down and rest. This essence will take them to the still, small place within where they can then relax

Boronia ... where the same thoughts about a problem or subject of interest keep repeating themselves over and over in the head and so prevent relaxation of the body and emotions

Crowea ... where constant worrying is preventing a person from relaxing. This essence can be of real help as it centres, calms and brings about balance. Crowea releases tension in the muscles and helps a person to unwind

Flannel Flower ... this essence will encourage real enjoyment in touching and being touched and relaxing into the physical—whether it be a professional massage or a hug from someone you love

Hibbertia ... for those with a tendency to always strive to be the best, to know everything, to be strict and fanatical with themselves; this essence will allow them to release all this effort and simply let go and relax a little, in the knowledge that their own inner wisdom knows more than they will ever find in a book

Jacaranda ... will help break the pattern of needing to react to every new stimuli so you can simply slow down, stay in the one place, in a calm state for an extended time

Little Flannel Flower ... for having fun, letting go of seriousness and adult things

Meditation Essence ... for stilling an over-active mind and body

Sundew ... once you stopped procrastinating and have addressed, commenced or completed a project, an immense sense of serenity ensues

Sexuality Essence ... enables the individual to be fully present, and to find relaxation and contentment in their sensuous play and lovemaking

Yellow Cowslip Orchid ... enhances the ability to detach from an emotionally intense involvement and see your situation from a more relaxed and objective state

relaxed with people (*see also* family and social interaction; immaturity)

Bauhinia ... to be able to embrace, accept and release the emotional charge around someone you don't like or towards whom you feel annoyance or irritation

Billy Goat Plum + Dog Rose + Kangaroo Paw ... for the shyness, self-consciousness and awkwardness you can feel when approaching someone to whom you are sexually attracted

Dog Rose ... this will help the shy person to overcome their fears and to interact more comfortably in social situations

Illawarra Flame Tree ... for the person who is tense or 'over the top' with others because of fear of rejection

Kangaroo Paw ... helps the socially gauche person to have more harmony and ease in their social interactions

Mountain Devil ... releases feelings of jealousy and envy when they are with others whom, they perceive, have more than they do or have possessions or qualities they want

Pink Mulla Mulla ... for the person who is constantly on guard and putting out prickles to keep others away, for they have an underlying fear of being hurt if others become close to them

Slender Rice Flower ... to be able to deal with an individual or a group against whom you have a strong prejudice

Tall Mulla Mulla ... is for those who prefer to be alone so there is less chance of conflict and disharmony

Tall Yellow Top ... allows you to have a sense of belonging, being part of a group

release *see* letting go emotionally

repetitiveness (*see also* addictions; boredom; obsessiveness)
Boronia ... for the thoughts that go over and over in the mind
Bottlebrush ... for breaking habits, letting go
Southern Cross ... for those who don't learn lessons from their past experience

repressed emotions *see* denial

repressed, held in personality *see* introversions

resentment (*see also* anger)
Alpine Mint Bush ... for those who see themselves forced into a situation where they have no alternative but to look after someone else, and who are in danger of burning out. The resentment could be directed towards the person for whom they are caring or to others who they think should be helping and supporting them more, but aren't

Bluebell ... when a feud arises over the issue of money or a will and there is a lack of generosity and sharing between the family members

Dagger Hakea ... where there is resentment towards close family and friends

Mountain Devil ... addresses more the general resentment against everyone and everything. These people can be full of anger and hostility as well as mistrust and envy towards others

Southern Cross ... for those who feel they are being used by others; for the 'poor me' type person

resignation

Boab ... daring to break the mould of how things have traditionally been done in the family

Kapok Bush ... giving up; not even trying because it seems too hard

Peach-flowered Tea-tree ... abandoning projects even though they are not yet completed, because there is no longer any challenge involved

Red Grevillea ... knowing what you want but not being able to see how to bring it about

Sunshine Wattle ... to release the attitude of being resigned to the fact that things will never change or get better

resilience

Alpine Mint Bush ... gives strength and renews enthusiasm for those in caring jobs who are in danger of burning out

Banksia Robur ... enhances recuperation back to vitality and full strength again

Black-eyed Susan ... helps the very busy, quick and speedy type from burning out

Illawarra Flame Tree ... exerts a specific influence on the thymus and boosts the immune system and sense of wellbeing, especially in response to chronic or serious acute disease

Macrocarpa ... for physical strength, endurance and stamina

Mint Bush ... maintains one's ability and capacity to go through extended periods of perturbation

Old Man Banksia ... enhances the tremendous capacity these people have for offering a shoulder for others to cry on and unburden their troubles

Waratah ... tenacity and adaptability in the face of great challenge and adversity

responsibility (*see also* commitment)

Bottlebrush ... for a couple entering into parenthood to help them deal with change and responsibility

Illawarra Flame Tree ... overwhelmed by thought of responsibility

Jacaranda ... fearful of making a decision in case it is wrong

Kangaroo Paw ... refusing to grow up and take on the responsibilities of adulthood

Southern Cross ... for those who blame others for life's difficulties; helps person take responsibility and control of their own life

Sturt Desert Rose ... helps an individual to remain true to their own personal integrity

Yellow Cowslip Orchid ... usually very responsible people who see it as their role to preserve the fabric of society as we know it by main-taining and upholding the existing laws, rules and regulations

restlessness *see* frustration; hyperactivity; stuck

restriction (*see also* stuck)
Bauhinia . . . clears restrictive self-imposed images an individual has built up about themselves because they believe they are not the type of person who does a certain activity, such as dancing or painting
Five Corners . . . for when you want to do something new but are afraid you are not good enough or will make a fool of yourself, so you don't attempt it
Old Man Banksia . . . when feeling sluggish, burdened or lacking in energy
Red Grevillea . . . when experiencing a sense of being 'trapped' but unable to initiate moves to a more desired state
Wild Potato Bush . . . eases the frustration of physical movement being restricted by pregnancy, obesity, injury or illness

retirement (*see also* aging; change)
Banksia Robur . . . if they do not establish activity that fulfils their need for contribution then these people will often feel tired and lethargic
Bauhinia . . . being open to new lifestyle ideas and possibilities
Bottlebrush . . . adapting to the changes and new beginnings that retire-ment brings
Five Corners . . . for an individual whose self-worth is derived from what they do and not who they are
Kapok Bush . . . only a few years ago the life expectancy for men after retirement in the USA and Australia was less than two years. This is an essence for someone who has lost interest in life, for this is the type of response that will usually lead to an early death if it is not arrested
Mint Bush . . . retirement often heralds a total re-evaluation of your beliefs and values and what you now consider to be the meaning of life
Silver Princess . . . for finding new direction in life when you have reached a crossroad. Some people focus so much on all the things they'll do when they retire that, when they get there, they feel quite flat and are not as interested in doing them as they had thought they would be. This essence removes that feeling of flatness and allows them to move on with motivation and interest once more
Tall Yellow Top . . . where a person's sense of identity, which has pre-viously been connected to their work role, no longer exists and they feel quite lost and isolated

retrieving forgotten skills
Angelsword . . . retrieving skills and gifts that were developed in previous

lifetimes if they are relevant to what you are doing now
Isopogon ... retrieving skills and knowledge forgotten this lifetime because of poor memory
Waratah ... retrieving forgotten survival skills in times of crisis

revenge *see* anger; resentment

revulsion *see* body image; shame

rigidity (*see also* change; flexibility)
Bauhinia ... for those resisting change or who are closed to new ideas
Boab ... hanging on to family patterns of behaviour that no longer fit
Boronia ... where there is obsessiveness
Bottlebrush + Boronia ... helps break addictive behaviour and habitual ways of doing things
Flannel Flower ... its relationship to rigidity is to engender a gentleness and a softness in the psyche
Hibbertia ... where there is excessive self-discipline and fanaticism
Isopogon ... controlling, rigid and stubborn personality
Little Flannel Flower ... for the individual who is lacking flexibility and is over-serious
Little Flannel Flower, Hibbertia ... a rigid mind will create a rigid body. These two essences create a lightness and flexibility in the person, their thinking and anywhere hardness is found in the body—for example, arthritis, arteriosclerosis
Yellow Cowslip Orchid ... a strong preference or insistence on old traditional values or ways of doing things

risk taking (*see also* cautious; responsibility; trust)
Dog Rose ... daring to confront one's fears
Freshwater Mangrove ... being willing to let go of old prejudices and beliefs, not really knowing what the consequences will be
Gymea Lily ... where a person shows off in order to be the centre of attention. On a positive note it also encourages someone to be different and to take risks in fulfilling themselves and achieving their goals
Illawarra Flame Tree ... putting aside the possibility of being rejected and going up and introducing yourself to new people
Kangaroo Paw ... for the immature or naive person whose behaviour can be risky and dangerous
Peach-flowered Tea-tree ... someone willing to take risks because it adds a bit of adrenalin and excitement when they are feeling bored
Pink Mulla Mulla, Sexuality Essence ... they both represent a person willing to once more take the chance of intimately opening themselves up to others after previously being hurt
Waratah ... to enhance courageous behaviour in dangerous or extremely challenging situations

rushing (*see also* impatience)

Black-eyed Susan ... for the busy over-committing individual whose quality of life is continually being eroded by this overlay of rush that permeates every aspect of their life and leads to intolerable stress

Jacaranda ... rushing from one thing to another, often before finishing the one in hand

sabotage

Dog Rose ... for fear of success, which will lead to failure and sabotage

Five Corners ... rather than seeing failure as a learning experience these people 'bash themselves up' and give themselves a really hard time and generally erode away their self-worth. When goals or projects into which a person puts a lot of effort don't succeed, this can often indicate that there is a subconscious sabotage occurring. The bottom line behind most sabotages is that the person doesn't believe that they are good enough to deserve the goal or project

Pink Mulla Mulla ... a very deep spiritual sabotage, stemming from the belief that following your spiritual path will lead to complete annhilation on all levels

Sunshine Wattle ... for when, after one or a series of failures, you feel as if nothing will succeed

sadness *see* grief

sarcasm (*see also* humour)

Little Flannel Flower ... using humour to gently send someone up or to show the absurdity of a situation

Rough Bluebell ... for the deliberately hurtful person who can be really cruel and cut people down with their sarcastic humour

Yellow Cowslip Orchid ... for those who exhibit a very dry, witty humour which can often be sarcastic in nature

scattered energies *see* focus

schizophrenia

Angelsword ... to remove negative energies or entities that have entered when the individual's aura has been opened, usually at a time when there has been loss of consciousness—either through drugs, general anaesthetic, alcohol, severe trauma or injury. 'Possession' refers, in actual fact, to this very same phenonomen. Some people are very psychic but at the same time have not been aware of how to protect and close themselves off to these entities or energies which, in turn, create many of the symptoms which we refer to as schizophrenia— confusion, multiple personality, delusional states, violent and self-destructive behaviour

Bush Fuchsia ... to help balance brain function, especially with the firing of the neurons and the reception of the neurotransmitters

Dog Rose of the Wild Forces ... should be thought of whenever there is a sense or possibility of losing control

Emergency Essence ... can be used in crisis situations for both the schizophrenic and the carers

Fringed Violet ... will repair and heal any damage to the aura

Mountain Devil ... for paranoia where there is the feeling that others are criticising and talking about you, even conspiring to take your possessions and rip you off

Red Lily ... can help reach schizophrenics who are in a catatonic state

Sundew ... where there is disassociatedness, vagueness or a sense of being split

Waratah ... for the hopelessness, despair and confusion associated with the loss of control

secretive *see* denial; trust

'seeker of knowledge'

Angelsword ... to open clear communication channels with your Higher Self and Angelic Being

Bush Iris ... allows you to go deeper in your spiritual and psychic understandings and perceptions

Hibbertia ... constantly acquiring and devouring new information and philosophies and spiritual teachings

Mint Bush ... helps person seeking knowledge to reach 'Halls of Knowledge' (rub into the 3rd eye)

self-assertion (*see also* confidence)

Bush Fuchsia ... speaking up, trusting and following your intuition

Dog Rose ... sticking up for yourself and not allowing yourself to be dominated or walked over by anyone

Five Corners, Confid Essence ... building self-esteem and daring to express the radiant being you really are

Gymea Lily ... daring to be different from others and from society in pursuing your highest path

Southern Cross ... moving into your own power and boldly stepping forth and creating your life and reality the way you want it to be

Sturt Desert Rose ... honouring and being true to yourself no matter what ripples this creates

self-conscious *see* shame

self-control (*see also* addictions)

Bottlebrush + Boronia ... to help break addictive behaviour

Dog Rose of the Wild Forces ... where you are in danger of being swept up into the surrounding emotional turmoil

Mountain Devil ... where there is a need for self-control when feeling anger, hatred, jealousy or the desire to hurt others. This essence helps to not only control but also transmute such feelings into love, compassion and forgiveness

Wedding Bush ... to strengthen your commitment and resolve, especially when the desire to do otherwise is strong

Yellow Cowslip Orchid ... helps you to step back from emotional intensity, maintain internal discipline and stay mentally in control of yourself—and hence the situation

self-denial *see* denial

self-destructive (*see also* abusing self; addictions; anorexia nervosa; confidence; love; suicide)

Five Corners ... for the person who self-sabotages their own goals and dreams

Isopogon ... not learning from past experiences

Waratah ... when a person is suicidal this remedy can quickly pull them back

self-effacing

Five Corners ... to break the pattern of constantly putting yourself down and apologising

Philotheca ... where a person gives easily but can't accept from others, especially acknowledgment and praise

self-esteem *see* confidence

self, fear of revealing *see* communication; fear; trust

selfishness

Bluebell ... for those who have difficulty sharing their love, themselves or their possessions with others

Bush Gardenia ... for the person caught up in their own world, with little time for, or unaware of, what is really happening with those other important people in their life

Gymea Lily ... for those who wield power without compassion

Isopogon ... for the stubborn, controlling person who is purely concerned with getting their way

Kangaroo Paw ... for those who are so focused on themselves that they are unaware of the needs of the people around them

Red Helmet Orchid ... for men who are so involved with their career or other activities in their lives that they neglect their relationship with their children

Rough Bluebell ... completely centred on own wants; deliberately manipulating or using others to achieve their own ends

Yellow Cowslip Orchid ... very conservative with money and can have trouble spending on others

self-pity

Peach-flowered Tea-tree ... for those who have a tendency to hypochrondria and excessive self-interest or pity; those who are frequently overly concerned about themselves

Southern Cross ... blaming others for own problems and frequently using the phrase 'it's not fair'

senility *see* aging

sensitivity to needs of others *(see also* selfishness)

Bauhinia ... engenders open-mindedness and the ability to embrace and accept differences, even if annoying, in others

Bluebell ... opens the heart to love and enhances the ability to share with others joyfully

Bush Fuchsia ... increases awareness of one's own inner guidance

Flannel Flower ... increases sensitivity and gentleness and helps people express these aspects in their physical and emotional interactions with others

Fringed Violet ... as a protection for people who are very sensitive and whose energy can become easily drained by others, or else take on other energies

Green Spider Orchid ... to increase sensitivity to and from other life forms

Gymea Lily ... for people who love to hop in and take charge of a situation and organise or order other people. This essence helps them to be aware of the contribution others have to offer and the need they have to contribute

Kangaroo Paw ... helps you to shift your attention from being purely on yourself so that you can become aware of the needs of others

Meditation Essence ... increases sensitivity to subtle energies and vibrations

Mulla Mulla ... for people who are overly sensitive to heat or fire

Pink Mulla Mulla ... for people who are overly sensitive to perceived hurts or abuse

Red Grevillea ... helps those who are very sensitive to and affected by criticism from unpleasant people

Red Helmet Orchid ... where, because of their careers, fathers give little consideration to the needs of their children

Rough Bluebell ... deliberately manipulating or using people to get your own way; being completely indifferent to their needs and wants

Slender Rice Flower ... helps arouse awareness of our oneness with others

sensuality *(see also* sexuality)

Billy Goat Plum ... to take pleasure and delight in your own body and beauty

Bluebell . . . to allow feelings to be felt

Flannel Flower . . . to heighten sensitivity in touch and to help show feelings that are felt but not expressed

Little Flannel Flower . . . to release the child within; to awaken a sense of play and fun

Turkey Bush . . . to observe the beauty and perfection in nature and the world and express this through your own creativity

Wisteria . . . to uncover the softer feminine sides of males and females, and to be open to and to enjoy sensuality

separation *see* grief; relationships

serenity *see* calmness

seriousness

Hibbertia . . . for the person who is driven by their intellect and fanatical about self-improvement!

Little Flannel Flower . . . allows a person to lighten up, have fun, play, enjoy life and others

Paw Paw . . . it is very easy to be too serious when you are in total overwhelm with activities and projects

Peach-flowered Tea-tree . . . they exhibit an excessive self-concern which can even result in hypochondria

Sunshine Wattle . . . for those who expect the grim struggle of their lives to continue in that vein without any brighter outlook or expectation

Yellow Cowslip Orchid . . . for the very dry, logical, rational, 'I am not amused' type of person who is usually out of touch with and uncomfortable with feelings

sexuality (*see also* abuse, victim of; infidelity; rape; relationships; also see the chapter on Sexuality in *Australian Bush Flower Essences* (1st edn))

Billy Goat Plum . . . to help you realise that sexuality is more than just about the physical; it encompasses the emotional and spiritual; transmutes feeling of shame and any associated feelings that sexuality, or their genitals, are dirty or unclean

Black-eyed Susan . . . so as to be more relaxed and still, and therefore fully present and able to enjoy the intimacy

Boab + Boronia + Bottlebrush + Bush Iris + Flannel Flower + Wedding Bush . . . for transforming and resolving sex addiction

Boronia + Crowea + Dog Rose + Five Corners + Flannel Flower + Sturt Desert Rose . . . very effective combination for reversing male impotence, and the common emotional reactions—namely guilt, worry, fear that it will happen again, doubts about their masculinity and self-worth—which men experience in this condition and which affects nearly all of them at some point in their lives

Bush Gardenia . . . for renewing passion and interest with your partner

Crowea ... removes the worry that perhaps you are not doing things right

Dog Rose ... for fear and insecurity associated with sexual activity

Flannel Flower ... to enhance and bring back the joy in physical and sexual activity while also developing gentleness and sensitivity in touching and caressing. Flannel Flower also allows you to feel comfortable with and accept your body. It enables you to be open to sensuality and touch and to enjoy physical and emotional intimacy

Flannel Flower + Fringed Violet ... to heal male sexual trauma and sexual abuse

Flannel Flower + Fringed Violet + Wisteria ... to heal female sexual trauma and sexual abuse

Kangaroo Paw ... to be very tuned into and aware of the needs of your partner

Little Flannel Flower ... to both enjoy and experience the fun, delight and spontaneous play that sexuality truly is, and can be

Paw Paw ... creates clarity if there is confusion about your sexual orientation

Spinifex ... to help heal and clear the sexually transmitted diseases chlamydia and herpes

Sturt Desert Rose ... releases sexual guilt and any associations linking sex to guilt. Whenever there is a contraction of a sexually transmitted disease, there is almost invariably a great deal of unresolved sexual guilt as a major predisposing factor

Sundew ... if one of the partners is very much in their head and fantasising during lovemaking, then there will be a very obvious missing component and destructive element entering the relationship

Wisteria ... transforms frigidity by allowing the woman to reconnect to and be open to the sensuality, passion and pleasure in her own body and her trust and willingness to share that with a partner

shame

Billy Goat Plum ... *the* remedy for shame, whether it be about your own body, sexuality, parents, job—anything!

Dog Rose ... when shy, fearful, insecure and self-conscious

Isopogon ... helps a person see that life's failures are not mistakes or something to be ashamed about, but rather are life's learning experiences

Red Grevillea ... when over-reacting to what others think or say about you

Sturt Desert Rose ... shame resulting from past actions where you have remorse and regret

sharing

Bluebell ... for those who find it difficult to share possessions, themselves or their feelings because of a belief in lack and the fear that there is just not enough to go around, so that they should hold on to what they have

Bottlebrush ... can help parents let go of and share their adolescent and adult children with others

Flannel Flower ... trusting that it is safe to share your innermost feelings and secrets

Green Spider Orchid ... knowing the appropriate time to share information or profound experiences with others

Mountain Devil ... resolving anger and suspicion can open a person to sharing love with others

Slender Rice Flower ... encourages group harmony, co-operation and sharing information and resources with others, especially in a group situation

shattered feelings *see* relationships; trauma, shock; turmoil

shift workers
Bush Iris ... by working on the pineal gland, this essence adjusts the body clock to help it adapt to changing time frames and body rhythms

shock *see* trauma, shock

shyness (*see also* anxiety; timidity)
Confid Essence ... helps combat shyness by building confidence and self-esteem

Dog Rose ... for people who are shy because they are apprehensive and fearful of other people

Five Corners ... for those lacking confidence about self and own body

Tall Mulla Mulla ... helps those who are apprehensive about social interaction and prefer to be alone, where there is less likelihood of conflict and disharmony

singing (*see also* music; speech problems)
Bush Fuchsia ... profound effect, enhancing the tone, timbre and quality of the voice while singing; it allows the ear to easily pick up melodies and rhythms while singing

Five Corners ... the confidence just to sing and enjoy your voice and be free of inhibitions. This is when your voice will really sound wonderful

Heartsong Essence ... frees your voice and opens your heart. Inspires creative and emotional expression in a gentle and calm way; provides courage and clarity in singing

Red Grevillea ... by working on the temporomandibular joint in the jaw, it facilitates full opening of the jaw and therefore much clearer and rounder notes while singing

sleep (*see also* dreams; insomnia; relaxation)
Black-eyed Susan ... will help break the pattern these people have of always staying up late, finding lots of things to do and invariably

leaving themselves an inadequate number of hours' sleep each night; unable to go off to sleep at night because they keep thinking and planning for all the things they feel they need to do

Boronia . . . where obsessive thoughts or ideas going round and round prevent the mind from switching off and surrendering to sleep

Bush Iris . . . helps your body clock to adjust to a different country's time zone when travelling

Bush Iris + Dagger Hakea + Fringed Violet + Isopogon + Old Man Banksia + Tall Mulla Mulla . . . this combination addresses the major causes of snoring, including such things as mouth breathing and blockages in the sinuses

Crowea . . . where a person can't sleep due to worry or when they just feel out of balance

Dog Rose + Red Helmet Orchid . . . for bedwetting: Dog Rose addresses the fear which triggers the reaction in the kidney, while Red Helmet Orchid addresses fear of the father or issues relating to the father, the most common fear affecting bedwetting

Emergency Essence . . . to ease and relax an individual during times of emotional or physical stress and allow them the nurturing qualities and blissful mercy of sleep to continue the healing process

Green Spider Orchid + Grey Spider Flower . . . fear of going to sleep because of recurring nightmares because it will help to stop the nightmares; allows a person to go back to sleep after a nightmare

Macrocarpa . . . of great benefit to people who are so exhausted and burnt out that, paradoxically, they are unable to sleep

Red Lily + Sundew . . . addresses the incidence of sleepwalking

Sundew . . . for the person who has an excessive need for sleep which can't be explained by any biological imbalance

Sundew + Tall Mulla Mulla . . . for sleep apnoea where a person readily falls asleep anywhere, any time and where they can stop breathing while sleeping

sluggishness *see* lethargy; tiredness

smoking, giving up *see* addictions

social skills *see* communication; family and social interaction

softness *see* sensitivity to needs of others; tenderness

soul, deep wound of
Pink Mulla Mulla . . . helps resolve deep hurts from a very early incarnation which has been carried in the psyche—usually at the level of the outer causal body—ever since

'spaced out' feeling (*see also* focus; reality)
Bush Fuchsia . . . for feeling of unreality after TV, computer games, etc.

Crowea ... helps bring about balance after a person has been disturbed during deep meditation or astral travelling

Red Lily ... keeping one's feet on the earth during intense or prolonged religious practice

Sundew ... being vague and 'spaced out' as a consequence of drugs, anaesthetic; for the vague, dreamy constitutional type

speech problems (*see also* communication; learning; singing; stuttering)

Bush Fuchsia ... helps with speech and co-ordination problems such as stuttering and 'word salad' (where people say words back to front); integrates left and right hemispheres of the brain so a person can focus on the individual words yet at the same time be aware of the overall meaning and context of the words. Consequently, while reading or speaking they know when to use tone and inflection in their voice rather than merely reading word after word in a monotonous drone, rarely remembering what they have just read

Red Grevillea ... works on and balances the temporomandibular joint (TMJ)—so an individual can open their mouth wide and speak more clearly and easily

spirituality (*see also* chakras; enlightenment; meditation)

Angelsword ... for spiritual discernment; allows access and retrieval of previously developed gifts and skills from past lives; releases negative energies and entities from the psyche; protects from outside influences and entities so you can receive clear information from your Higher Self without interference

Angelsword, Mint Bush, Red Lily ... for clearing confusion and fogginess in spiritual life

Black-eyed Susan ... helps you to find your still, quiet place within, where spiritual guidance and direction can be found

Bluebell ... opens the heart to unconditional love

Boab ... sends earth-bound spirits to the Light. This essence can also help where the energy of trying to conform to your traditional family way of religion or spiritual practice is stunting your own spiritual growth and energy

Boronia ... greatly improves your ability to concentrate and hold steady a vision or image in manifestation and creative visualisation

Bush Fuchsia ... to listen to and follow your intuition

Bush Iris ... for awakening your spirituality to realise that there are ways beyond the perception of the five senses by increasing faith and trust as well as awareness of spirituality. It acts to release any fear of death. It clears blocks in the base, the fifth chakra or trust centre and the third eye or sixth chakra

Crowea ... aligns the subtle energy bodies (being suddenly disturbed while astral travelling, either in deep sleep or meditation, will usually be the cause of this imbalance)

Five Corners, Pink Mulla Mulla, Red Grevillea, Waratah ... helps to prevent sabotaging your spiritual growth

Fringed Violet ... will heal any breaks or holes in the aura and should be thought of automatically for spiritual protection and guarding against psychic attack or energy drain by others

Green Spider Orchid ... enables spiritual teachers to impart their knowledge non-verbally; tunes a person to be more receptive and telepathic with other life forms

Green Spider Orchid, Kapok Bush, Red Lily ... for opening, balancing and harmonising the higher chakras above the crown

Gymea Lily ... for spiritual humility when recognising and contemplating the vastness, perfection and complexity of the spiritual world and your role within it. Such humility will allow you to humbly ask for guidance and direction when working with Spirit and to not come from your ego

Kangaroo Paw ... addresses the feelings of naivety and awe you can have when first entering upon and contemplating the vastness, perfection and complexity of the spiritual world

Little Flannel Flower ... helps children to reconnect with their spirit guides if this ability has been lost through criticism or negative reaction by unaware parents, teachers or other influential adults

Meditation Essence ... a wonderful combination to awaken your spirituality and allow you to go deeper into any religious or spiritual practice; enhances access to your Higher Self while providing psychic protection and healing of the aura

Mint Bush ... for the trials and perturbations preceding spiritual initiation and the moving on to a higher level

Paw Paw ... for contacting your Higher Self and own inner wisdom in order to find the best solution when faced with a choice of two or more things

Red Lily ... opens the crown and higher chakras above the crown, and helps you to remember that you are the loving child of a loving God; for spirituality and connection to God in a grounded, centred way

Rough Bluebell ... helps us to release more and more of our inherent love vibration

Transition Essence ... for spiritual death and re-birth; where there is fear of, or resistance to, transformation

split, emotionally (*see also* focus; schizophrenia)
Bluebell ... for an individual who goes in and out of being emotionally split, rather than leaving their body, due to severe emotional pain. Frequently they deal with the pain by totally closing down their emotions and feelings

Crowea ... helps to realign the subtle bodies which, when out of kilter, can lead to severe psychic disturbance and feeling split. At the same time it will bring a person back into emotional balance

Pink Mulla Mulla, Sturt Desert Pea ... both essences work to resolve and heal deep emotional hurt and psychic wounding but the latter addresses more the grief and sadness, the principal cause of an individual being emotionally split, which is another way of saying mental illness

Red Lily ... for any individual choosing to avoid feelings and emotions by pursuing their spiritual or religious practice to such a point that they become ungrounded, impractical and live with their 'heads in the clouds'. This essence will keep them in touch with the earth and themselves, here on a physical level, while still working with Spirit

Sundew ... when there is severe deep or excessive emotional pain, a person may choose to 'split off'. This essence will help bring their spirit back into their body

spontaneity

Illawarra Flame Tree ... encourages emotional spontaneity—dealing with things when they come up—passionately, openly and honestly

Little Flannel Flower ... to release the child within and live life with fun, joy and playfulness, and not be suppressed and restricted by society's conventions and rules

sport

Bauhinia ... to be open to new techniques, strategies and concepts involving the sport you are playing

Bush Fuchsia ... by integrating the hemispheres of the brain and balancing the hypothalamus, which affects spatial orientation, this remedy enhances, fine tunes and noticeably improves physical co-ordination, skill, timing and sharpness

Crowea ... assists to heal sore, tired and damaged muscles and tendons; also helps a sportsperson to be calm and centred before participating in competitive or challenging sport

Dynamis Essence ... aids stamina and endurance while training and performing

Emergency Essence ... addresses any injuries or trauma while training for or participating in a sport

Flannel Flower ... allows you to enjoy your body and the physical expression of it. Encourages you to be a participant rather than viewing sport on TV; also increases physical energy

Little Flannel Flower ... to not lose the appreciation and sense of fun and play involved in sport

Macrocarpa ... engenders stamina and endurance and is of great help when there is physical exhaustion or danger of burnout

Slender Rice Flower ... encourages group harmony and co-operation from individuals so they can successfully play and perform as a team

Sturt Desert Rose . . . for personal integrity and playing by the rules in any sporting activity

Waratah . . . for great courage, strength and tenacity. Also a good one for dealing with the despair of 'losing'

Wedding Bush . . . for total commitment to training and preparation for sport, especially when played at a high level

Wild Potato Bush . . . helps you to deal with any frustration associated with injuries that stop you from competing or performing at all or in the way that you want to. It can also be used to address frustration regarding any limitations in ability, or conditioning that stops you performing as you would like

stability

Crowea . . . for calming and centring when one is feeling 'not quite right' or a little out of balance

Dog Rose of the Wild Forces . . . helps a person who is surrounded by chaos or very intense emotions to stay calm and not be carried away by the agitated environment in which he finds himself

Jacaranda . . . when there is a sense of being scattered, dithering and 'all over the place', rarely finishing one thing before starting another

Mint Bush . . . when there is tremendous confusion, change and perturbation going on in life and your usual 'security blankets' and sense of support and stability have been pulled asunder

Peach-flowered Tea-tree . . . for people whose moods tend to swing. Such people often lose interest in a project once the initial challenge has dissipated and it is becoming mundane but well before completion

Red Lily . . . if you are on a spiritual path this essence can help you move into your spirituality while remaining very much in touch with the practicalities of your life

Sundew . . . is for the dreamy person who is vague and disconnected. This will help bring them back into the present moment

stage fright (see also confidence; fear)

Bush Fuchsia . . . for developing and enhancing your ability to project your voice, sing and speak with greater melody, clarity, feeling, tone and inflection

Crowea . . . worrying about how the show or event will go

Dog Rose . . . feeling anxious and shy before performing

Grey Spider Orchid . . . for the paralysing fear that can sometimes accompany speaking or performing in public

stamina, endurance (see also exhaustion; strength; tiredness)

Macrocarpa . . . works on adrenals to maintain strength and stamina and to help overcome exhaustion and physical burnout

standing out from crowd see courage; enlightenment; fear

stiffness *see* flexibility

street kids (*see also* abuse, victim of; adolescence; family and social inter-action; fatherhood; motherhood)
Bluebell ... can help those who work with such children to open their hearts to them
Boab ... these kids no longer fit into their family patterns of behaviour. This essence can break the family patterns they can no longer tolerate, without anger. It is also very good for the parents so they, in turn, can change the traditional principles of their parenting and so be more effective parents
Dog Rose of the Wild Forces ... where there is danger of taking on the emotional agitation of those around them and going out of control themselves
Five Corners ... to boost their self-esteem, self-worth
Grey Spider Flower ... for the extreme fear and terror these kids can experience when they are living on the streets
Macrocarpa ... gives them the physical strength and endurance when living in what are often far from ideal conditions
Red Helmet Orchid ... for the teenager or child who has a problem dealing with authority figures. Much teenage rebellion stems from a poor father–child relationship, which this essence can heal
Rough Bluebell ... this essence helps kids to know that they can be loved, loving and lovable
Sexuality Essence ... many of these children and adolescents ran away from their family homes because of the physical or sexual abuse they suffered there. It is the sad but stark truth that such abuse is just as prevalent, if not more so, on the streets than in their homes. This essence addresses such sexual abuse
Silver Princess ... will help them find a sense of direction and purpose rather than feeling aimless and lost
Slender Rice Flower ... can clear any tendency for them to feel totally separate from and hostile towards mainstream society
Southern Cross ... empowers a street kid to see themselves not as victims, but as one who can mould and shape their life with vision and purpose to create the destiny they desire
Sunshine Wattle ... addresses their sense of struggle, difficulty and, in many cases, their lack of hope or optimism
Tall Mulla Mulla ... some street kids have such a difficult time with confrontation and social skills that they choose to live alone on the streets, away from their family and society
Tall Yellow Top ... for healing their sense of alienation from both family and society
Waratah ... will give courage to keep going in difficult circumstances. It also helps to draw on forgotten survival skills

strength (*see also* commitment; endurance)

Crowea ... works on muscles and tendons and so can help to improve physical strength

Gymea Lily ... gives strength to those who are ahead of their peers and helps them to stay at the top of their chosen life path

Macrocarpa ... because this essence boosts the adrenal glands it is very effective in improving physical stamina. When a person is in danger of burning out physically this essence can bring about renewed enthusiasm, endurance and inner strength

Sturt Desert Rose ... is about having the strength and courage to adhere to your own morality and beliefs

Waratah ... will give the strength and fortitude to keep going even in very, very difficult circumstances

stress (*see also* calmness; change; environment; relaxation)

Alpine Mint Bush ... for the stress of having to care for or constantly make decisions about the welfare and wellbeing of others

Bauhinia ... can be effective when stress is a consequence of resisting change

Black-eyed Susan ... *the* stress essence for when you are constantly feeling rushed, that there is never enough time to do things. It is especially effective if you are a very active and enthusiastic person who doesn't know how or when to stop and rest—and a great remedy for those who have to work with them!

Boronia ... the stress of not being able to close the mind off from constant and repetitive thoughts

Cognis Essence ... for the stress associated with an educational environment in which an individual is battling with learning difficulties

Crowea ... where stress is resulting from chronic worrying, this essence can help to centre, calm and relax

Dog Rose ... will relieve anxiety, shakiness and niggling fears which rob a person of their vital life force

Emergency Essence ... should be taken frequently when a person is in a very tense situation or when unexpected shock or trauma is creating stress in their lives. Can be used for all emotional stress, trauma or crises

Jacaranda ... for the stress that arises when a person who is indecisive and scattered has to make a decision, for they have a real fear of making the wrong one and so get very uptight and jittery

Kapok Bush ... for breaking the pattern of giving up when stress gets too high

Mint Bush ... deals with the intense stress associated with perturbation and confusion

Paw Paw ... where there is stress about decision making or in coping with a large quantity of work to be completed or information to be assimilated, especially when there is limited time in which to do it

Red Suva Frangipani . . . this nurtures and soothes an individual experiencing stress and pain in relationships when they are at a crisis point

Sturt Desert Pea . . . for the tension associated with deep hurt or personal loss

Transition Essence . . . addresses and eases all the stresses of major change

strictness *see* discipline

struggle (*see also* apathy; optimism; victim)
Sunshine Wattle . . . engenders an awareness that life doesn't always have to be grim and hard

stubbornness
Bauhinia . . . where there is resistance to embracing new ideas and different ways of doing things

Freshwater Mangrove . . . for those who are closed to new experiences because of often unjustified prejudice

Isopogon . . . for the controlling personality who often uses stubbornness to try to control others, but without any malice

Rough Bluebell . . . this essence is for the deliberately hurtful and manipulative person who stubbornly pursues, on many levels, the suppression of their inherent love vibration. On a positive note this essence engenders compassion, sensitivity and, of course, love

stuck (*see also* frustration; restriction)
Alpine Mint Bush . . . for the person in the position of caring for another who, after a time, feels trapped. This essence will renew enthusiam, joy and compassion in what they are doing

Bauhinia . . . for those who are resistant to new ideas; where there is an unwillingness to venture into new areas of life

Boab . . . where negative family patterns are preventing action or personal growth or where a person is so controlled by traditional family values that they are unable to do things any other way

Five Corners . . . for the person who sabotages their own goals. They know what they want to do and how to do it but almost unconsciously they allow things to happen in their lives which prevent them achieving their dreams, because at the bottom level they believe that either they are not good enough or they don't deserve it

Kapok Bush . . . this type of person stays stuck where they are because any change in their status quo seems just too hard and too much effort

Mint Bush . . . can be really helpful when you hit the proverbial brick wall in your spiritual growth. It helps burn off the dross so you can move through to a new level of awareness. Or alternatively, it can help when you feel that you have been stuck in that process of burning off the dross for far too long and there is no end in sight

Red Grevillea ... when a person knows exactly what they want to do but can't see how they can possibly do it. They are stuck! This essence will help them see the way through—often in a manner that is unique, and different from what others had imagined

Sunshine Wattle ... where negative past experiences leave a person unable to even consider a more positive future, this essence will help them see the beauty, joy and excitement in the present, and optimistically anticipate life ahead

studying *see* adolescence; focus; learning

stuttering (*see also* speech problems)
Bush Fuchsia ... for any speaking and voice problems, but also specifically for stuttering

Dog Rose ... where the person who stutters is feeling shy, anxious or fearful

Five Corners ... stuttering frequently occurs when a person doubts themselves or is not feeling self-confident

subconscious mind (*see also* dreams)
Ninety per cent of our beliefs—which are stored in the subconscious mind—were formed between conception and three years of age, at a time when our cognitive processes and intellect were very immature and far from being fully formed. These beliefs, formed when we were so young, continue to direct and affect our conscious behaviour way into adulthood, for we are constantly creating situations to reinforce the particular beliefs that we hold. We rarely have a conscious awareness formulated early in our lives. One of the main actions of the Australian Bush Flower Essences is to release and clear any such negative beliefs that we are holding in our subconscious mind. All sixty-two of the Bush Essences work powerfully on the subconscious mind in their specific sphere of action. The following examples are in no way exhaustive but rather highlight some of the more frequently used essences due to their general across the board or critical action on the subconscious mind

Boab ... one of the most powerful essences in that it clears the subconscious mind of the tremendous amount of patterning arising from your chosen family, down which excess and deleterious emotional baggage has been flowing generation after generation. After such repatterning by Boab, more of the true essence of the individual can awaken and emerge

Five Corners ... aligns the conscious with the subconscious mind, thereby clearing any sabotage while you are working towards your goals. A Universal lesson we have all come here to learn is self-love and acceptance. The most common and core negative belief must be that 'I'm not good enough, I'm unlovable'. Five Corners works to restore the rightful awareness of yourself as being loving, unique and Divine, and full of self-love and acceptance.

Waratah ... transmutes any suicidal or death wish in the subconscious mind into an appreciation and love of life

success (*see also* confidence; courage; goal setting; perseverance)

Bauhinia ... opens one to the gifts and abundance of the Universe that come as rewards for success

Boab ... to be used whenever there is a lack of history or reference to success by either parent or in the family as a whole

Boronia ... strengthens and sustains your focus and vision of being successful which is an important precursor to actually achieving success

Five Corners ... helps you attain success by clearing sabotage and boosting your self-worth and your belief that you deserve to be successful

Gymea Lily ... will give the strength to stay successful and be a peer leader without any arrogance or feelings of superiority

Peach-flowered Tea-tree ... supports someone who has already overcome the difficulties and challenges of starting a project but who has a tendency not to successfully follow it through to completion because it feels too easy or boring

Silver Princess ... after a goal is reached there is often a feeling of flatness. Silver Princess will give a sense of what is next and allow you to enjoy the journey while striving for the new goal

Wedding Bush ... for deepening commitment to a scheme or project

suicide (*see also* depression; hope)

Angelsword ... any internal voice telling us to hurt or kill ourselves is not that of our Higher Self but rather an attached negative psychic entity. Angelsword is the remedy to cut out, literally, such energies or entities from the psyche

Emergency Essence ... to help deal with the trauma of an attempted suicide—both for the individual who has tried to take his own life and for those who are supporting him. It addresses the shock of those finding the dead body or friends and relatives hearing about the suicide or suicide attempt

Red Grevillea ... where the feeling of being trapped in a situation can lead to thoughts of suicide as a way of escape

Southern Cross ... supports us to realise that we are not victims of fate and that we can take charge of and responsibility for our lives and create them to be meaningful and desirable

Sturt Desert Rose ... will ease the guilt of those who felt they should have been more aware of what was happening to the person who suicided, or who could have done more beforehand to have stopped it from occurring

Sunshine Wattle ... for the person with a grim past who has great trouble seeing any likelihood of a bright future

Tall Yellow Top . . . a feeling of total isolation and abandonment and of never really fitting in can frequently give rise to either a conscious or subconscious death wish

Waratah . . . this powerful essence will quickly pull a person back when they are feeling suicidal and going through a 'dark night of soul'. It works incredibly quickly, as indeed it needs to if a person is suicidal. Rarely will it take more than three or four days to take effect. It helps us to realise that we are never given anything in life with which we can't cope and allows us to draw on spiritual faith and trust to get through the crisis. By also retrieving and activating any forgotten survival skills, it further gives us the courage to cope with any crisis

sulky, sullen, whining *see* complaining

superficial

Jacaranda . . . for the scattered, dithering type of person who finds it hard to get deeply involved

Kangaroo Paw . . . in interaction and conversation they will rarely, or only tokenly, ask about the other party: all they are really interested in is themselves

Peach-flowered Tea-tree . . . this sort of person starts off on a scheme with great excitement and drive but quicky loses interest after the initial enthusiasm

Rough Bluebell . . . an individual who attempts to con or trick others, pretending to be who they aren't or feigning love and affection as a way of manipulating others to get what they want

Sturt Desert Rose . . . to help people adhere to their own morality and not try to live their lives by other's standards

superiority (*see also* arrogance; racism)

Gymea Lily . . . removes the need and tendency for arrogance and feeling of superiority towards others

Hibbertia . . . for the strict and exacting personality who is constantly striving to improve himself and acquiring information and knowledge, and who feels mentally superior to others with less knowledge or to those who aren't following or pursuing what he does

Slender Rice Flower . . . where just being a member of a different race or religion is enough for this person to judge another as inferior

Yellow Cowslip Orchid . . . they feel superior to those who don't do the right thing, or break the rules and regulations, and are therefore not pulling their weight for the common good or to help society function

suppressed feelings (*see also* denial)

Bluebell . . . helps a person to be aware of suppressed or cut-off feelings

Bottlebrush + Boronia . . . for people who use addictive behaviour or substances to alter their mood, thereby suppressing or blocking painful or uncomfortable feelings—the 'hole in the soul'

Flannel Flower ... for those who feel emotions but have difficulty expressing or communicating them

Flannel Flower + Fringed Violet + Wisteria ... where a person has suppressed their need for emotional and physical intimacy as a result of sexual abuse or trauma

Philotheca ... for people who play down their achievements and successes

Pink Mulla Mulla ... puts a brave or tough front on to cover deep hurt and pain

Rough Bluebell ... for those who have forgotten or have chosen not to express the love vibration within them. This is why they can maliciously hurt others and be indifferent about it

Sundew ... people who 'space out' when feelings become too intense

Tall Mulla Mulla ... they act or say what they think other people will want to hear, so as to avoid conflict

Yellow Cowslip Orchid ... when emotions become too intense they close down to go away to think about them; in times of danger and chaos they have the necessary strength and discipline to allow their mind to stay in control of their emotions

survival skills
Bush Fuchsia ... to be open to and trust your intuition, which can be crucial for survival

Dog Rose of the Wild Forces ... allows you to stay calm and in balance in a crisis situation where to lose your head could literally mean your demise

Flannel Flower ... helps to set up and establish healthy boundaries and therefore a much safer environment

Yellow Cowslip Orchid ... in times of danger and chaos it enables you to have the necessary strength and discipline to allow your mind to stay in control of your emotions and make clear, beneficial choices

Waratah ... helps retrieve old forgotten survival skills and gives the person courage and the ability to work through very difficult experiences or crises

suspicious (*see also* aggressiveness; fear; trust)
Mountain Devil ... for the very suspicious and wary person who is always on their guard, expecting the worst of everyone they meet, and not trusting others. This essence can bring through unconditional love, forgiveness and happiness

Pink Mulla Mulla ... they remain suspicious of and cautious in opening up to others in case they are abused or hurt

Slender Rice Flower ... when you have had a negative experience at the hands of one or more individuals of a clique, culture, religion or nationality that now makes you suspicious of anyone from that same group

Yellow Cowslip Orchid ... intellectual people who are very suspicious of emotions and especially of 'overly emotional' people

switched off, feeling *see* focus; 'spaced out' feeling

synergy (*see also* harmony)
Slender Rice Flower . . . the sum of the whole is always greater than the
sum of the individual parts. This remedy helps to bring about unity,
group harmony and co-operation where individuals can put aside their
egos for the common good of the group. It can be very effective when
sprayed around a meeting room or wherever people, especially com-
mittees, assemble

tactless *see* sensitivity to needs of others

taking on energy of others (*see also* protection)
Fringed Violet . . . gives protection against unconsciously taking on board
the negative energies of others

'tall poppy' syndrome
Gymea Lily . . . helps support those who are willing to go out on a limb
to achieve what is dear to their hearts or their life's passion, even when
some of the people around them are trying, subtly or openly, to bring
them down—solely because of the greatness or uniqueness of the
person they perceive to be a 'tall poppy'
Mountain Devil . . . for the envy and jealousy that is felt towards others
by those who are not fulfilling themselves
Rough Bluebell . . . addresses the part in individuals where they have
trouble expressing their love but no trouble maliciously putting
someone down

tantrums (*see also* anger; children; temper)
Dog Rose of the Wild Forces . . . where a person, when surrounded by
others who are out of control emotionally, is in danger of losing their
self-control completely and becoming caught up in it as well
Kangaroo Paw . . . an immature or naive person can sometimes display
tantrum-like behaviour without realising that it is not the appropriate
way to behave in the circumstances
Moutain Devil . . . this can help the person who thinks the only way to
express feelings of anger is by emotional outbursts and violence
Red Helmet Orchid . . . for the rebellious, hot-headed person who will
put on a tantrum as an act of defiance
Rough Bluebell . . . for the controlling adult who is capable of putting on
a tantrum or playing the martyr in order to get their own way

teariness (*see also* depression; fear; grief; hormonal imbalance;
overwhelm)
Bottlebrush . . . the process of letting go can entail, and be helped by, a
good cry

Crowea + Peach-flowered Tea-tree + She Oak ... for the teariness that sometimes accompanies premenstrual syndrome in women

Dog Rose of the Wild Forces ... for hysteria

Flannel Flower ... trusting that it is safe and OK to express and let out your feelings, including tears and sadness

Fringed Violet ... after any shock or trauma when there is a sense of being very vulnerable

Peach-flowered Tea-tree ... for the person who has mild or even excessive mood swings, when they are feeling low and teary

Red Suva Frangipani ... during any relationship break-up or turmoil when a person is feeling emotionally very fragile and raw

Sturt Desert Pea ... when there is a release of deeply felt pain and hurt which has often been long held. This need to cry is a very important part of the healing process. Conversely this is the essence to think of for individuals who have difficulty crying or feel they can't cry. Give them this remedy and a box of tissues, and wait for the results

teeth grinding (*see also* addictions; boredom; repetitiveness)

Black-eyed Susan ... helps to reduce the stress that is behind the action

Boronia ... helps break habitual behaviour

Dagger Hakea, Mountain Devil ... anger, according to Chinese medicine, is traditionally held in the jaw

Dog Rose ... grinding teeth in children is sometimes a sign of an ongoing, but frequently unexpressed, fear

Red Grevillea ... corrects any imbalance in the TMJ, the underlying causes of which can be a common cause of teeth grinding

telepathy (*see also* clairaudience)

Green Spider Orchid ... this essence assists in working with telepathy. To attune a person to be more receptive to not only other people but also to other species and kingdoms. It allows anyone teaching spiritual subjects or matter to impart that knowledge non-verbally and intuitively as well

temper (*see also* anger; tantrums)

Black-eyed Susan ... for those who feel annoyed and irritated at others who can't work at the same frenetic pace as themselves

Dagger Hakea ... lets resentment and irritation slowly bubble and brew in a cold, sharp, subtle temper, hostility or prickliness

Dog Rose of the Wild Forces ... for situations where emotions are in danger of running out of control because of the intense energy of others

Kangaroo Paw ... for immature or inappropriate expressions of anger or irritation

Mountain Devil ... for those expressing anger, sometimes violently, because of hatred, jealousy or simple rage

Pink Mulla Mulla ... for someone very quick to anger or temper as a protective mechanism to stop them coming too close to others and to keep others at a distance, the bottom line being they are afraid of being hurt if they get close to other people

Rough Bluebell ... someone who allows themselves to hurt and affect others by choosing not to suppress or withhold their anger, temper or rage

tenderness (*see also* sensuality; sexuality)

Alpine Mint Bush ... re-establishing the joy and tenderness of caring for others, when there has been a danger of compassion burnout

Bluebell ... opening heart to joyful sharing of unconditional love

Bush Gardenia ... for deepening communications and drawing together those in a relationship who are tending to move away from each other

Flannel Flower ... this essence engenders gentleness and sensitivity in touching. It helps a person trust and express their inner feelings and be vulnerable

Kangaroo Paw ... of great benefit to the individual who is awkward, clumsy and all thumbs

Wisteria ... benefits the 'macho male' personality by allowing him to be more aware of his softer, feminine nature; to be open to, enjoy and express one's sensuality and sensual feelings

tension *see* relaxation; stress

terror (*see also* fear)

Emergency Essence ... to be used frequently after a person has experienced terror or a shocking trauma

Green Spider Orchid ... for the terror, nightmares and phobias which have their origins in a past life experience. This essence is also for those who are terrified by the sight of blood

Grey Spider Flower ... can help with terror and nightmares relating to present life or sudden unexpected horrors which occur in our lives. Some terrors come from in-womb experiences and this essence can be of benefit in treating them

thoughts, obsessive *see* obsessiveness

thoughts, putting into words *see* communication; speech problems; learning

tight with money, love, feelings (*see also* abundance, lacking; love; trust)

Bluebell ... for those unable to share their love, feelings, money or material goods because they operate from a subconscious fear that there is just not enough

Dagger Hakea ... where there is a tendency to allow resentment and old grudges to stop them from sharing themselves or their belongings with others

Flannel Flower ... encourages a person to trust that it is safe to let out their feelings and express themselves

Mountain Devil ... their anger, suspicion and lack of trust prevent them from opening up and being loving and generous with others

Pink Mulla Mulla ... they are very reluctant to show their sensitivity and vulnerability to others

Sunshine Wattle ... is for the person who has no optimism about their financial situation and so hangs on grimly to what they've got

Yellow Cowslip Orchid ... these rational, logical people, who tend to be out of touch and disconnected from their feelings, are very conservative and cautious by nature. They generally store or bank their money, saving it for a rainy day, being more concerned about the future and possible threats. They are not known for being spendthrifts or buying on the spur of the moment. They would be most unlikely to squander the proceeds of an unexpected windfall on a no-expenses-spared night on the town

timidity (*see also* confidence; fear; shyness)

Bauhinia ... people who shy away from having any contact with new technology because they feel it is all too complicated and difficult and beyond them, or who just don't want to trouble themselves having to learn something new

Dog Rose ... for those shy people who have niggling fears and are apprehensive around other people

Five Corners ... if you are feeling good about yourself then others will not intimidate you

Kapok Bush ... very intimidated and reluctant to play around with anything electrical or mechanical that is broken because they don't have much of an idea about machines or technology. This remedy helps give an overview as well as knowledge of the specific step by step functioning of how these things work

Sundew ... because of their dreaminess, indecision and lack of focus this person is often reluctant to take action

Tall Mulla Mulla ... for those who feel unsafe mixing with people and who would much rather be by themselves. They fear that if they do socialise with others then disharmony could result which would make them very uncomfortable, so they usually keep their distance

Waratah ... this very powerful essence will give a timid person the courage to get through a difficult experience

tiredness (*see also* exhaustion)

Alpine Mint Bush ... where the continued hearing of people's problems;

caring for them or having the constant responsibility of making decisions day in, day out for the health and wellbeing of other people can lead to exhaustion

Banksia Robur . . . for the normally energetic person who is temporarily lacking enthusiasm and energy, usually as a result of illness or setback

Black-eyed Susan . . . for the tiredness that comes from frenetic activity and intensity; for the sort of person who doesn't know how to slow down and rest, and can sometimes end up burning out

Bluebell . . . by opening up and getting in touch with previously suppressed feelings and memories, one generates vitality and energy

Fringed Violet . . . for sensitive people who find their energy easily being drained by others

Macrocarpa . . . when someone is tired, exhausted and burnt out. Physically this essence can bring about renewed enthusiasm, endurance and inner strength. It can also be beneficial to women during a long labour when they need physical stamina to get through the birthing process

Old Man Banksia . . . for the slower, phlegmatic constitutional type when weary or tired or run down. These very family-minded people tend to be the ones to whom everyone turns for a shoulder to cry on; they are usually there for everyone else

Peach-flowered Tea-tree . . . when tiredness is the result of low blood sugar

Pink Mulla Mulla . . . where old emotional or spiritual pain and blockages are preventing a normal or adequate flow of energy

Silver Princess . . . if there is no sense of purpose, direction or passion for what you are doing, you usually have low energy

tolerance (*see also* acceptance; impatience; racism)

Bauhinia . . . encourage one to accept and tolerate the differences, idiosyncrasies and peculiarities in people

Black-eyed Susan . . . for the very active, energetic and efficient person who has a low tolerance for any perceived incompetence or slowness in others

Boab . . . helps parents become more tolerant of their children, because it serves to stop them from projecting all of their unfulfilled desires and expectations on to their children and then reacting because the children want to do their own thing and lead their own lives

Hibbertia . . . for the very self-disciplined and well informed person who feels a sense of superiority to other 'lesser' beings

Slender Rice Flower . . . acts to remind an individual that ultimately there is no separation and that all people are equal, no one is better than anyone else, even though some may be evolving at a higher rate

Yellow Cowslip Orchid . . . these air or intellectual types have a tendency to be very critical and judgmental of others, especially if they are out of balance

touch, uncomfortable with *see* sexuality

tranquillity *see* calmness

transformation (*see also* spirituality)
Bauhinia ... where there is resistance to any new ideas or ways of thinking or doing things
Dog Rose ... for niggling fears about new experiences and knowledge
Mint Bush ... for difficult periods in spiritual growth when dross has to be burnt off before you can emerge to a higher spiritual level
Transition Essence ... can help a person to let go, to 'die' at some level, and so have a clear path before them on which to move forward

trapped *see* stuck

trauma, shock (*see also* abuse, victim of; accident)
Emergency Essence ... administer frequently during or immediately after physical or emotional shock or trauma, when there is panic, distress, fear or an inability to cope
Fringed Violet ... for healing the aura which is damaged by trauma. It has a particular use for people who have had a cathartic experience after re-birthing or past life regression, whenever a person has gone back a long way in time during a healing session
Green Spider Orchid ... where nightmares or terrors result from traumatic happenings in past lives
Grey Spider Flower ... for terror from nightmares or other horrific occurrences
Pink Mulla Mulla ... this essence can clear residual trauma from an horrific experience in a very early incarnation, which has been blocking personal and spiritual growth

trust
Black-eyed Susan ... encourages super active people to realise the world will not fall down if they stop and rest occasionally; helps people to delegate
Bluebell ... helps a person trust that it is OK to give out and share their love because this is not a finite resource. The more you give out, the more you will receive
Bush Fuchsia ... increases awareness and trust in own intuition
Flannel Flower ... allows one to trust that it is safe to be physically or emotionally intimate with another person or people
Hibbertia ... for the person who doesn't trust their own inner wisdom but instead relies on obtaining knowledge from books or philosophies
Mountain Devil ... it clears anger, hatred and suspicion, making way for trust and love
Pink Mulla Mulla ... lacking trust in others because of fear of the repetition of a past hurt

Southern Cross ... trusting that we are not merely victims of fate, during our time on earth; that there is a reason behind everything that happens to us; even the most challenging and difficult experience is an invaluable lesson to be learnt

Spinifex ... trusting that there is a message—which we need to learn—behind each illness

Sturt Desert Rose ... encourages trust in own standards and morality

Tall Mulla Mulla ... where there is fear of interaction with others because of fear of conflict and disharmony

Waratah ... helps restores faith and trust that we are never given anything in life with which we can't cope

truth (*see also* honesty; spirituality)

Angelsword ... for discernment in identifying what is the truth for us among a plethora of spiritual teachings and channelled information

Hibbertia ... to realise that you can never find total truth in outside sources, that it is also interwoven with your own inner wisdom and experiences

Spinifex ... to be able to read the truth that your physical symptoms are attempting to reveal to you

Sturt Desert Rose ... enables a person to honour their own truth

Red Lily ... to know and understand Universal truths

turmoil (*see also* calmness; fear; trauma, shock)

Black-eyed Susan ... these people have a tendency to burst on to a scene like a whirlwind—departing just as quickly—and leaving family members, work colleagues or friends dazed and stunned

Crowea ... this remedy calms, mellows and helps balance very intense people who are often seething beds of emotions and who frequently attract—and enjoy—drama

Dog Rose of the Wild Forces ... for where a person has a fear of losing total control because the emotions they are feeling within themselves or immediately around them are very intense

Emergency Essence ... for use during any fearful, stressful or chaotic situations. Take it frequently as it will allay your distress and create an ability to cope

Jacaranda ... these people often create turmoil and havoc due to their chaotic, scattered approach to life

Red Suva Frangipani ... for the initial grief, emotional upheaval and rawness which comes with the break-up of, or turmoil within, a relationship

TV, videos, computers, after long periods watching *see* 'spaced out' feeling

unaware (*see also* awareness; focus; spirituality)

Bush Gardenia ... in relationships when there is lack of awareness of what is really going on with those close to them. They are also often unaware that their actions and words are not being perceived in the same manner as they were conveyed

Bush Iris ... can help to awaken a spiritually unaware person

Freshwater Mangrove ... to become aware of different ways of seeing and perceiving reality, and to be open to new paradigms of thinking

Kangaroo Paw ... for the socially unaware person who hurts and offends others without either intending to or noticing that they have because they are so self-focused

Spinifex ... where there is a lack of awareness as to the significance behind your set of physical symptoms and what message your Higher Self is attempting to convey to you

Sundew ... for the dreamy, unfocused person who can be completely unware of what is going on around him

unborn child *see* pregnancy and birth

uncentred, ungrounded *see* focus

unconditional love *see* love

unrealistic *see* immaturity; practicality

unreliable (*see also* stability; trust)

Jacaranda ... one can never be sure whether agreed upon or intended tasks or projects will be completed as these people are so easily distracted and sidetracked

Peach-flowered Tea-tree ... this sort of person will start off full of energy and enthusiasm, but once the initial excitement has passed, they are likely to grow bored and lose interest

Rough Bluebell ... there can be a level of dishonesty in what they say and what they do

Sturt Desert Rose ... will help those who are easily led by others to stick to their own principles

Sundew ... they agree to do something but procrastinate for so long that it is never completed, sometimes not even started; or they are so vague and dreamy that they forget all about it

Tall Mulla Mulla ... they will make commitments they have no intention of fulfilling but which at the time gets them out of potentially uncomfortable situations

used, feeling, by others *see* stuck; victim

vagueness *see* aging; focus

vanity (*see also* arrogance; superiority)

Gymea Lily ... addresses the desire for glamour and to be the centre of attention, love and adoration from others

Hibbertia . . . they can be fanatically driven to improve themselves simply for the sake of wanting to look good to others

Illawarra Flame Tree . . . the very visual individual who is extremely conscious of how they look and appear so as to make as big an impression as possible, much preferring to be noticed than to be ignored or be in the background

Kangaroo Paw . . . they are totally preoccupied with their own selfish needs and wants

veterans of war

Alpine Mint Bush . . . for the mental and emotional exhaustion of those who had the responsibility of giving orders, knowing that their choice affected the lives of their men

Bluebell . . . where there has been multiple repression of emotions and experiences connected with the horror of war: for many it was the only way they could survive

Dog Rose of the Wild Forces . . . where there can be traumatic stress disorder as a result of all the previously repressed feelings and experiences coming to the surface and threatening to totally engulf them

Emergency Essence . . . for dealing with the nightmares and flashbacks arising from their experiences

Fringed Violet . . . to remove the effects of shock and trauma that warfare inflicts on its soldiers, even though the war may have finished decades ago

Silver Princess . . . to help re-establish a sense of life direction after such a shocking interruption to day-to-day life

Slender Rice Flower . . . where there is a total hatred of or intolerance towards the nations they were fighting

Sturt Desert Pea . . . for the deep hurt and pain that comes from seeing your best friends or family killed around you

Sturt Desert Rose . . . to alleviate any guilt and remorse resulting from actions they committed, or failed to commit, in the war

Tall Yellow Top . . . where there is a sense of alienation and aloneness as a result of knowing that what was experienced during the war is not understood or appreciated by friends, family and the country in general. Also for the alienation that many Vietnam veterans experienced on their return home where, by and large, they didn't have the support of the community to validate what they had done or to help them readjust to civilian life as all Australian soldiers from previous wars had had. Nor later from the politicians who ignored and tried to cover up the obvious physical and emotional scars the veterans brought home with them (e.g. the denial that Agent Orange had anything to do with their multitude of health problems, including birth defects in their children)

Wild Potato Bush . . . to help deal with the restriction and frustration of war wounds, especially where they left permanent damage

Wisteria + Flannel Flower . . . to help an individual become aware of and express once again their gentle, softer nature which can so easily be hardened and lost as a result of the experiences of war

victim (*see also* abuse, victim of; sexuality)

Confid Essence . . . helps build confidence in the ability to take responsibility for yourself and everything that occurs in your life

Flannel Flower, Philotheca, Sturt Desert Rose . . . all three help those who, for varying reasons, can have a problem saying 'no', which can lead to a feeling of powerlessness, and not being in control of how they want things to be

Southern Cross . . . feeling others are to blame for your own life situation. It is the words, thoughts and actions that you put out that will come back to you in the creation of your reality. This essence enables you to realise it is *you* who create your reality, not fate, nor is it out of your hands to create what in fact you do want

Spinifex . . . To help anyone suffering with a so-called incurable condition—such as AIDS, hepatitis C, herpes or 'terminal' cancer—to understand what may be the underlying emotional trigger or cause behind the illness. The continual reappearance of any illness or symptom picture is an indication that they have not learnt the lesson of the illness

visualisation *see* meditation

vitality (*see also* exhaustion; tiredness)

Little Flannel Flower . . . brings about joy and vitality and an excitement about living

Silver Princess . . . when you are doing what really makes your heart sing, you will always have plenty of 'juice' and vitality

Turkey Bush . . . when expressing your creativity and tapping into creative energy, you become quite energised, vital and alive

voice (*see also* learning; music; speech problems)

Bush Fuchsia . . . for expressing verbally in speech or in song. This essence helps with the projection and timbre of the voice

Heartsong Essence . . . for opening the heart and using your voice to sing with joy

vulnerability (*see also* sensitivity to needs of others; trust)

Emergency Essence . . . to help get through shock, stress or a crisis situation when a person can feel very vulnerable

Flannel Flower . . . this brings an ease with intimacy and a trust that it is safe to let out and share your innermost feelings, thoughts and secrets to another—to really let them know what is going on with you

Fringed Violet ... for the times when a person has experienced great shock or trauma and is feeling fragile

Mint Bush ... for anyone going through tumultuous change or confusion and feeling very sensitive and vulnerable

Red Suva Frangipani ... for the extreme feeling of rawness which comes when a person is going through the upset of a relationship at rock bottom or a relationship break-up

Sturt Desert Rose ... the vulnerability that comes from honestly owning up to mistakes you have made and which you feel embarrassed about

weighed down, feeling (*see also* overweight; restriction; tiredness)

Alpine Mint Bush ... when feeling weighed down by the constant caring for a family member or in a job that involves caring and being responsible for others

Old Man Banksia ... for the Water or phlegmatic type who feels sluggish, weary and weighed down by the demands of life, family and friends

Paw-Paw ... for the sense of overwhelm when making decisions, taking on new information or coping with a large work load

Wild Potato Bush ... being weighed down by your body which, because of accident, illness, pregnancy or obesity, is not functioning as you would like it to

wisdom (*see also* awareness; spirituality)

Angelsword ... enables you to receive clear information and spiritual insight from your Higher Self without interference from outside influences or entities

Bush Fuchsia ... for hearing and trusting your own intuition and inner wisdom

Freshwater Mangrove ... a wise individual is one who can perceive and accept new understandings and theories, or see a new reality by looking from a new perspective

Green Spider Orchid ... enables a person to know when the time is right to share information, knowledge or experiences with others

Hibbertia ... when the intellect is connected to the heart, then true wisdom occurs

Paw Paw ... helps with getting in touch with your own Higher Self and own inner wisdom

Red Lily ... opens the crown and higher chakras to spiritual truths and insights

withdrawal (*see also* fear; confidence; depression)

Dog Rose ... for those who withdraw from others because of shyness and fear

Flannel Flower ... helps a person who pulls back from intimacy because of discomfort with physical or emotional closeness

Pink Mulla Mulla ... for the loner who puts out prickles to keep people away because of a fear of being hurt again after a previous wounding

Southern Cross ... where there is a tendency to withdraw and sulk, with the attitude that 'it is just not fair'

Tall Mulla Mulla ... this person keeps away from others because they basically fear that social interaction might result in conflict or turmoil and loss of peace

Tall Yellow Top ... for the 'stranger in a strange land' who feels lonely and alienated. Frequently, as a result of their pain being too great, they disconnect from their heart and feelings and live in their head or intellect

Yellow Cowslip Orchid ... the intellectual who tends to stay aloof from others or who emotionally withdraws when there is too much intensity in interactions with others. During a fiery argument, for example, they will want to 'put up the shutters' and go off by themselves to think about it rather than stay in the heat

workaholic (*see also* addictions; frenetic)

workshop 'junkies'
Hibbertia ... where there is a constant search for new knowledge, but often it is not integrated or there is little application of it in day-to-day life

worry (*see also* anxiety; fear; relaxation; stress)
Alpine Mint Bush ... worrying about the people under your care or whether the decisions you are making for them, or on their behalf, are the best that can be made

Angelsword ... for worry and concern that arises when a spiritual teacher or piece of channelled information goes against your understanding or intuition. This essence allows for discernment as to the best course of action and to help find the truth for you

Banksia Robur ... addresses the worry and concern associated with an illness, especially a chronic and debilitating one such as chronic fatigue syndrome or ME where an individual wonders if and when they will ever be well again

Billy Goat Plum ... concern about a part of yourself that you really dislike

Bluebell ... worry about just how much love can be given and shared before it 'runs out'

Crowea ... *the* worry essence. For those who always feel there is something to worry about and who are constant 'worry warts'

Illawarra Flame Tree ... they are often worried that people won't like them

Isopogon ... for the worry that follows the realisation that your memory is declining

Little Flannel Flower ... letting worry about what other people think of you stop you from being playful, having fun and even being a little bit silly!

Peach-flowered Tea-tree ... for those hypochondriacal types who are always worried about and preoccupied with their own health

Transition Essence ... for when you are worried about what will unfold as you enter into a new phase of life

Repertory
of Physical
—Conditions—

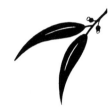

Throughout this book much emphasis has been placed on the connection between emotional patterns and imbalances and physical illness. The purpose of this Repertory of Physical Conditions is to give further insight into emotional patterns and other factors that can lead to disease. The Repertory contains a listing of illnesses and specific anatomical features.

Use the Repertory in the following way: find the illness, note the essence or essences recommended in treatment and refer to the description of the essence in the text. For example, under the heading **blood pressure, high** the following essences are listed: Bluebell, Crowea, Five Corners, Hibbertia, Little Flannel Flower, Mountain Devil and Mulla Mulla. Anyone suffering from high blood pressure can read the material on each of those seven essences, decide which is, or are, the most suitable and work with that essence or essences to help resolve that pattern. In no way should this Repertory be seen as a claim that the essences will cure the disease. They should never replace the services of a qualified practitioner.

abdominal distension (see also
   digestion; irritable bowel
   syndrome)
Crowea
Green Essence

Paw Paw
Peach-flowered Tea-tree

abscess
Billy Goat Plum

Dagger Hakea
Mountain Devil
Sturt Desert Pea

accidents, shock after
Emergency Essence
Fringed Violet

accidents, head injuries
Bush Fuchsia
Emergency Essence
Sundew

aches
Bluebell
Emergency Essence
Five Corners
Tall Yellow Top

acidity
Crowea
Dog Rose
Pink Mulla Mulla

acne
Billy Goat Plum
Detox Essence
Five Corners
Red Lily
Rough Bluebell
Spinifex
Sundew

ADD (attention deficit disorder)
Black-eyed Susan
Boab
Bush Fuchsia
Crowea
Flannel Flower
Fringed Violet
Jacaranda
Kangaroo Paw
Paw Paw
Red Lily
Sundew

addictions
Boab
Boronia + Bottlebrush
Dog Rose of the Wild Forces + Mint
    Bush
Five Corners
Flannel Flower

Fringed Violet
Red Lily
Southern Cross
Sturt Desert Rose
Sundew
Waratah
Wedding Bush

adenoids
Dagger Hakea
Red Helmet Orchid

adhesions, scars
Bush Iris + Slender Rice Flower (both
    internally and topically rubbed into
    scars)

adrenals
Black-eyed Susan
Dog Rose
Kapok Bush
Macrocarpa

aging, acceptance of
Bottlebrush

aging, rejuvenate skin
Mulla Mulla
She Oak

aging, slowing the process of
Bauhinia
Dagger Hakea
Little Flannel Flower
Mountain Devil
Peach-flowered Tea-tree

agoraphobia
Boab + Flannel Flower
Dog Rose
Emergency Essence
Grey Spider Flower

AIDS (*see also* chronic disease;
    depression; immune system, boost)
Billy Goat Plum
Detox Essence
Illawarra Flame Tree
Macrocarpa + Five Corners
Peach-flowered Tea-tree + Spinifex
Sturt Desert Pea
Sturt Desert Rose
Waratah

allergic reaction, to decrease
Emergency Essence
Fringed Violet

allergies
Bauhinia
Bush Iris + Dagger Hakea + Fringed
  Violet
Crowea + Paw Paw + Peach-
  flowered Tea-tree
Dog Rose
Freshwater Mangrove
Tall Mulla Mulla

Alzheimer's disease
Cognis Essence
Isopogon
Red Lily
Rough Bluebell
Sundew

amenorrhoea
Billy Goat Plum
Five Corners
She Oak
Wisteria

amnesia
Emergency Essence
Isopogon
Little Flannel Flower
Red Lily
Sundew

amputation, phantom limb pain
Fringed Violet

anaemia
Bluebell
Five Corners
Kapok Bush
Little Flannel Flower
Pink Mulla Mulla
Red Grevillea
Waratah

anaesthetic, aftereffects
Angelsword + Fringed Violet +
  Macrocarpa + Sundew

anal disorders
Black-eyed Susan
Bottlebrush
Mountain Devil

Peach-flowered Tea-tree
Sturt Desert Rose

ankle problems
Flannel Flower
Isopogon
Sturt Desert Rose

ankles, swollen
Bush Iris
Dog Rose
Philotheca
She Oak
Wild Potato Bush

anorexia nervosa
Crowea + Dog Rose + Paw Paw +
  Peach-flowered Tea-tree
Dagger Hakea
Five Corners
Grey Spider Flower
Paw Paw
Pink Mulla Mulla
Waratah
Wild Potato Bush

antibiotics, after taking
Bush Iris
Crowea
Illawarra Flame Tree
Kapok Bush
Peach-flowered Tea-tree + Spinifex
Philotheca

aorta
Bluebell
Waratah

appetite disorders (*see also* anorexia
  nervosa; bulimia; digestion)
Bluebell
Crowea
Dog Rose
Five Corners
Paw Paw

arm pain
Bottlebrush
Flannel Flower
Paw Paw
Philotheca

arteries
Bluebell

Tall Mulla Mulla

arteriosclerosis
Bauhinia
Bluebell
Bottlebrush
Flannel Flower
Hibbertia
Isopogon
Little Flannel Flower
Tall Mulla Mulla
Yellow Cowslip Orchid

arthritis (*see also* rheumatism;
  rheumatoid arthritis)
Bauhinia
Boab
Dagger Hakea
Detox Essence
Flannel Flower
Hibbertia
Isopogon
Little Flannel Flower
Mountain Devil
Pink Mulla Mulla
Southern Cross
Sturt Desert Pea
Sundew + Tall Mulla Mulla
Yellow Cowslip Orchid

assimilation of nutrients
Crowea
Dog Rose
Paw Paw
Peach-flowered Tea-tree

asthma
Bluebell
Boab + Illawarra Flame Tree
Bush Iris + Dagger Hakea + Fringed
  Violet
Crowea
Flannel Flower
Red Grevillea
Sturt Desert Pea
Tall Mulla Mulla
Tall Yellow Top

asthma, during acute attack
Emergency Essence
Grey Spider Flower (rub in behind
  the sternal notch)

**asthma, to remove body and
  medicinal toxins**
Detox Essence (look for original
  cause)

athlete's foot
Bush Iris
Spinifex

aura, broken
Angelsword + Fringed Violet

aura, misaligned
Crowea

autism
Bluebell
Boronia
Bush Fuchsia
Flannel Flower
Green Spider Orchid
Red Lily
Sundew

babies, 'floppy'
Emergency Essence or Sundew

back, general
Emergency Essence added to a
  sorbolene cream and applied
  topically
Gymea Lily
Paw Paw
Sunshine Wattle
Waratah

back, cervical, neck
Bluebell
Crowea
Five Corners
Isopogon
Kangaroo Paw
Paw Paw
Sturt Desert Rose
Tall Yellow Top

back, thoracic area
Bottlebrush
Crowea
Sturt Desert Pea
Sturt Desert Rose

back, lumbar/sacral-iliac
Bluebell

Boab
Crowea
Flannel Flower + Wisteria
Gymea Lily
Southern Cross
Sunshine Wattle
Tall Yellow Top

back, coccyx
Tall Yellow Top

bacterial infection
Black-eyed Susan
Dagger Hakea
Mountain Devil
Spinifex
Sturt Desert Pea

bad breath *see* halitosis

balance
Bush Fuchsia
Crowea
Jacaranda

balance, major organs
Crowea (one-off dose will balance 14 major organs and nervous system)

baldness
Boab
Dog Rose
Hibbertia
Tall Mulla Mulla
Yellow Cowslip Orchid (frontal)

bed wetting
Dog Rose + Red Helmet Orchid

birth control pill, to balance hormones after long use
Bush Fuchsia + She Oak

bites, insect
Emergency Essence
Mountain Devil
Spinifex

blacking out, fainting
Dog Rose
Emergency Essence
Five Corners
Peach-flowered Tea-tree
Sundew

bladder infection
Bottlebrush
Dagger Hakea
Dog Rose
Mountain Devil
Peach-flowered Tea-tree (internally and added to bath water)

blisters
Fringed Violet
Mulla Mulla
Spinifex

bloating *see* abdominal distension; candida; digestion

blood disorders
Bluebell
Bottlebrush
Dog Rose
Little Flannel Flower
Pink Mulla Mulla

blood pressure, high
Bluebell
Crowea
Five Corners
Hibbertia
Little Flannel Flower
Mountain Devil
Mulla Mulla

blood pressure, low
Five Corners
Kapok Bush
Southern Cross
Tall Mulla Mulla

blood vessels, hardening *see* arteriosclerosis

body clock
Bush Iris

body odour
Billy Goat Plum
Bush Iris
Dog Rose
Five Corners

body type, air
Yellow Cowslip Orchid

body type, earth
Macrocarpa

body type, fire
Illawarra Flame Tree

body type, water
Old Man Banksia

boils
Billy Goat Plum
Dagger Hakea
Mountain Devil
Sturt Desert Pea

bone fracture
Fringed Violet
Gymea Lily
Red Helmet Orchid
Sturt Desert Rose

bone marrow
Five Corners

bones
Gymea Lily
Sturt Desert Rose

bowel
Bauhinia
Bottlebrush
Kapok Bush

brain, better functioning of (*see also* arteriosclerosis)
Bottlebrush
Bush Iris
Cognis Essence
Dog Rose
Gymea Lily
Old Man Banksia
Peach-flowered Tea-tree
She Oak
Tall Mulla Mulla
Yellow Cowslip Orchid

brain damage (*see also* stroke)
Bush Fuchsia
Emergency Essence
Isopogon
Sundew

brain tumour
Bush Iris + Cognis Essence + Dagger Hakea

brain tumour, pituitary
Yellow Cowslip Orchid

breasts
Alpine Mint Bush
Bluebell
Bottlebrush
Flannel Flower
Philotheca

breathing problems
Five Corners
Sundew + Tall Mulla Mulla
Sunshine Wattle
Tall Yellow Top

bronchioles, spasm
Crowea

bronchitis
Dagger Hakea
Red Suva Frangipani
Spinifex
Sturt Desert Pea

bruising
Bluebell
Five Corners
Flannel Flower

bulimia
Billy Goat Plum
Crowea + Paw Paw
Five Corners
Grey Spider Flower
Meditation Essence
Sturt Desert Rose

bunions
Boab
Bottlebrush + Emergency Essence
Hibbertia

burning sensations
Mulla Mulla

burns
Dagger Hakea + Mountain Devil
Mulla Mulla (can be taken internally or topically, either sprayed directly on the skin or on the dressings)

calcification in body
Dagger Hakea
Hibbertia
Little Flannel Flower
Sturt Desert Pea

calluses
Bauhinia
Spinifex
Yellow Cowslip Orchid

cancer (*never treat cancer without medical supervision*)
Bottlebrush
Dagger Hakea
Detox Essence
Flannel Flower + Fringed Violet + Wisteria
Kapok Bush
Mountain Devil
Slender Rice Flower
Southern Cross
Sturt Desert Pea

cancer, skin
Mulla Mulla

cancer, treating side effects of chemotherapy
Detox Essence

cancer, treating side effects of radiation therapy
Fringed Violet + Mulla Mulla

candida
Bottlebrush
Green Essence
Kangaroo Paw
Peach-flowered Tea-tree
Spinifex

carpal tunnel syndrome
Bottlebrush
Crowea
Southern Cross

car sickness *see* motion sickness

cardiac problems *see* heart

cataracts
Red Suva Frangipani
Sunshine Wattle
Waratah

catatonic schizophrenia
Angelsword + Bush Fuchsia + Fringed Violet + Sundew
Grey Spider Flower
Red Lily

catarrh *see* allergies; sinusitis

cellulite
Billy Goat Plum
Bottle Brush
Bush Iris
Dagger Hakea
Tall Mulla Mulla

cerebral palsy
Bush Fuchsia + Crowea + Fringed Violet + Spinifex

chicken pox
Boab
Dagger Hakea
Dagger Hakea + Fringed Violet + Spinifex
Spinifex

childbirth *see* pregnancy, labour

childbirth, to prevent premature
Emergency Essence
She Oak + Yellow Cowslip Orchid

chilblains
Mulla Mulla + Tall Mulla Mulla

chin
Five Corners
Gymea Lily
Tall Yellow Top

chiropractic, to assist or alleviate any reaction to
Emergency Essence
Gymea Lily

chlamydia
Spinifex

cholesterol imbalance
Black-eyed Susan
Bluebell
Boab
Flannel Flower
Little Flannel Flower
She Oak

chronic disease
Bauhinia
Dog Rose
Illawarra Flame Tree
Kapok Bush
Sunshine Wattle

circulation problems
Bluebell
Five Corners
Flannel Flower
Pink Mulla Mulla
Tall Mulla Mulla

claustrophobia
Bottlebrush
Dog Rose
Emergency Essence
Flannel Flower
Grey Spider Flower

cleansing and detoxifying
Detox Essence (Bottlebrush + Bush
    Iris + Dagger Hakea + Dog Rose +
    Wild Potato Bush)

coccyx *see* back

cold hands and feet
Tall Mulla Mulla

colds and flu
Black-eyed Susan
Bush Iris
Illawarra Flame Tree
Jacaranda
Mulla Mulla
Paw Paw

cold sores
Mulla Mulla + Spinifex (topically
    and/or internally)
Spinifex

colic
Black-eyed Susan
Crowea + Paw Paw
Emergency Essence

colitis
Bottlebrush
Dog Rose
Red Suva Frangipani
Crowea
Kapok Bush

colon
Bottlebrush
Kapok Bush
Peach-flowered Tea-tree
Spinifex

colon spasm
Bottlebrush + Crowea
Grey Spider Flower

coma
Emergency Essence
Red Lily
Sundew

compulsive eaters *see* addictions

conjunctivitis
Mountain Devil
Sunshine Wattle

constipation
Bauhinia
Bluebell
Bottlebrush
Flannel Flower

convalescence
Alpine Mint Bush
Banksia Robur
Black-eyed Susan
Dynamis Essence
Kapok Bush
Macrocarpa

co-ordination, physical
Bush Fuchsia
Kangaroo Paw

corns
Bauhinia
Isopogon
Spinifex

coughs
Dagger Hakea
Emergency Essence (rubbed behind
    sternum notch)
Illawarra Flame Tree
Red Helmet Orchid

cramps, muscle
Black-eyed Susan + Bottlebrush +
    Crowea + Grey Spider Flower +
    Tall Mulla Mulla
Crowea

cuts, fine
Spinifex
Sturt Desert Rose

cystic fibrosis
Boab
Bush Iris
Peach-flowered Tea-tree
Southern Cross

cystitis
Bottlebrush
Dagger Hakea
Dog Rose
Mountain Devil
Mulla Mulla

cysts
Dagger Hakea
Mountain Devil
Slender Rice Flower
Sturt Desert Pea

dandruff
Black-eyed Susan
Crowea
Tall Mulla Mulla

deafness
Black-eyed Susan
Bush Fuchsia
Green Spider Flower
Illawarra Flame Tree
Isopogon
Red Grevillea
Tall Yellow Top

dehydration
She Oak (2 drops in water 2–3 times daily)

dental work, to recover from (see also teeth)
Emergency Essence
Red Grevillea

depression
Alpine Mint Bush
Black-eyed Susan
Flannel Flower + Kapok Bush
Red Grevillea
Tall Yellow Top
Waratah
Wild Potato Bush

dermatitis (see also cleansing)
Dagger Hakea + Mulla Mulla + Rough Bluebell

Rough Bluebell (internally and topically)

detoxification
(Detox Essence) Bottlebrush + Bush Iris + Dagger Hakea + Dog Rose + Wild Potato Bush

dexterity
Bush Fuchsia

diabetes (always in conjunction with medical supervision)
Peach-flowered Tea-tree
Peach-flowered Tea-tree + Sunshine Wattle

diaphragm
Black-eyed Susan
Crowea
Paw Paw
Tall Mulla Mulla

diarrhoea
Black-eyed Susan
Bottlebrush
Kapok Bush
Paw Paw

digestion
Black-eyed Susan
Boronia
Crowea
Dog Rose
Paw Paw
Peach-flowered Tea-tree

discharges of the body, unpleasant (see also cleansing)
Billy Goat Plum
Peach-flowered Tea-tree

disks, intervertebral
Crowea
Gymea Lily
Tall Yellow Top

disorientation
Bush Fuchsia
Red Lily
Sundew

diverticulitis (see also irritable bowel syndrome)
Bottlebrush
Tall Mulla Mulla

dizziness
Bush Fuchsia
Crowea
Hibbertia
Jacaranda
Pink Mulla Mulla
Yellow Cowslip Orchid

drained of energy
Dynamis Essence
Fringed Violet

drowsiness *see* tiredness

**drugs, grounding after
    hallucinogenic**
Red Lily
Sundew

**drugs, to remove toxins from
    body**
Bottlebrush + Bush Iris + Dagger
    Hakea + Dog Rose + Wild Potato
    Bush

dry skin
Dog Rose
Old Man Banksia
She Oak

duodenal ulcer
Crowea
Crowea + Paw Paw

dural torque
Tall Yellow Top (for several weeks)

dwarfism
Boab
Yellow Cowslip Orchid

dying, fear of
Bush Iris
Transition Essence

dyslexia
Bush Fuchsia
Jacaranda
Sundew
Tall Yellow Top

dysmenorrhoea
Crowea + She Oak
Billy Goat Plum
Wisteria

ear infections
Bush Fuchsia + Bush Iris + Spinifex
Emergency Essence

eating disorders *see* anorexia
    nervosa; bulimia; digestion

eczema
Billy Goat Plum
Dagger Hakea
Freshwater Mangrove
Fringed Violet (when delayed
    reaction to trauma)
Mulla Mulla
Rough Bluebell
Spinifex

elbow
Bauhinia
Bottlebrush

electromagnetic radiation
Bush Fuchsia + Crowea + Fringed
    Violet + Mulla Mulla + Paw Paw +
    Waratah

elimination *see* cleansing

emphysema
Crowea + Tall Mulla Mulla +
    Sundew
Five Corners

endocrine system
pineal: Bush Iris
hypothalamus: Bush Fuchsia
pituitary: Yellow Cowslip Orchid
thyroid: Old Man Banksia
parathyroids: Hibbertia
thymus: Illawarra Flame Tree
adrenals: Macrocarpa
pancreas: Peach-flowered Tea-tree
ovaries: She Oak
testes: Flannel Flower

endometriosis
Illawarra Flame Tree
Peach-flowered Tea-tree + She Oak

endurance, physical
Banksia Robur
Macrocarpa

energy lack
Alpine Mint Bush

Banksia Robur
Crowea
Dog Rose
Dynamis Essence
Jacaranda
Kapok Bush
Little Flannel Flower
Macrocarpa
Old Man Banksia
Sunshine Wattle

epilepsy (treat epilepsy only with
  medical supervision)
Black-eyed Susan
Bush Fuchsia
Emergency Essence (when acute)
Grey Spider Flower
Sundew
Wild Potato Bush

Epstein-Barr virus
Banksia Robur
Detox Essence
Macrocarpa
Peach-flowered Tea-tree
Sturt Desert Pea

exhaustion
Banksia Robur
Kapok Bush
Macrocarpa

eyebrows
Dagger Hakea
Mountain Devil

eyes
Bush Fuchsia
Freshwater Mangrove
Mountain Devil
Red Suva Frangipani
Sunshine Wattle
Waratah

eyes, pupils unequal
Fringed Violet

face
Billy Goat Plum + Five Corners

fainting
Dog Rose
Dog Rose of the Wild Forces
Emergency Essence
Sundew

Fallopian tubes
She Oak
Spinifex

fatigue, chronic (*see also* ME)
Banksia Robur
Crowea
Detox Essence
Fringed Violet

feeling 'out of sorts'
Crowea

feet
Bauhinia
Bottlebrush
Dog Rose
Red Grevillea
Silver Princess
Sundew
Sunshine Wattle

feet, cracked skin on soles
Bottlebrush + Kapok Bush
Spinifex in sorbolene cream (apply
  topically)

fertility *see* infertility

fevers
Mountain Devil
Mulla Mulla

fibroids, adhesions
Bush Iris
Mountain Devil
Slender Rice Flower
Sturt Desert Rose

finger pain (*see also* arthritis)
Kapok Bush
Paw Paw
Sundew

finger and toe nails
Fringed Violet
Green Essence
Peach-flowered Tea-tree
Spinifex

flatulence (*see also* abdominal
  distension)
Bottlebrush + Crowea + Paw Paw

flu *see* influenza

fluid retention
Bottlebrush
Bush Iris
Dog Rose
Philotheca
Pink Mulla Mulla
She Oak

food poisoning
Crowea + Paw Paw
Dagger Hakea + Fringed Violet +
　Kapok Bush

frigidity
Sexuality Essence

frozen shoulder
Dagger Hakea
Emergency Essence (topically)
Little Flannel Flower
Paw Paw
Sunshine Wattle

fungal infections
Green Essence
Peach-flowered Tea-tree
Spinifex

gallstones, gall bladder
Dagger Hakea
Illawarra Flame Tree
Slender Rice Flower
Southern Cross

glandular fever *see* Epstein-Barr
　virus

glaucoma
Waratah

glue ear
Bush Fuchsia
Bush Fuchsia + Bush Iris

golden staph infection
Red Grevillea

gout
Black-eyed Susan
Gymea Lily
Mountain Devil
Mulla Mulla

growths *see* cancer; cysts

gum boils
Dagger Hakea
Mountain Devil

gum problems
Jacaranda
Kapok Bush
Peach-flowered Tea-tree

haemophilia
Boab
Jacaranda
Kapok Bush

haemorrhoids
Black-eyed Susan
Bottlebrush
Dagger Hakea

hair follicles, infection of
Spinifex + Tall Mulla Mulla

hair loss *see* baldness

halitosis (*see also* gum boils)
Black-eyed Susan
Crowea
Jacaranda
Mountain Devil
Paw Paw
Peach-flowered Tea-tree
Rough Bluebell

hands
Bush Fuchsia
Flannel Flower
Kapok Bush
Paw Paw
Sundew

hay fever
Black-eyed Susan
Bush Iris + Dagger Hakea + Fringed
　Violet
Hibbertia

headaches
Black-eyed Susan
Boronia
Bottlebrush
Crowea
Dagger Hakea
Emergency Essence
Five Corners

Paw Paw
She Oak
Sturt Desert Rose

head, fullness, pressure
Boronia + Crowea

head injuries
Emergency Essence
Sundew
Bush Fuchsia
Spinifex
Gymea Lily

healthy lifestyle
Bottlebrush
Five Corners
Flannel Flower
Wedding Bush (helps with
    commitment to diet, exercise)

hearing
Black-eyed Susan
Bush Fuchsia
Green Spider Orchid
Illawarra Flame Tree
Isopogon
Kangaroo Paw
Tall Yellow Top

heart
Alpine Mint Bush
Black-eyed Susan
Bluebell
Little Flannel Flower
Old Man Banksia
Philotheca
Rough Bluebell
Tall Mulla Mulla
Waratah

heart attack, during (*always get
    medical attention immediately*)
Bluebell + Emergency Essence

heart attack, after
Waratah

heart, valve, ventricles
Waratah

heat, fluctuations in body
Old Man Banksia
Peach-flowered Tea-tree

heat, problems with
Mulla Mulla

heat rash
Dagger Hakea + Mulla Mulla

heavy metal detoxification
Bottlebrush + Bush Iris (Detox
    Essence) + Dagger Hakea + Dog
    Rose + Wild Potato Bush

hepatitis (*see also* liver; infections)
Dagger Hakea
Mountain Devil
Rough Bluebell

hepatitis C
Billy Goat Plum
Dagger Hakea
Freshwater Mangrove
Mountain Devil
Rough Bluebell

hereditary illness
Boab
Dog Rose of the Wild Forces
Green Spider Orchid

hernia (*see also* hiatus hernia)
Black-eyed Susan
Crowea
Dagger Hakea + Mountain Devil
Jacaranda

herpes
Billy Goat Plum
Mulla Mulla
Spinifex
Sturt Desert Rose

herpes blisters
Spinifex (use topically)

hiatus hernia
Jacaranda

hiccups
Black-eyed Susan + Crowea + Paw
    Paw

hip problems (*see also* osteoporosis)
Dog Rose
Silver Princess
Sundew
Sunshine Wattle

hives
Dagger Hakea
Dog Rose
Fringed Violet
Yellow Cowslip Orchid

homoeostasis
Bauhinia
Crowea
Old Man Banksia

hormone imbalance *see* endocrine
system

**hormone imbalance from HRT or
the contraceptive pill**
Bush Fuchsia
She Oak
Yellow Cowslip Orchid

hyperactivity (*see also* allergies)
Black-eyed Susan
Jacaranda
Red Helmet Orchid
Sundew

hypochondria
Peach-flowered Tea-tree

hypoglycaemia
Kapok Bush
Paw Paw
Peach-flowered Tea-tree

hypothalamus
Bush Fuchsia

ileocaecal valve
Bauhinia
Red Grevillea

illness, long
Banksia Robur
Illawarra Flame Tree
Kapok Bush
Sunshine Wattle
Wild Potato Bush

immune system, boost
Bush Iris
Illawarra Flame Tree + Southern
Cross
Philotheca

impetigo
Billy Goat Plum
Dagger Hakea
Green Essence (topically)
Spinifex

impotence
Boronia + Crowea + Five Corners +
Flannel Flower

incontinence
Bottlebrush
Crowea
Dog Rose
Dog Rose of the Wild Forces

indigestion
Black-eyed Susan
Crowea + Dog Rose + Paw Paw +
Peach-flowered Tea-tree
Jacaranda

infection, bacterial and viral
Black-eyed Susan
Dagger Hakea
Illawarra Flame Tree
Mountain Devil
Spinifex
Sturt Desert Pea

infection, fungal and parasitic
Green Essence
Peach-flowered Tea-tree
Spinifex

infection, golden staph
Red Grevillea

infertility
Flannel Flower
She Oak (4 weeks on, 2 weeks off,
for up to 6 months)
Turkey Bush

inflammation
Black-eyed Susan
Dagger Hakea
Mountain Devil
Mulla Mulla

influenza
Black-eyed Susan
Bush Iris
Flannel Flower

Illawarra Flame Tree
Jacaranda
Mulla Mulla
Paw Paw

injuries *see* accidents; shock; trauma

insect bites
Emergency Essence (topically and/or
    internally)
Mountain Devil

insomnia
Black-eyed Susan
Boronia
Crowea
Emergency Essence
Green Spider Orchid + Grey Spider

intestine, small
Bauhinia
Crowea
Paw Paw
Peach-flowered Tea-tree

intestine, large
Bottlebrush
Kapok Bush

intestinal ulcer
Crowea

iris markings (iridology)
brown colon and disturbed liver:
    Bottlebrush + Mountain Devil +
    Dagger Hakea
fibres scrunched: Jacaranda
gaps in nerve wreath: Sundew
green or yellow colouration: Dog
    Rose
irregular pupil: Sundew
lymphatic rosary: Bush Iris,
    Philotheca
nerve rings: Black-eyed Susan,
    Crowea, Gymea Lily, Meditation
    Essence
sodium ring: Bluebell, Dagger Hakea,
    Hibbertia, Isopogon, Sturt Desert
    Pea, Tall Mulla Mulla

irritable bowel syndrome (*see also*
    candida; colitis)
Bauhinia
Black-eyed Susan

Bottlebrush
Crowea
Kapok Bush
Paw Paw

itching
Black-eyed Susan
Dagger Hakea
Fringed Violet
Red Grevillea
Rough Bluebell

jaundice
Dagger Hakea
Mountain Devil
Pink Mulla Mulla (haemolytic
    jaundice)

jaw problems
Dagger Hakea
Mountain Devil

jaw, TMJ
Red Grevillea

jet lag
Travel Essence

joints
Bauhinia
Bottlebrush
Crowea
Gymea Lily
Hibbertia
Tall Mulla Mulla

kidney
Dog Rose
Grey Spider Flower

knee problems
Bauhinia
Freshwater Mangrove
Gymea Lily
Isopogon

labour *see* pregnancy, labour

laryngitis
Flannel Flower
Red Helmet Orchid
Bush Fuchsia
Mountain Devil

legs

Bottlebrush
Kapok Bush
Red Grevillea
Sundew
Sunshine Wattle

lesions and rashes
Billy Goat Plum
Detox Essence
Green Essence
Rough Bluebell

ligaments and bones
Gymea Lily

light-headed
Bush Fuchsia + Sundew

lips, cracked
Flannel Flower + Spinifex + Wisteria

liver
Dagger Hakea
Mountain Devil
Slender Rice Flower
Sunshine Wattle

low blood sugar
Peach-flowered Tea-tree

low sperm count
Flannel Flower

lung problems
Red Suva Frangipani
Sturt Desert Pea
Tall Mulla Mulla + Sundew

lymphatic system
Bush Iris
Philotheca

malabsorption of food
Black-eyed Susan + Crowea + Dog
    Rose + Paw Paw + Peach-flowered
    Tea-tree

malaria
Green Essence
Mulla Mulla
Paw Paw (apply topically along lung
    meridian)
Spinifex

ME (post-viral fatigue syndrome)
Banksia Robur

Detox Essence
Dynamis Essence
Fringed Violet (look for cause)

measles *see* fever; lesions and
    rashes

memory failure
Isopogon

meningitis (*see also* inflammation)
Emergency Essence
Illawarra Flame Tree + Mulla
    Mulla

menopause
Bottlebrush
Femin Essence
Illawarra Flame Tree
Macrocarpa
Mulla Mulla
Peach-flowered Tea-tree
She Oak

mental retardation
Boab
Bush Fuchsia
Fringed Violet
Sundew
Yellow Cowslip Orchid

meridians, imbalances in
Crowea
Five Corners
Slender Rice Flower

metabolic rate
Black-eyed Susan
Crowea
Mulla Mulla
Old Man Banksia

miasms
Boab

migraine
Bauhinia
Black-eyed Susan
Emergency Essence
She Oak

morning lethargy (*see also* energy
    lack)
Banksia Robur

morning sickness
Bottlebrush
Dagger Hakea
Dog Rose
She Oak

motion sickness
Bush Fuchsia + Crowea + Paw Paw
Dog Rose
Red Grevillea
Spinifex + Tall Mulla Mulla
Travel Essence

mouth problems
Bauhinia
Isopogon

multiple sclerosis
Bluebell
Gymea Lily
Hibbertia
Isopogon
Rough Bluebell
Southern Cross
Spinifex

mumps (*see also* inflammation; infections)
Hibbertia + Red Grevillea + Peach-flowered Tea-tree

muscle cramps
Bottlebrush
Crowea
Grey Spider Flower
Tall Yellow Top

muscle pain
Crowea (use externally, frequently)

muscular dystrophy
Crowea
Dog Rose of the Wild Forces
Flannel Flower
Waratah

nails *see* finger and toe nails

nail biting
Boronia + Bottlebrush
Crowea

nausea
Crowea
Dagger Hakea

neck
Dog Rose
Paw Paw

neck
Black-eyed Susan
Bluebell
Crowea
Five Corners
Gymea Lily
Isopogon
Kangaroo Paw
Paw Paw
Sturt Desert Rose
Tall Yellow Top

nephritis
Dog Rose
Emergency Essence
Grey Spider Flower
Mulla Mulla

nerves, central nervous system
Bush Fuchsia
Crowea

nerve damage, pain
Bush Fuchsia + Emergency Essence + Spinifex
Sturt Desert Rose

nervous breakdown
Angelsword
Black-eyed Susan
Dog Rose of the Wild Forces
Fringed Violet
Jacaranda
Old Man Banksia
Paw Paw

nervous exhaustion
Alpine Mint Bush
Banksia Robur
Macrocarpa
Paw Paw

nervousness
Black-eyed Susan
Dog Rose
Jacaranda

neuralgia *see* nerve damage, pain

neurological development
Bush Fuchsia

nose bleeds
Fringed Violet
Illawarra Flame Tree

nose, blocked
Bush Iris
Crowea + Tall Mulla Mulla
Dagger Hakea
Fringed Violet

nose, running
Flannel Flower

numbness
Bluebell + Flannel Flower + Kapok
    Bush

obesity *see* overweight

oedema
Bush Iris
Dog Rose
Old Man Banksia
She Oak

organ transplant rejection
Waratah

osteoporosis (*see also* aging;
    assimilation of nutrients; bone
    fracture)
Gymea Lily
Hibbertia
She Oak
Tall Yellow Top

out of sorts
Crowea

ovarian cysts
Dagger Hakea
Mountain Devil
She Oak Sturt
Desert Rose

ovaries
She Oak

overweight
Bluebell
Bush Iris
Crowea
Dog Rose
Five Corners
Fringed Violet
Old Man Banksia

oxygenation of tissues
Dog Rose
Mulla Mulla
Tall Mulla Mulla

pain
Bluebell
Bottlebrush + Emergency Essence
Bush Iris
Dog Rose of the Wild Forces
Five Corners
Spinifex
Sturt Desert Rose

pain, cellular level memory
Boab
Dog Rose of the Wild Forces
Fringed Violet

palpitations
Bluebell
Bush Fuchsia
Crowea
Jacaranda
Waratah

pancreas
Peach-flowered Tea-Tree

paralysis
Bauhinia
Bush Fuchsia
Grey Spider Flower
Wild Potato Bush

**paralysis, immediately after
    accident or trauma**
Emergency Essence

parasites
Billy Goat Plum
Bottlebrush
Green Essence
Kapok Bush
Peach-flowered Tea-tree
Rough Bluebell
Southern Cross
Spinifex

Parkinson's disease
Bush Fuchsia + Crowea + Dog Rose
    + Jacaranda
Gymea Lily
Yellow Cowslip Orchid

pelvic inflammation (*see also* inflammation)
Billy Goat Plum
Spinifex
Wisteria + Fringed Violet

peptic ulcer
Crowea

period pain
Crowea
She Oak

perspiration, excessive
Bush Iris
Dog Rose
Macrocarpa
She Oak

physical growth
Yellow Cowslip Orchid

pimples *see* acne

pineal gland
Bush Iris

pituitary gland
Yellow Cowslip Orchid

pleurisy
Sturt Desert Pea
Red Suva Frangipani

PMS (premenstrual syndrome)
Crowea + Peach-flowered Tea-tree + She Oak

pneumonia
Black-eyed Susan
Macrocarpa
Mountain Devil
Sturt Desert Pea
Waratah

polio
Jacaranda

pollution, protection from
Detox Essence + Fringed Violet

post-nasal drip
Flannel Flower
Southern Cross
Sturt Desert Pea

pregnancy
Bottlebrush
Fringed Violet
She Oak
Wild Potato Bush
Wisteria
Yellow Cowslip Orchid

pregnancy, labour
Bauhinia
Billy Goat Plum
Bush Fuchsia
Crowea
Emergency Essence
Fringed Violet
Kapok Bush
Macrocarpa
Red Grevillea
Slender Rice Flower (for incised wounds or tears)
Yellow Cowslip Orchid

premature ejaculation
Macrocarpa
Sturt Desert Rose

prostate gland
Billy Goat Plum
Flannel Flower
Freshwater Mangrove
Fringed Violet
Sturt Desert Rose

psoriasis
Billy Goat Plum (topically or internally)
Flannel Flower
Green Essence
Peach-flowered Tea-tree (if yeast component)
Pink Mulla Mulla

puberty
Adol Essence
Billy Goat Plum
Bottlebrush
Five Corners
Flannel Flower (for boys)
She Oak (for girls)

radiation
Mulla Mulla
Radiation Essence

radiation therapy, combat side effects of
Mulla Mulla
Radiation Essence

rape
Billy Goat Plum
Emergency Essence
Flannel Flower + Fringed Violet (for males)
Flannel Flower + Fringed Violet + Wisteria (for females)

rash *see* lesions and rashes

reflexes
Bush Fuchsia
Jacaranda

respiratory system *see* breathing problems; lung problems

rheumatism (*see also* arthritis)
Bluebell
Dagger Hakea
Isopogon
Southern Cross
Yellow Cowslip Orchid

rheumatoid arthritis (*see also* immune system, boost)
Bluebell
Dagger Hakea
Hibbertia
Red Helmet Orchid
Southern Cross
Sturt Desert Pea

ribs
Fringed Violet + Red Helmet Orchid

Ross River virus *see* infections; ME

round shoulders
Dog Rose
Five Corners
Sunshine Wattle
Waratah

RSI (repetitive strain injury)
Crowea
Red Grevillea
Silver Princess
Southern Cross

'run down'
Banksia Robur
Crowea
Macrocarpa

running nose
Flannel Flower

scars
Bush Iris + Slender Rice Flower (internally and topically)

scars from burns
Mulla Mulla (internally and topically, in a cream, twice daily for two weeks, then once daily for as long as needed)

sciatica (*see also* inflammation)
Crowea
Dog Rose
Spinifex

scleroderma
Flannel Flower
Fringed Violet
Spinifex
Tall Mulla Mulla

scoliosis
Crowea
Gymea Lily
Red Helmet Orchid
Tall Yellow Top

sea sickness *see* motion sickness

senility
Isopogon
Red Lily
Sundew

sexually transmitted disease (*see also* AIDS)
Billy Goat Plum
Spinifex
Sturt Desert Rose

shingles
Spinifex
Billy Goat Plum
Five Corners
Black-eyed Susan

shock
Emergency Essence
Fringed Violet

shock, electric
Radiation Essence
She Oak

shortness of breath
Black-eyed Susan + Jacaranda
Tall Mulla Mulla

shoulders
Dog Rose
Five Corners
Kapok Bush
Paw Paw
Sunshine Wattle
Waratah

sinusitis
Bush Iris + Dagger Hakea + Fringed
   Violet

skin cancers
Mulla Mulla (internally and applied
   to skin)

skin problems
Billy Goat Plum
Detox Essence
Five Corners
Fringed Violet
Mulla Mulla
Old Man Banksia
Rough Bluebell
Spinifex

skin, weeping, itchy
Five Corners
Freshwater Mangrove
Fringed Violet
Green Essence (applied topically)

sleeping, difficulty see insomnia

sleep apnoea
Sundew + Tall Mulla Mulla

sleep, need lots
Macrocarpa
Red Lily
Sundew

smoking, difficulty quitting (see
   also addictions)
Boronia + Bottlebrush

smoking, effects see of addictions;
   breathing problems; detoxification;
   lung problems

snoring
Banksia
Bottlebrush
Bush Iris + Dagger Hakea +
   Fringed Violet + Isopogon + Old
   Man

somnambulance
Red Lily + Sundew

**'spaced out', after too much TV,
   etc.**
Bush Fuchsia
Sundew

speech problems
Bush Fuchsia
Red Grevillea

spleen
Boronia
Dog Rose
Pink Mulla Mulla

spinal cord
Gymea Lily
Tall Yellow Top

spine see back

sprains
Bauhinia
Black-eyed Susan
Crowea
Emergency Essence
Gymea Lily

sternum
Bluebell
Fringed Violet
Red Helmet Orchid

stiffness
Bauhinia
Hibbertia
Isopogon
Little Flannel Flower

Pink Mulla Mulla
Yellow Cowslip Orchid

sting, insect
Emergency Essence
Mountain Devil
Spinifex

stomach problems (*see also* digestion)
Bauhinia
Crowea

stomach ulcers
Crowea
Paw Paw

stress, tension
Black-eyed Susan
Crowea
Emergency Essence
Flannel Flower
Paw Paw

stroke
Bauhinia
Bush Fuchsia
Emergency Essence
Isopogon
Kapok Bush
Mountain Devil
Red Lily + Sundew

stuttering
Bush Fuchsia
Five Corners

suicidal
Waratah

sunburn
Mulla Mulla (use topically and internally before and after sun exposure)

sun spots
Mulla Mulla (internally and topically 3 times a day for at least 3 weeks)

surgery, beforehand
Emergency Essence (for 2 days)

surgery, afterwards
Angelsword + Emergency Essence +

Slender Rice Flower + Macrocarpa (for 1–2 weeks)

sweating, excessive *see* perspiration

swelling *see* oedema

teeth
Jacaranda
Paw Paw
Sundew

teeth grinding
Black-eyed Susan
Dagger Hakea
Red Grevillea

teething, babies
Emergency Essence

temporomandibular joint (TMJ)
Dagger Hakea
Mountain Devil
Red Grevillea

tendons and muscles
Crowea

terminal illness
Transition Essence

testicles
Flannel Flower
She Oak (only if Flannel Flower has not corrected the problem)

throat problems
Bush Fuchsia
Bush Iris
Flannel Flower
Mountain Devil
Old Man Banksia
Turkey Bush

thrombosis, deep venous
Bluebell
Red Grevillea
Sunshine Wattle
Tall Mulla Mulla

thrush
Green Essence
Peach-flowered Tea-tree
Spinifex
Sturt Desert Rose

thymus
Confid Essence
Illawarra Flame Tree
Mountain Devil

thyroid
Old Man Banksia

thyroid, over-active
Black-eyed Susan + Jacaranda + Old
   Man Banksia

tinea
Green Essence
Peach-flowered Tea-tree
Spinifex

tinnitus
Bush Fuchsia

tiredness *see* energy lack

tiredness, temporary
Banksia Robur

tissue rejection
Waratah

toenails
Fringed Violet

tongue, red patches on
Crowea

tonsillitis
Bush Fuchsia
Bush Iris
Flannel Flower

toxicity *see* detoxification

transplant surgery, rejection
Waratah

trauma, acute
Emergency Essence
Fringed Violet
Sundew

travel sickness
Crowea
Emergency Essence
Paw Paw
Travel Essence

tremor
Bush Fuchsia + Crowea + Dog Rose
   + Jacaranda + Spinifex

tuberculosis
Sturt Desert Pea
Sunshine Wattle
Waratah

ulcers, digestive system
Crowea
Paw Paw

ulcers, skin
Billy Goat Plum
Green Essence
Spinifex
Tall Mulla Mulla

ulcers, mouth
Mulla Mulla + Spinifex

urinary infections (*see also* bladder
   infection; kidney)
Dagger Hakea
Dog Rose
Mountain Devil
Spinifex

uterus
Crowea
She Oak
Turkey Bush

vaginitis
Dagger Hakea
Sturt Desert Rose

vaginitis, burning
Mulla Mulla

varicose veins
Five Corners
Paw Paw
Red Grevillea
Tall Mulla Mulla

veins
Five Corners
Tall Mulla Mulla

venereal disease *see* sexually
   transmitted disease

venous thrombosis
Bluebell
Five Corners
Little Flannel Flower
Red Grevillea
Sunshine Wattle
Tall Mulla Mulla

vertigo *see* dizziness

viral infections *see* infection

vitiligo
Bush Iris
Tall Yellow Top

vomiting
Bauhinia
Bottlebrush
Crowea
Paw Paw

warts
Billy Goat Plum + Five Corners

wasting diseases
Crowea + Paw Paw + Peach-
  flowered Tea-tree
Kapok Bush
Southern Cross
Waratah

Australian Bush Flower Essences and the Related Subtle —Bodies—

by Erik Pelham

As well as the more obvious physical body, you have surrounding you a number of subtle bodies, these being in order as they are found from the physical body outwards: the etheric, the emotional, the astral, the mental and the causal body. I am very grateful to be able to include Erik Pelham's wonderful research as to which specific subtle body each Bush Essence has its major sphere of action on. I hope that it may be of relevant application and benefit for you.—Ian White

Alpine Mint Bush . . . Mental, Astral

Angelsword . . . Soul, Etheric, Mental, Astral

Banksia Robur . . . Soul, Astral, Etheric

Bauhinia . . . Mental, Astral

Billy Goat Plum . . . Mental, Physical

Black-eyed Susan . . . Mental, Emotional

Bluebell . . . Mental

Boab . . . Mental, Astral, Etheric

Boronia . . . Mental

Bottlebrush . . . Mental, Physical

Bush Fuchsia . . . Causal, Etheric

Bush Gardenia . . . Mental, Astral, Emotional

Bush Iris . . . Soul

Crowea . . . Astral, Emotional

Dagger Hakea . . . Mental, Emotional

Dog Rose of the Wild Forces . . . Causal, Astral, Etheric

Dog Rose . . . Causal, Astral, Etheric

Five Corners . . . Causal, Emotional, Physical

Flannel Flower . . . Soul, Astral

Fringed Violet . . . Astral, Etheric

Green Spider Orchid . . . Mental, Astral

Grey Spider Flower . . . Soul, Astral

Gymea Lily . . . Mental, Astral

Hibbertia . . . Mental, Emotional

Illawarra Flame Tree . . . Causal, Astral

Isopogon . . . Mental

Jacaranda . . . Mental, Astral

Kangaroo Paw . . . Causal, Astral, Physical

Kapok Bush . . . Mental, Causal

Little Flannel Flower . . . Mental, Astral, Physical

Macrocarpa . . . Physical

Mint Bush . . . Mental, Astral

Mountain Devil . . . Emotional

Mulla Mulla . . . Astral, Physical

Old Man Banksia . . . Soul, Astral, Etheric

Paw Paw . . . Soul, Mental

Peach-flowered Tea-tree . . . Causal, Physical

Philotheca . . . Mental

Pink Mulla Mulla . . . Causal, Physical

Red Grevillea . . . Causal

Red Helmet Orchid . . . Causal, Emotional

Red Lily . . . Soul, Astral, Physical

Red Suva Frangipani . . . Soul, Astral, Etheric

Rough Bluebell . . . Mental, Physical

She Oak . . . Causal

Silver Princess . . . Causal

Slender Rice Flower . . . Emotional, Causal

Southern Cross . . . Mental, Astral

Spinifex . . . Physical

Sturt Desert Pea . . . Causal, Emotional

Sturt Desert Rose . . . Mental, Emotional

Sundew . . . Mental, Astral, Etheric

Sunshine Wattle . . . Causal, Emotional

Tall Mulla Mulla . . . Causal, Physical

Tall Yellow Top . . . Mental, Causal, Emotional

Turkey Bush . . . Mental, Astral, Emotional

Waratah . . . Mental, Causal, Emotional

Wedding Bush . . . Causal, Emotional

Wild Potato Bush . . . Mental, Etheric

Wisteria . . . Causal, Emotional

Yellow Cowslip Orchid . . . Mental, Causal

—Bibliography—

Arroyo, Stephen. *Astrology, Psychology and the Four Elements*. CRCS Publications, Sebastopol, California, 1975.

Baker, Margaret, Corringham, R. & Dark, J. *Native Plants of the Sydney Region*. Three Sisters Productions, Sydney, 1986.

Brennan, Kym. *Wildflowers of Kakadu*. G. Brennan, Jabiru, 1986.

Brock, John. *Top End Native Plants*. John Brock, Darwin, 1988.

Caddy, Eileen. *Footprints on the Path*. Findhorn Press, Findhorn, 1976.
——*God Spoke to Me*. Findhorn Press, Findhorn, 1971.

Carter, Rita. *Mind Mapping*. Weidenfeld & Nicolson, 1998.

Chopra, Deepak. *Quantum Healing*. Bantam, New York, 1990.

Cunningham, Donna. *Flower Remedies Handbook*. Sterling Publishing Company Inc., 1992.

Dyer, Wayne W. *Everyday Wisdom*. Hay House, Inc., Carson, 1993.

Eggenberger, Richard & Mary Helen. *The Handbook on Plumeria Culture*. The Plumeria People, Houston, Texas, 1988.

Gardener, C.A. *Wildflowers of Western Australia*. St George Books, Perth, 1959.

Gerber, Richard, MD. *Vibrational Medicine*. Bear & Co., Sante Fe, 1988.

Gibran, Kahlil. *The Prophet*. Random House Inc., New York, 1923.

Goodman, Linda. *Linda Goodman's Sun Signs*. Pan Books, London, 1972.
——*Star Signs: The Secret Codes of the Universe*. St Martins Press, New York, 1987.

Guttman, Ariel & Johnson, Kenneth. *Mythic Astrology: Archetypal Powers in the Horoscope*. Llewellyn Publications, St Paul, Minnesota, 1993.

Hand Clow, Barbara. *Chiron: Rainbow Bridge between the Inner and Outer Planets*. Llewellyn Publications, St Paul, Minnesota, 1994.

Hawkins, Gerald S. *Stonehenge Decoded*. Dorset Press, New York, 1965.

Hay, Louise. *Heal Your Body*. Specialist Publications, Sydney, 1976.
——*You Can Heal Your Life*. Hay House, Santa Monica, 1984.

Hayward, Susan (ed.). *A Guide for the Advanced Soul*. In-Tune Books, Sydney, 1985.
—— & Cohan, Malcom (eds). *A Bag of Jewels*. In-Tune Books, Sydney, 1988.

Johnson, Roberts. *Owning Your Own Shadow*. Harper, San Francisco, New York, 1991.

Krystal, Phyllis. *Cutting the Ties that Bind*. Element Books Ltd, Shaftesbury, 1989.

Kushi, Michio. *Oriental Diagnosis*. Sunwheel Publications, London, 1978.

Lofthus, Myrna. *A Spiritual Approach to Astrology*. CRCS Publications, Sebastopol, California, 1983.

Maltz, Maxwell. *Psycho-Cybernetics*. Prentice-Hall, Inc., New Jersey, 1960.

Mann, A.T. *Astrology and the Art of Healing*. Unwin Hyman Ltd., London, 1989.

Nixon, Paul. *The Waratah*. Kangaroo Press, Sydney, 1987.

Noontil, Annette. *The Body is the Barometer of the Soul*. Noontil, Nunawading, 1994.

Odent, Michel. *Birth Reborn*. Pantheon Books, New York, 1984.

Pelham, Erik. Devic Analyses. Unpublished paper.

Ray, Sondra. *Ideal Birth*. Celestial Arts, Berkeley, 1985.

Ramtha. *Ramtha* (ed. S. L. Weinburg). Sovereigny Inc., Washington, 1986.

Roberts, Jane. *The Nature of Personal Reality*. Prentice-Hall, New Jersey, 1974.

Ruhela, S.P. (ed.). *Immortal Quotations of Bhagavan Sri Sthya Sai Baba*. BR Publishing Corporation, Delhi, 1996.

Sagan, Samuel. *Planetary Forces, Alchemy and Healing*. Clairvision School Foundation, Sydney, 1996.

Sams, Jamie & Carson, David. *Medicine Cards*. Bear & Company, Santa Fe, 1998.

Setzer, Claudia. *The Quotable Soul*. The Stonesong Press Inc., USA, 1994.

Sharamon, Shalila & Baginski, Bodo J. *Cosmobiological Birth Control*. Lotus Light Publications, Wilmont, USA, 1989.

Stevenson, Ian. *Children Who Remember Past Lives: A Question of Reincarnation*. University Press, Virginia, 1987.
—— *Twenty Cases of Reincarnation* (2nd edn). University Press, Virginia, 1980.
—— *Where Reincarnation and Biology Intersect*. Praeger, 1997.

Trenorden, Jan. *The Essences and Chironic Healing*. Chironic Enterprises Pty Ltd, Warrnambool, Victoria, 1991.

Urban, Anne. *Wildflowers and Plants of Central Australia*. Southbank Editions, Melbourne, 1990.

Valles, C.G. *Unencumbered by Baggage*. X. Diaz del Rio, Gujarat, India, 1987.

Verny, T. *The Secret Life of the Unborn Child*. Sphere Books, London, 1981.

White, Ian. *Australian Bush Flower Essences*. Bantam, Sydney, 1991.
—— *Australian Bush Flower Remedies* (revd edn). A.B.F.E., Sydney, 1996.

Wilde, Stuart. *The Force*. Wisdom Books, Toos, New Mexico, 1984.

Zolar. *The History of Astrology*. W. Foulsham & Co. Ltd, London, 1972.

The Australian Bush Flower Essence Society

The Society has been formed to provide you with the most up to date information on the Bush Essences. There is a minimal annual subscrition fee for which members receive four newsletters per year containing updates on essences, details of workshops and many special offers. It also provides a forum, through the publication of case histories, to share your knowledge and experience of the Bush Essences.

For information please contact:
Australian Bush Flower Essences, 45 Booralie Road, Terrey Hills NSW 2084, Australia.
Phone (02) 9450 1388; Fax (02) 9450 2866
Email: info@ausflowers.com.au
Web site: www.ausflowers.com.au